THE BIOCULTURAL BASIS
OF HEALTH

EXPANDING VIEWS OF MEDICAL ANTHROPOLOGY

THE BIOCULTURAL BASIS OF HEALTH

EXPANDING VIEWS OF MEDICAL ANTHROPOLOGY

LORNA G. MOORE, Ph.D.

Associate Professor of Anthropology, University of Colorado;
Assistant Professor of Preventive Medicine,
University of Colorado Health Sciences Center, Denver, Colorado

PETER W. VAN ARSDALE, Ph.D.

Assistant Professor of Anthropology,
University of Denver, Denver, Colorado

JoANN E. GLITTENBERG, R.N., Ph.D.

Associate Professor of Nursing,
University of Colorado Health Sciences Center, Denver, Colorado

ROBERT A. ALDRICH, M.D.

Professor of Preventive Medicine and Pediatrics,
University of Colorado Health Sciences Center, Denver, Colorado

with 88 illustrations

The C. V. Mosby Company

ST. LOUIS • TORONTO • LONDON   1980

Cover adapted from Sun and Moon with Mountains,
a Sandpainting of the Hailway. Used by permission of the
Wheelright Museum of the American Indian,
Santa Fe, New Mexico.

Copyright © 1980 by The C. V. Mosby Company

Printed in the United States of America

The C. V. Mosby Company
11830 Westline Industrial Drive, St. Louis, Missouri 63141

Library of Congress Cataloging in Publication Data

The Biocultural basis of health.

    Bibliography: p.
    Includes index.
    1. Medical anthropology. 2. Health.
I. Moore, Lorna G., 1946-   [DNLM: 1. Health.
2. Environmental health. 3. Anthropology.
4. Cross-cultural comparison. 5. Adaptation,
Physiological. QT140 B615]
GN296.B56   362.1'042   80-11554
ISBN 0-8016-3481-4

GW/VH/VH 9 8 7 6 5 4 3 2 1   02/A/245

Foreword

This book, written by three anthropologists and a physician, is about human health. It deals with the fundamental question of where responsibility rests for maintaining wellness or for preventing illness in individuals as well as in society. This is a subject whose time for attention has arrived, as is reflected in the public debate about health in the United States. Although this has become a national economic and political issue, it is, nevertheless, of special significance for contemporary college and university students who will be the parents of the next generation, for whom this subject will be of particular concern because of the unprecedented demographic changes occurring both in the developed and the developing countries. A growing number of scientists and other scholars perceive, as evolutionary phenomena, changes in attitudes and practices for health and health enhancement as distinct from disease and medical care.

Biological knowledge, which has expanded so rapidly during the past four decades, has been incorporated only incompletely into a science of health—personal and social. Since biological factors have psychosocial effects and psychosocial factors have biological effects, a better understanding of health depends on expanding knowledge of the interaction of biological and psychosocial processes. Research in this relatively unexplored area will clarify many important questions regarding human health.

Insights about the way in which our earliest ancestors lived in prehistoric times are being provided by archaeological and anthropological studies. Much is now known about their villages, dwellings, water supplies, food sources, and life-styles. Historical records of early Egypt, Greece, and other civilizations are replete with detailed written descriptions of life in later times. Monuments and other structures that still remain add to our knowledge and appreciation of these cultures and the way in which they manipulated their environment to meet the needs created by their ever changing lives. In our times, sophisticated technology, intended to provide advantages for humankind, sometimes has had unforeseen adverse effects on human health. This is evident in the debate about environmental pollution, which threatens human and planetary health. The latter must also be added to the consideration of biological and sociocultural influences on health throughout the human life span.

The authors have approached their subject from the premise that the capacity for health and wellness is built in, so to speak, and that humans still possess the great adaptability that enabled them to survive the adverse circumstances that existed in earlier evolutionary times. Homo sapiens, being the last survivor of the hominids that coexisted prehistorically, must, according to the authors, possess a high inborn capacity for health and wellness; and they have considered the influence of cultural and environmental factors on this natural attribute. Since human beings have survived previous environments, importance is placed on the homo sapiens—environmental relationship that may be crucial for a continuing future of humankind. The homology of humans as both experimenters and guinea pigs on planet Earth suggests caution in the experiments they carry out.

The authors consider the full human life span from before conception through birth, infancy, childhood, and adolescence, and then into the several stages of adulthood, ending in the later years and dying. Throughout the book the processes of life are traced as they flow and change continuously under the influence of cultural and biological factors, in harmony or in dissonance with the myriad of life events that leave an imprint on later years. The authors discuss the human life span in a way that considers similarities and differences for women and men and that can be used in cross-cultural comparisons. In this way, comparisons of attitudes and practices surrounding conception, birth, puberty, maturity, and death—which are common to all—are made to illustrate how various cultures perceive and adapt to the various stages of life.

Adaptation also varies, as is reflected in the means of transportation, dress, housing, food, and life-style of different cultures. Changes in these may have adverse as well as beneficial effects on the lives of individuals. Changes with great impact that occur too close together in time can overwhelm our adaptive capacity and can contribute to a breakdown in health. This is evident in morbidity and mortality at stages of the life span when such events usually occur and in the sex primarily affected. Men and women do not necessarily experience the same life events, and those that are the same do not

necessarily occur at the same stages of life. Thus health is influenced biologically, culturally, and environmentally and is affected by experiences in the course of the life span. Health is a complex phenomenon related to all these factors and to adaptability to change.

Modern technology facilitates human adaptation in overcoming limitations, as aided by the availability of eyeglasses, dentures, hearing aids, wheelchairs, oxygen tents, elevators, refrigerators, and other items. The authors have shown the role of "habitat" on biological and social processes in the course of the life span. Habitats have different influences at each stage of life, and in this sense their effects also enter into the process of life itself. The term "ekistic development" is used to express this process. The term ekistics was coined by the late Constantinos Doxiadis, who proposed that the "built environment," as in cities, should have design characteristics appropriately adapted to the different periods of the life span and should respect human scale and cultural values for families as well as for children, teenagers, adults, and the elderly, separately.

While health is the primary focus of this work, it succeeds in seeing humans as persons in their context and illustrates how later phases of life are affected by earlier events in ways that had not previously been foreseen. The book does not try to tell readers how to live their lives, but instead offers a way of thinking about their own health and that of their families and friends. It provides a most useful perspective for students, professionals in health, and anyone personally interested in the importance of health in all its dimensions.

Jonas Salk

Preface

An Egyptian philosopher of science, Hermes Trismegistres, believed that "everything is mind" and visualization of perfect health could cure disease.* Using a very different set of assumptions, Carl and Stephanie Simonton** have been working to clarify the role of visualization in terms of psychotherapy, attitudinal change, and biofeedback in an attempt to restore health in cancer patients. These two brief examples illustrate ways in which persons have thought about the influence of beliefs on health. These and other approaches—not all of which are equally effective in curing sickness or restoring health—illustrate a facet of medical anthropology that is explored in this book; namely, that the basis of human health is rooted in the traditions and dynamics of cultural belief systems as well as in the biological attributes of human beings that have evolved over the millenia of human existence.

This book emphasizes the role of adaptation in the processes of health and sickness. Our purpose is to introduce the reader to the many facets of medical anthropology through a perspective that is both evolutionary and contemporary, biological and cultural, comparative and holistic. Health care systems are compared cross-culturally, while special attention is devoted to the strengths and weaknesses of Western systems. The biocul-

tural basis of health is surveyed across the human life cycle to emphasize the importance of retaining both a biological and a cultural perspective for assessing individual well-being. Likewise, the analysis of belief systems in western and nonwestern cultures points to the importance of the interaction of cultural factors with biological processes in the attainment of health. Our hope is that readers will come to recognize the important role of anthropology in the study of health and sickness, while at the same time recognizing that this discipline represents far more than the study of so-called exotic cultures. Expanding the view of medical anthropology in the manner we propose leads to recommendations for change in the present system of health care in the United States. Such recommendations are offered in the final chapter.

The book is designed to reach an audience of advanced undergraduate and graduate students in anthropology, medical and nursing students, and practicing professionals in these fields. Students in the social, behavioral, and health sciences and in the humanities, as well as a broad readership among educated laymen, may also find it of use as a means of tying together the diverse fields pertaining to health and sickness.

We would like to express our gratitude to the many people who aided us as the book passed through its formative, transitional, and final stages. Superb assistance in editing the manuscript was provided by Salvinija G.

---

*Samuels, M., and Samuels, N. *Seeing With The Mind's Eye*, Castro Valley, Calif., 1975, p. 22.
**Simonton, O. C., and Simonton, S. *Getting Well Again*, Los Angeles: J. P. Tarcher, Inc., 1978.

Kernaghan. Organization and style were much improved as a result of her patient yet demanding efforts. Dr. George Armelagos and Dr. Cheryl Ritenbaugh kindly served as manuscript reviewers. Their comments were exceedingly helpful, and many of their suggestions are included. Dr. Theresa Graedon, Dr. Linda Gerber, and an anonymous individual also reviewed selected portions of the book and made valuable suggestions. Melinda Lewis and Jonathan Sheldon served as research assistants, performing such varied and crucial tasks as finding references and other substantive materials in the library and securing permissions for the use of previously published illustrations. Vicki Collette, Judy Hertz, and Greg Jouflas provided creative interpretations of data, without which several sections of the book would have been much less complete and less interesting. Carole Campbell, Evelyn Eller, Linda Fenton, Glenn Fieldman, Sue Gilday, Leona Rozinski, Dorothy Singer, and Joanne Smith typed—and in many cases were patient enough to retype—the manuscript. Their efforts and encouragement are greatly appreciated. Special thanks are given to Bill Moore, Kathy Van Arsdale, Don Glittenberg, and Marge Aldrich for their ongoing and enthusiastic support through a trying period encompassing some 2 years.

Lorna G. Moore
Peter W. Van Arsdale
JoAnn E. Glittenberg
Robert A. Aldrich

Contents

CHAPTER 1

A new way of looking at health

THE HEALTH CARE CRISIS

Health care delivery in the United States is beset with a variety of problems, ranging from high costs to shortages of trained personnel in rural areas. Numerous and obvious causes are frequently identified when blame is being laid for these problems. One cause that is often overlooked is our society's straying from human scale in the organization of institutions and the construction of cities and towns. Individual capabilities, limitations, and needs can become lost in the rush of technological development. Industrialization and its handmaiden urbanization have generally been led by technological advances without penetrating consideration of their full range of human impact. For example, the construction of freeways after World War II, prompted by the proliferation of high-speed automobiles, has offered time-saving convenience but also has resulted in the splintering of once cohesive neighborhoods, significant air pollution, and dwindling fuel supplies. Thus, health and the need for medical care in cities have been influenced by such factors as increasing air pollution, noise, and vehicular traffic; at the same time, obtaining health care is complicated. Transportation to see the physician at an office, clinic, or hospital requires time, money, and even partial self-diagnosis if the appropriate specialist is to be reached. Appointments must be scheduled days or even weeks in advance, and even then the delays at the appointed time may be long and inconvenient. Having

reached the hospital or clinic, the patient needs a guide to get through the maze of insurance forms and admission papers. Attrition among the ranks of general practitioners who once practiced in urban centers has been great both because those who have died have seldom been replaced and because many have abandoned the inner city for more lucrative suburban practices. As a result, hospital emergency room services are the only accessible and immediate health care that is available around the clock to many inner-city dwellers and mobile suburbanites. No wonder the use of emergency rooms has risen at a dizzying rate since the 1950s; the emergency room *is* the access to medical care for millions of people (Mills, 1978).

The presence of problems in the current delivery of health care does not mean that the Western health care system does not offer benefits. Once dreaded diseases such as diphtheria, typhoid, and rheumatic fever have nearly disappeared; and smallpox appears to have been eliminated worldwide. Advances in medical research for understanding disease mechanisms have led to control of tuberculosis, measles, poliomyelitis, chicken pox, and mumps through immunization. Steps toward the control of chronic cardiovascular and respiratory diseases and cancers have been taken with the recognition of early warning signs and improved means of treatment, but the uncertainty surrounding the mechanisms respon-

1

sible for these diseases so far has prevented their complete control and cure.

Furthermore, the nature of the health care system itself is changing and in some instances demonstrates evidence of improvements in both its formal and informal structures. Movements toward increasing access to health care have occurred, with a resurgence of interest among physicians in the areas of general practice and family medicine and with the emergence of nurse practitioners, child health associates, and physicians' assistants. Another phenomenon that points to the dynamic nature of Western health care is the number of health and healing modes that have emerged during the past 2 decades as alternatives or complements to hospital- and clinic-based systems. In addition, there has been the efflorescence of such subdisciplines as medical anthropology. Health food stores, exercise spas, life-style changes, and biofeedback and relaxation techniques are growing in popularity within the broader context of a movement called "holistic health." Holistic health recognizes the importance of the whole person—including lifestyle, attitude, diet, and self-awareness—in addressing health care needs. Clearly visible among the individuals attracted to these resources and approaches is a questioning attitude toward the traditional role of physicians in meeting health needs. There is a "do-it-yourself" attitude, a searching for self-care, and an acceptance of responsibility for one's own health. The physician continues to be valuable for intervention at times of serious medical need, but is not regarded as a general guide to a life-style that promotes good health. In addition, more and more people are turning to non-Western systems in search of viable health and healing alternatives (Mattson, 1977).

Despite these changes in the health care system in the United States, health care costs, in terms of absolute dollars and per-cent of the gross national product, have risen and continue to rise dramatically (Fig. 1-1). Expenditures in 1980 are currently estimated to amount to $226.4 billion, more than a threefold increase over 1970 dollar amounts. From 1975 to 1977, costs for medical services rose at a rate that was more than one and one half times the overall rate of increase for all consumer prices (Culliton, 1978). The high costs appear to result from "the basic structure of the hospital industry and not to some one-shot causal factor such as wage 'catch-up' by hospital workers" (Council on Wage and Price Stability, 1977). The high costs of medical care clearly benefit physicians, drug companies, hospitals, medical schools, and other powerful groups in American society who continue to resist governmental efforts to control costs. The "spare-no-expense" attitude of the American patient when faced with the need for care, "the permissive atmosphere in which . . . medical workups are elaborated without much benefit to the patient" (Feingold, 1978), and the necessity of ruling out other diagnoses for protection against malpractice suits further adds to the resistance against reductions in health care costs.

Americans are not getting healthier as a result of paying more than ever before for health care (Knowles, 1977). Life expectancy is lower, and both infant and maternal mortality are higher than in the Scandinavian and several other western European countries. Within the United States, the poor and nonwhite are subject to considerably higher mortality than residents of the country as a whole. Causes of the poorer health status of Americans are thought to reside in behavioral, nutritional, and environmental characteristics. Yet these and other factors that affect the prevention of illness receive comparatively little attention. Increasing amounts of medical expenditures are for episodic care for the sick, while the proportion

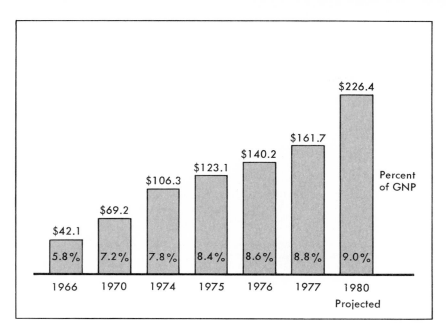

Fig. 1-1. National health expenditures in the United States and percent of gross national product (GNP) in selected years from 1966 to 1980 (billions of dollars). (From Feingold, 1978:2.)

spent on illness prevention has actually been decreasing (Feingold, 1978).

Spiralling costs, the unequal distribution of health care resources, and the lack of emphasis on preventing illness all contribute to the crisis—but whose crisis is it? Is it the crisis of the health care professions, the public, or individual sectors of the population, such as the aged and the poor? Who or what is responsible for the crisis? Some arguments point to the degree of specialization of health care personnel. Other arguments implicate collective bargaining, malpractice insurance, health insurance programs, and the duplication of expensive equipment in neighboring hospitals. Too, the intense concern of the adult American public over maintaining a state of near-perfect health leads to a demand for treatment when no treatment may be available or necessary.

Unraveling the causes of the crisis at a societal level is complicated by the knowledge that the United States is not a simple, homogeneous culture. Rather there are widely diverse subcultures that have become partially integrated into the dominant Western European matrix established by the early pioneers. Health beliefs and practices of our nation's founders largely reflected Western European notions of scientific methodology and relied on a model of specific cause and effect relationships for understanding health. As a result, many Americans subscribe to the belief that in order to achieve good health they must either ingest a variety of medications to destroy germs or have a diseased organ removed surgically.

Diverse subcultures remain within American society whose health belief systems vary from those of the dominant culture. A significant minority subscribe to folk practices and beliefs that are clearly of non-Western origin. Causes of illness are seen as related to strained or severed social relationships, and cures are sought in reestablishing the relationship or ingesting a range of balancing substances. Health care practitioners who originate in the dominant culture should be aware of the variant health beliefs of their clients and of the public at large. While the beliefs may be phrased in ways that are unacceptable to the Western practitioner, understanding the beliefs and the importance placed on the natural, physical, and social environments can complement and expand the Western notions of health and illness. In fact, Western scientists are beginning to develop theories of illness that parallel some non-Western beliefs in which, for example, life crises are seen as contributing to the cause of illness (Holmes and Masuda, 1973).

Thus, there are powerful yet conflicting health-related processes occurring in American society. Simultaneously, we are witnessing the long-term effects of urbanization and industrialization, a changing perception by the public about the physician's capabilities and roles, increasing costs of Western medicine, and a renewal and discovery of alternative means of health care.

What directions can we take to resolve this crisis? How can we place individuals in a position to promote their own health effectively? Where are there models that promote health and minimize risks? Living on a human scale offers a key to understanding these questions. By human scale, we refer to the size and the complexity of the culture in which the individual lives. Solutions to problems such as health care delivery need to be considered in terms of their impact on the individual rather than solely in terms of groups or systems. Reliance on technology has permitted human beings to modify their natural and physical environments throughout human existence. Yet within industrialized and urbanized countries, ramifications for health of the increasing scale of technological accomplishments, such as high-rise

office buildings and the automobile, begin to limit their advantages. Technological advances usually address a particular need and are judged on the basis of how well they meet that need. We must start looking at such changes in a broader context, including identifying their trade-offs for health. A human scale is one in which technological requirements (such as energy, space, density) are dealt with in such a way that the environmental modifications introduced do not threaten health. It is essential that health be sustained throughout the life span of individuals and that our human-built environments promote health and the overall human condition.

Recognition of the importance of the human scale in the maintenance of health has been acquired in large part through the work of medical anthropologists. Their efforts and those of related scientists in conducting comparative examinations of the biocultural basis of health and disease across the human life cycle and throughout many different cultures are the foundation for our discussions of health and health care in the subsequent chapters.

ANTHROPOLOGICAL VIEWS OF HEALTH

The term "medical anthropology" has become widespread in the short span of 15 years. The term first originated in the early 1960s (Scotch, 1963), paralleling developments in sociology that had led to the formulation of medical sociology. Yet the concepts of medical anthropology predate the early 1960s and are a part of the history of anthropology itself. Without always having been called "medical" this new subspeciality is, in fact, as old as anthropology itself.

To introduce medical anthropology, then, requires first the introduction of the field of anthropology as a whole. Anthropology has a broad scope that lends it a great deal of flexibility and potential for integrating information. A main purpose of anthropology is to enable us to escape the confines of our own individual culture. Each of us, by definition, acquires culture by virtue of being alive in a particular environment. Anthropologists have long tried to escape the bonds of ethnocentrism—the judgment of other cultures imposed by the norms and values of one's own particular culture—and to realize some additional dimensions of growing up and of being human. Anthropology tries to make other cultures accessible in ways that outsiders can understand, although recognizing that people who themselves grow up in another culture may possess a degree of familiarity with that culture that may exceed that of the investigator. At the broadest level, anthropologists try not only to understand cultures as they exist in the present or in the recent past but also to understand the processes by which human beings evolved.

Anthropology has twin dimensions: (1) time, past and present, and (2) the particular focus, cultural and biological. Anthropology's uniqueness lies in these two dimensions. Looking at past cultures is the domain of archaeology. Looking at present cultures is the concern of cultural anthropology. Likewise, the study of our past biological attributes is subsumed by paleoanthropology and paleontology. The study of our present biological condition by anthropologists is the concern of biological anthropology. Human ecology synthesizes aspects of cultural and biological anthropology concerning the ways in which contemporary or recent human populations have adapted to their environments. The scope of the natural sciences expands in many directions but without attempting to combine the cultural and behavioral aspects of humankind, as anthropology does. Likewise, other social sciences and humanities are not as concerned with the biological dimension of humankind as is anthropology.

Consequently, the discipline of anthropology aids in integrating the natural sciences, the social sciences, and the humanities.

Themes and methods of anthropology

The central themes that unite anthropology are culture and evolution. Culture is a simple concept when viewed at the general level, yet is subtly profound in its complexity when considered in more detail. Literally hundreds of definitions of culture have been put forth over the past century, but one that contributes to a clear understanding of biocultural interactions in an evolutionary perspective is the following: culture is the humanmade environment, encompassing the physical space in which humans are located, the behavioral patterns that contribute to their utilization of and interaction with the natural environment, the intangible outgrowths of such behavioral patterns (such as language and ritual), and the tangible products used to further modify or interact with the environment (such as tools, weapons, and buildings).

Culture is uniquely human. No other species has developed a system of this sort, although many exhibit one or more elements of the pattern (for example, even fire ants use small twigs as tools). All human groups exhibit culture, but it is in the analysis of detailed differences at the local level that the subtle complexities emerge. The traditional culture of the lowland Asmat hunter-gatherers in New Guinea is different from that of the highland New Guinea Dani horticulturalists and is also different from that of transitional Asmat being subjected to rapid change by outside agents, such as government officials and missionaries (Van Arsdale, 1975). Local adaptation patterns, necessitated by differences in the natural environment and a group's own traditions, are the keys to understanding culture at the microlevel. In turn, an understanding of health is a direct correlate of this same ecological perspective. At the macrolevel, general human health can be discussed as it is manifested by most members of our species, and at the microlevel can be discussed as characteristic of the adaptations of a particular group.

Evolution, the other unifying theme of anthropology, provides a means of integrating its biological and cultural dimensions. Evolution is a process of gradual change through time in the inherited characteristics of a population. Factors that facilitate the production of surviving offspring will be selected for, that is, they will become increasingly more common in future generations. Biological characteristics, such as resistance to disease, constitute adaptations that, if inherited, can influence the course of evolution. Likewise, cultural features can influence the production of surviving offspring and, hence, the direction of evolution. Thus, both biological and cultural traits are involved in evolution. Until recently, it was assumed that only biological traits could be directly transmitted by genes from generation to generation. However, sociobiologists have proposed that behavior may also be controlled by genes (Wilson, 1975), creating the possibility that cultural adaptations may also have genetic roots.

The methods, like the themes, of anthropology are distinct from those of other disciplines because they are comparative and holistic. The holistic approach considers things as wholes. If it is necessary to break them into parts in order to grasp them more directly, the ultimate aim is still to try to put them back together, to try to reassemble the pieces of the puzzle. In so doing, the anthropologist may use the same methods as other scientists, but the distinction arises in the conceptual use to which the methods are put. For example, the nutritionist and the anthropologist may use the same techniques to assess diet, but the goal of the anthropologist

is likely to concern a more general problem, such as the effect of culture change on diet, whereas the nutritionist may be trying to determine simply whether dietary needs are being met.

The term "comparative" refers to concerning oneself with diversity when trying to learn about a particular phenomenon and then attempting to generalize from the information obtained. Diversity can be visualized across space, looking at the different ways roughly contemporary but distinct cultures have molded a particular life event. For example, to compare burial customs, one could consider different ceremonies in contemporary cultures, examining the particular funeral practices, forms of ritual that are expressed at the time of a person's death, the way the grief is handled, the way the families are affected, the kind of relationships between the community and family, and the ways in which the body is prepared for burial (Mandelbaum, 1959). Diversity can also be visualized as variation across time. If one were interested in variation in burial customs through time, it might be helpful to know that the first evidence of what appear to be burial customs—evident in the still visible stains of red ocher on the fossilized bones of a Neanderthal man—appeared over 50,000 years ago (Solecki, 1975). There are a variety of possibilities, but each is comparative, and each uses information from several circumstances that is then integrated to infer the way people have dealt with life events—in this instance, death.

Development of medical anthropology

Medical anthropology relies on the following central attributes of anthropology: the themes of culture and evolution, the dimensions of time and space, concern with human cultural and biological variability, and the methods of comparative and holistic analysis. More specific consideration of the anthropological approach to understanding health and illness requires reviewing the history and continuing traditions of medical anthropology.

The emergence of medical anthropology occurred as a result of historical developments in Europe and the United States that originated in the 1600s and continue through the present (Fig. 1-2).

During the 1600s and 1700s, extensive overseas exploration and trade provided information on previously unknown peoples and diseases (Fig. 1-2). Western physicians, such as Jacobus Bontius, Francisco Hernandez, and Willem Piso, gave detailed descriptive accounts of diseases and medical customs of tropical peoples, since in fact the overseas explorations by European powers were aimed almost exclusively at tropical and semitropical areas. Western medicine did not have its natural science base well developed, so analytical studies of what were then considered dangerous diseases of tropical origin were not possible (Fig. 1-2). The absence of analytical studies also hindered the development of effective therapeutic measures. Yet, apart from the limited attempts made by some missionaries and explorers, application of Western medicine to tropical

peoples generally was not acceptable to early colonial administrations being set up in the Americas, Africa, south Asia, southeast Asia, and Oceania. It was not until the late 1800s that comprehensive systems of health care were introduced under some colonial regimes (Van Amelsvoort, 1964:10) (Fig. 1-2). One reason is that bacteriological discoveries, facilitated by the invention of the microscope, and epidemiological studies permitted progress to be made against tropical diseases. In Indonesia, for example, a hierarchy of hospitals and outpatient clinics was introduced in the late 1800s for care of the local population (Van Amelsvoort, 1964:10).

Developments within social philosophy paralleled overseas exploration and later introduction of Western medicine. During the 1600s and 1700s, social issues, such as the nature of human beings and of society, were being raised by philosophers such as John Locke (Fig. 1-2). These inquiries fostered the recognition that sociocultural phenomena were a legitimate field of inquiry and contributed to the emergence of sociology and anthropology in the 1800s and early 1900s. Theory building within anthropology utilized the information being provided by overseas exploration to reconstruct culture history in

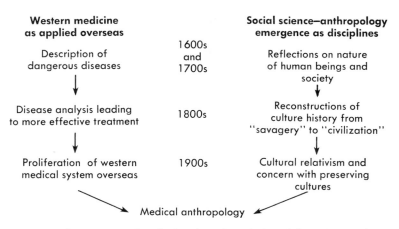

Fig. 1-2. The historical emergence of medical anthropology. (Adapted from Van Amelsvoort, 1964:9).

often grandiose terms, such as Lewis Henry Morgan's formulation of the stages of savagery, barbarism, and civilization through which cultures were expected to pass (Fig. 1-2).

An applied Western health ethic was emerging during the late 1800s, a point worth mentioning here because it bore on the general treatment of indigenous peoples and because of the subsequent close association between medical and applied anthropology. By the late 1800s, world exploration had been completed, and colonial regimes had become sufficiently entrenched and began to permit appreciation of local cultures to emerge among some administrators. In anthropology, cultural relativism—an affirmation of the uniqueness and the value of every culture—was emerging and replacing the earlier, ethnocentric descriptions of other cultures (Fig. 1-2). Smallpox, malaria, and other devastating diseases introduced to North America had devastated the settlements of many native Americans, and this recognition, combined with an increased sense of confidence on the part of well-to-do persons of European heritage that indigenous peoples no longer posed a threat to their own existence, caused some to speak out in behalf of better health care. Similarly, in the nineteenth century an Aborigines Protection Society was founded in London (Reining, 1970:3; McNickle, 1972).

Cross-cultural ethics were closely intertwined with a general paternalistic attitude on the part of colonialists, neocolonialists, and others engaged in the delivery of services to indigenous peoples. By the 1920s, complex educational systems had been established for local inhabitants in most of the colonial tropics. In west Africa, where the system of instruction paralleled that found in England, education was patterned after that of the mother country under the assumption that Europeans knew what Africans needed.

Other than observations recorded by anthropologists and other scientists on traditional cures and religious practices (for example, Rivers, 1924), these data were not being applied, and native people's knowledge of health and disease was not being incorporated into the colonial educational and medical systems.

Early twentieth century European observers of medical practices in non-Western cultures were often physicians themselves and hence were trained in the traditions of Western medical science (such as Rivers and Ackerknecht, whose work is reviewed in Chapter 6). They described their counterparts in other societies and the medical practices used. Great diversity in native medical systems was recorded, but these systems were assumed to depend on unreliable techniques of witchcraft and sorcery. On the other hand, both Rivers and Ackerknecht recognized the substantive nature of non-Western medical beliefs. According to Rivers, medical practices comprised a set of coherent beliefs, "inspired by definite ideas concerning the causation of disease" (1924: 51). The theoretical orientation of these early observers emphasized the importance of belief systems underlying the concepts of disease and medical practices to the virtual exclusion of considering biological factors affecting disease (Wellin, 1978). It was assumed that the biological factors were the same in all populations and, hence, were not subject to influences of local culture or conditions.

Subsequent impetus to the study of the cultural dimension in medical anthropology came from developments in the 1930s and 1940s (Foster, 1978). The culture and personality school of thought in anthropology was formulated in the 1930s by Ruth Benedict and others. Their idea that people living in a given culture are likely to share a common personality led to a union between anthropological and psychiatric understanding of mental illness that is still prevalent. Continuing contact between anthropologists and health professionals was also facilitated during World War II and afterward with the international public health movement. Public health workers expected non-Western cultures to adopt the medical practices they introduced. When the expected failed to occur, health workers turned to the writings and knowledge of anthropologists about indigenous sociocultural practices and beliefs that might affect the acceptance of Western medical practices. The resultant cooperation between anthropologists and health care workers remains one of the most successful enterprises in applied anthropology (Foster, 1978).

Contemporary studies in medical anthropology that rely on a cultural approach have continued the interests of earlier observers of the sociocultural belief systems that affect concepts of disease causation and the acceptance of treatment. In addition, concern in contemporary studies extends to the behavioral response that the disease elicits and to the human meaning of illness. Answers are sought to questions such as, what is it like to be ill? When disease occurs, who treats it? What forms of treatment are recognized as therapy? Do particular forms of illness fall within the aegis of particular kinds of healers? What kinds of interactions occur between the healer and other persons? When a choice must be made between forms of therapy, what kind of treatment is accepted? Sometimes in situations of culture contact, a fine distinction is made between the kinds of illnesses for which one goes to native practitioners and the kinds of illnesses for which one goes to Western medical practitioners. A number of interesting studies have documented the processes employed in the treatment of disease, their interaction, and the relative successes of the various methods employed (as in Landy, 1977; Logan and Hunt, 1978; Bauwens, 1978).

While not broadly recognized, the history of medical anthropology also extends to concern with the biological dimension of health and disease. There has been a longstanding alliance between the interests of basic medical sciences and students of human evolution. Anatomy has been a province of anthropologists interested in human evolution. Their approach, which continues today, has emphasized comparative and functional dimensions of anatomy. Geneticists and physiologists have cooperated with anthropologists in the exploration of genetic diversity and adaptation to environmental conditions. Nutrition, public health, and social and preventive medicine have all been areas of cooperation between medical scientists and anthropologists through the identification of broader dimensions of disease. The histories of nursing and anthropology overlap significantly. An important link is the common focus on the patient and the major factors that affect the disease experience.

Ecological framework

Increasing interest in human variation, stimulated by advances in genetics and evolutionary biology in the last few decades, has led to a contemporary synthesis of the cultural and biological dimensions of medical anthropology within an ecological framework. The ecological approach is concerned with factors underlying the incidence of disease. The factors are attributes of culture—such as urbanization and industrialization—and of biology that have major consequences for broad categories of disease, such as infectious ailments. In an ecological approach particular environmental circumstances are also recognized as important contributors to the kinds of disease endemic to a region.

The ecological approach is also concerned with the effects of disease and health practices on the culture itself. For example, what is the impact on a society of having 30% of its children die before the age of 1 year, as is true among the Amsat (Van Arsdale, 1978)? Some diseases that are endemic throughout much of the tropical world, such as schistosomiasis, are not usually fatal but do reduce the level of well-being and energy within a population.

The combination of biological and cultural dimensions of health and disease makes the ecological approach biocultural in nature. As the concept is discussed in this book, health is considered a reflection of an individual's ability to adapt to the environment by biological or behavioral means. Disease is defined as a reflection of failure to adapt to the environment and is usually manifested by abnormalities in the structure and function of body organs and systems. Disease and illness are often used interchangeably but may be considered to have slightly different meanings. Illness refers to the experience of "disvalued changes in states of being and social function" (Eisenberg, 1977:11). Illness thus includes those social and psychological aspects of a disease that not only affect the ill person, but also may affect the person's family and friends. As exemplified elsewhere in this volume, non-Western healers often focus their attention on illness, whereas Western healers tend to pay more attention to disease. Finally, sickness is a more general term with a less specific meaning and can be used to encompass both disease and illness.

THE BIOCULTURAL APPROACH TO HEALTH

Concepts of health and disease are a part of every culture and thus are themselves variable. Western culture has emphasized a specific mechanistic, causal explanation in trying to understand disease, while other societies have identified causes in a range of what might be termed systemic factors. Western medicine traces its formal origins to post-Renaissance Europe, a time when infectious diseases were prevalent. Under the leadership of scientists, such as Louis Pasteur and Robert Koch, advances were made in understanding diseases that were transmitted by microbes. The tradition subsequently developed whereby the understanding of disease meant an understanding of its cause, referred to by Dubos (1965) as the "doctrine of specific etiology." The doctrine was especially applicable to infectious diseases and was also in keeping with the prior cultural belief that disease was an interruption of a state of equilibrium. The disease vector could be isolated, external to the organism; and by its removal, the state of health could be restored. Adherence to the doctrine of specific etiology has impeded the acceptance of an ecological view founded on the more general notion that disease results from adaptive failure. When viewing the contemporary disease picture of the Western world, one that is replete with chronic disorders for which no single pathogen has yet been identified, some believe that attachment to the doctrine of specific etiology has slowed the search for a broader range of causal factors that may eventually lead to effective treatment of chronic disease such as cancers (Kelman, 1977).

In contrast to the doctrine of specific etiology, in other cultures the cause of disease may be thought to include an array of natural, social, or supernatural agents. Among the Kolongo-speaking Abran of Ghana, there are ten reported kinds of causes of disease, including natural causes, breaches of taboo or social regulation, and the actions of ghosts, witches, gods, or malevolent spirits (Alland, 1970:138). A study of Israeli mothers who had given birth to children with Down's syndrome revealed an array of factors that the mothers thought were responsible, including the effects of the Arab-Israeli war, bad dreams, and quarrels with family members, but almost no mention was made of the factor that Western medicine considers the cause, an extra twenty-first chromosome (Chigier, 1972). These examples illustrate two types of causal explanations: proximate and ultimate. The proximate cause is the agent (bacteria, virus, twenty-first chromosome) that accounts for the specific condition. Ultimate cause is less objectively ascertained. The question of ultimate cause seeks answers to questions such as "Why me?" or "Why now?" Western medicine can frequently identify proximate cause but often totally ignores questions of ultimate cause; other cultures emphasize ultimate cause and consider proximate cause as incidental or of secondary importance.

The effects of disease and their interpretation also vary according to cultural circumstance. The introduction of measles by an external agent to a previously unexposed South American Indian group, the Yanomama, occasioned significant mortality because of the disruption created for social and family life, whereas measles is rarely fatal in Western cultures (Neel, 1970). In parts of Mexico and Guatemala, mortality from measles is as much as 250 times greater than in the United States because of the influence of nutritional and other factors affecting resistance (Graedon, 1978). Another example concerns the incidence of albinism among the Hopi Indians of northern Arizona. Albinism is produced by a genetic defect in the enzyme responsible for producing pigmentation in the skin, hair, and eyes. In a study of the factors responsible for the higher than normal incidence of albinism among the Hopi, greater cultural acceptance and protection for the albinos was considered the most likely explanation (Woolf and Dukepoo, 1969). Thus, differences in cultures can act both to increase and to decrease the severity of disease.

A conception of diseases as fixed entities fails to recognize that diseases themselves evolve. In particular, viruses, bacteria, and parasites have a shorter generation time and therefore can accomplish genetic changes much more quickly than can their human hosts. The "new" influenza virus of a particular year may be the descendant of the virus of the previous year after a hundred generations of evolutionary change. In addition to recognizing that human beings have been adapting throughout their evolutionary history, we must also recognize that human beings have had diseases throughout their existence. The first human diseases were likely to have been caused by lice, intestinal worms, and protozoa, since these were shared with the animals hunted by early human beings and with other animals in the environment. Infectious diseases were not likely to have prevailed until agriculture and urbanization provided a sufficiently dense population base (Armelagos and Dewey, 1970).

Therefore, along with the evolution of disease has occurred the evolution of human adaptation to disease. Because the diseases faced by a population have varied according to environmental and cultural circumstance, human populations are characterized by adaptations to different kinds of diseases. Adaptation to malaria provides one of the most detailed examples. An inherited hemoglobin variant, hemoglobin S, is found in much higher frequency throughout tropical regions. The high frequency of hemoglobin S is surprising insofar as individuals who are homozygous for hemoglobin S (having received an S gene from each parent) have a usually fatal disease, sickle cell anemia. Trauma, injury, and other poorly understood causes can bring about a sickling crisis in these individuals, during which the hemoglobin inside red blood cells becomes locked into a rigid shape that in turn causes the red blood cells to assume an irregular or sickle shape. Blood capillary vessels in which the sickling occurs become jammed, preventing oxygen supply to vital organs, such as the brain; this can be fatal. The observation that malaria was common in areas where hemoglobin S was found led to the hypothesis that hemoglobin S, when present in the heterozygous condition (having received an S gene from one parent and the common form of hemoglobin from the other parent), conferred immunity to malaria (Allison, 1954). The immunity appears to result from biochemical features of red blood cells containing hemoglobin S that are incompatible with the nutritive requirements of the malaria parasite (Eaton and Brewer, 1969). Anthropological research indicating that malaria became prevalent after the introduction of agriculture had led to clearing the tropical forest and creation of standing pools of water pointed to a role played by culture in instigating the disease process (Livingstone, 1958). Recently nutritional deficiency of vitamin E also has been reported to protect against malaria (Eckman, Eaton, and Berger, 1976). Thus, cultural and other factors that lead to low dietary levels of vitamin E or that restrict the amount of vitamin E absorbed would be adaptations to disease in a fashion analogous to the genetic adaptation conferred by the hemoglobin variant.

Health and disease, then, far from being unchanging phenomena, are intrinsically variable. They vary as a result of a society's interpretation of health and disease, through changes in the biological and cultural factors causing the disease, and through biological and cultural adaptations conferring health. Too, the variation affecting health and disease is ongoing. Changes in biological factors are not easily observed over the short run, but, nonetheless, can be expected to occur. Changes in culture lead to advances in forms of therapy available to restore health and to create conditions that facilitate the maintenance of health. Culture can also further the spread of disease as illustrated by the malaria example. Critics of the nuclear power industry point to the likelihood that the proliferation of radioactive materials (from leaks and nuclear accidents, such as the March 1979 mishap near Harrisburg, Pennsylvania) will lead to increased incidence of leukemia and other cancers. Air pollution, another by-product of culture, is also linked to the frequency of respiratory and cardiovascular disorders. Thus, the analysis of biological and cultural factors must take into account the dynamic aspects of health and disease.

We develop the concept of the biocultural basis of health and disease and its implications for improving the current health care delivery system in the following six chapters. In Chapter 2, we develop in greater detail the ecological approach to understanding health and disease by presenting a model of the various factors that influence the health-sickness process; we then apply the model to three case studies taken from our research. Chapter 3 demonstrates the applicability of the model to large and small population groups through time. In it we examine the theoretical processes by which adaptation is achieved and the patterns of adaptation that are found in the evolutionary record and during later phases of human history, in particular during the period of colonialism in the Americas and Oceania.

Chapters 4 and 5 demonstrate the applicability of the model to the individual by charting the determinants of health through the human life cycle and by emphasizing the constant interplay between cultural and biological forces. Highlights include the critical role played by culture in ensuring that parents bond with their infants after birth, the impact of chronic disease on families and of families on chronic disease, the cultural changes in American society that are affecting the future of its children, and the biological and cultural factors associated with aging, dying, and death.

In Chapter 6, we examine more closely the impact of one aspect of culture—a society's belief system—on the manner in which disease is defined and treatment is applied. A comparison is made between the belief systems that have engendered primitive health care practices and those that have given rise to the varieties of health care currently practiced in Western society.

Chapter 7 draws from the previous chapters in an attempt to forecast the future of health. Questions regarding unequal distribution of worldwide resources are discussed and special issues facing developing countries and the United States are raised. Recommendations for achieving a humanistic health care system are made along with suggestions for the directions that such a system might take. Having described in Chapter 1 the crisis facing Western medicine and giving our view of the basis of human health and disease in subsequent chapters, we offer our interpretation of what desirable future health care policies should be.

REFERENCES

Alland, A. *Adaptation in Cultural Evolution*. New York: Columbia University Press, 1970.

Allison, A. C. Protection afforded by sickle-cell trait against subtertian malarial infection. *British Medical Journal*, 1954, *1*, 290-294.

Armelagos, G. J., and Dewey, J. R. Evolutionary response to human infectious diseases. *Bioscience*, 1970, *157*, 638-644.

Bauwens, E. E. (ed.). *The Anthropology of Health*. St. Louis: The C. V. Mosby Co., 1978.

Chigier, E. *Down's Syndrome: A Cross Culture Study of Child and Family in Israel*. Lexington, Mass.: Lexington Books, 1972.

Council on Wage and Price Stability. Executive Office of the President, Washington, D.C., January 1977.

Culliton, B. J. Health care economics: the high cost of getting well. *Science*, 1978, *200*, 883-885.

Dubos, R. *Man Adapting*. New Haven, Conn.: Yale University Press, 1965.

Eaton, J. W., and Brewer, G. J. Red cell ATP and malaria infection. *Nature*, 1969, *222*, 389-390.

Eckman, J., Eaton, E., and Berger, H. J. Role of vitamin E in regulating malaria expression. *Transactions of the Association of American Physicians*, 1976, *89*, 105-115.

Eisenberg, L. Disease and illness: distinctions between professional and popular ideas of sickness. *Culture, Medicine and Psychiatry*, 1977, *1*, 9-23.

Engel, G. L. The need for a new medical model: a challenge for biomedicine. *Science*, 1977, *196*(4286), 129-136.

Feingold, E. The crisis in health care. *Rackham Reports*, 1978, *4*, 1-3.

Foster, G. M. Medical anthropology: some contrasts with medical sociology. In Logan, M. H., and Hunt, E. E., (eds.). *Health and the Human Condition*. North Scituate, Mass.: Duxbury Press, 1978, pp. 2-11.

Graedon, T. F. Personal communication, 1978.

Holmes, T. and Masuda, M. Life changes and illness susceptibility. In *Separation and Depression*, American Association for the Advancement of Science, 1973, pp. 161-186.

Kelman, S. The social nature of the definition of health. In Navarro, V. (ed.) *Health and Medical Care in the U.S.: A Critical Analysis*. Farmingdale, N.Y.: Baywood Publishing Co., 1977.

Knowles, J. (ed.). *Doing Better and Feeling Worse: Health in the United States*. New York: W. W. Norton & Co., Inc., 1977.

Landy, D. (ed.). *Culture, Disease and Healing: Studies in Medical Anthropology*. New York: The MacMillan Co., 1977.

Livingstone, F. B. Anthropological implications of sickle cell gene distribution in west Africa. *American Anthropologist*, 1958, *60*, 533-562.

Logan, M. H., and Hunt, F. F. (eds.). *Health and the Human Condition*. North Scituate, Mass.: Duxbury Press, 1978.

Mandelbaum, D. G. Social uses of funeral rites. In Feifel, H. (ed.). *The Meaning of Death*. New York: McGraw-Hill Book Co., 1959.

Mattson, P. Holistic health: an overview. *Phoenix: New Directions in the Study of Man*, 1977, *1*, 36-43.

McNickle, D. Indian and European: Indian-white relations from discovery to 1887. In Walker, D. E. (ed.). *The Emergent Native Americans: A Reader in Culture Contact*. Boston: Little, Brown and Co., 1972.

Mills, J. D. Introduction. In Jenkins, A. D. (ed.). *Emergency Department Organization and Management, ed. 2*, St. Louis: The C. V. Mosby Co., 1978, pp. 1-7.

Neel, J. V. Notes on the effects of measles and measles

vaccine in a virgin-soil population of South American Indians. *American Journal of Epidemiology*, 1970, *91*, 418-429.

Reining, C. C. A lost period of applied anthropology. In Clifton, J. A. (ed.). *Applied Anthropology: Readings in the Uses of the Science of Man*, Boston: Houghton Mifflin Co., 1970.

Rivers, W. H. R. *Medicine, Magic, and Religion*. New York: Harcourt Brace Jovanovich, Inc., 1924.

Scotch, N. Medical anthropology. In Siegel, B. J. (ed.). *Biennial Review of Anthropology*. Stanford, Calif.: Stanford University Press, 1963, pp. 30-68.

Solecki, R. S. Neanderthal is not an epithet but a worthy ancestor. In Hunger, D. E., and Whitten, P. (eds.). *Anthropology: Contemporary Perspectives*. Boston: Little, Brown and Co., 1975.

Van Amelsvoort, V. F. P. M. *Early Introduction of Inte-grated Rural Health Into a Primitive Society*. Assen, Netherlands: Van Gorcum, 1964.

Van Arsdale, P. W. *Perspectives on development in Asmat*. In Trenkenschuh, F. A. (ed.). *The Asmat Sketch Book Series*. Asmat Museum, Agats, Irian Jaya, 1975.

Van Arsdale, P. W. Population dynamics among Asmat hunter-gatherers of New Guinea: data, methods, comparisons. *Human Ecology*, 1978, *6*, 435-467.

Wellin, E. Theoretical orientations in medical anthropology. In Logan, M. H., and Hunt, E. E. (eds.). *Health and the Human Condition*. North Scituate, Mass.: Duxbury Press, 1978, pp. 23-39.

Wilson, E. O. *Sociobiology: The New Synthesis*. Cambridge, Mass.: Harvard University Press, 1975.

Woolf, C. M., and Dukepoo, F. C. Hopi Indians, inbreeding, and albinism. *Science*, 1969, *169*, 30-37.

CHAPTER 2

The human ecosystem and human adaptation—a contemporary view

Human populations, just as other forms of life, undergo a continual process of adaptation to disease. Archaeological and paleo-anthropological studies illustrate the dynamics of human adaptation to a variety of environmental stresses throughout the millions of years of human evolution. In more recent times, written and spoken accounts of historical events allow us to examine more closely and to evaluate the effects of disease and illness on human populations. As we move into the last decades of the twentieth century, it is clear that the disease process has become increasingly complex.

In underdeveloped countries infectious diseases, such as pneumonia, tuberculosis, and diarrheal diseases, still are the primary causes of death, but in developed industrialized countries, environmental selective pressures are more complex. In developed countries, changes in demography, epidemiology, and technology have increased the complexity of the human ecosystem. A multifactorial analysis of many interacting variables is now necessary to understand the disease process, as opposed to the unicausal system that grew out of the nineteenth century Koch postulates, known as the "one germ—one disease" theory. Today's environment may be too intricate for the traditional "doctrine of specific etiology" to be useful. For example in contemporary epidemiological studies, single host, vector-carrier, and vic-

tim explanations do not go far enough in examining disease causation. A multiple-variable model of the human ecosystem is necessary to analyze and explain the various causes of injury, illness, and disease.

MODEL OF THE HUMAN ECOSYSTEM

The model we believe best represents the interrelationships and dependencies of the human ecosystem (Fig. 2-1) consists of two major subsystems. Subsystem I covers environmental factors and includes two levels of analysis, the macro- and microlevel environmental variables, which in turn include inorganic variables, all living matter, and humanmade sociocultural factors. Subsystem II—the individual—is the organismic level. The factors that are included in this subsystem represent a holistic view of an individual's adaptive capacity in the health-sickness process.

Subsystem I

The macrolevel. The macrolevel unit of analysis of Subsystem I involves large aggregates of populations—societal, national, hemispheric, or even global. In the larger of these groups, it is unlikely that all individuals share a common environment. Widely separated populations around the globe adapt to different physical factors: a hot, dry desert; a cold, cloud-layered mountainous region;

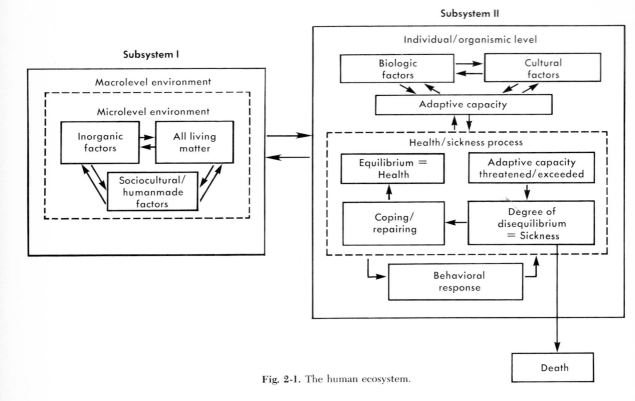

Fig. 2-1. The human ecosystem.

a fertile valley in a temperate zone; or a multitude of other climatic and geographic elements (Fig. 2-2). Likewise, the diversity found among all living matter is clear evidence of the variety of flora and fauna that are best adapted to each ecological niche. Certainly the diets of both human and animal populations are largely influenced by the prevalent food supplies in their area.

Humanmade environments are also diverse and have innumerable physical and cultural manifestations. The great variety of cultural patterns found throughout the world reflect the human ability to develop behavior patterns that enhance the probability for survival in each ecological niche.

The microlevel. The microlevel, in contrast to the macrolevel, is composed of smaller population aggregates that may share an

inorganic, organic, and humanmade environment. The distinction of the microlevel is the fact that the aggregate population is a common mating pool. The reasons for the common mating pool are varied; but foremost among them is that the physical environment imposes geographical restraints that limit the sharing of mates. Other factors also may limit the exchange of mating partners through the cultural rules and taboos that are associated with choosing partners from another class, ethnic group, or religion. For example, in the Mayan Indian town of Patzun, Guatemala, the 8000 inhabitants share a mountainous, high-altitude ecological niche. Their chief food supply consists of corn, beans, and wheat, and their chief occupation is subsistence farming. There is little migration away from the community among the townspeo-

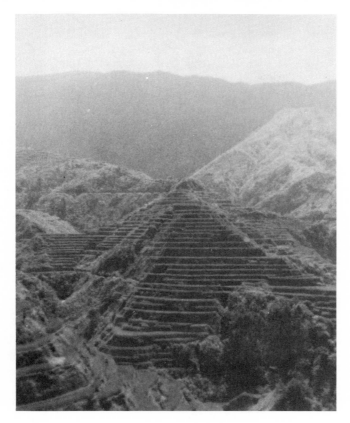

Fig. 2-2. Terraced fields accommodate the need for raising crops in mountainous settings in the Phillipines. (Courtesy M. B. Drysdale.)

ple. *Patzuneros* cultural norms require them to marry within their own town; in fact, it is preferred that mates be chosen from a designated section of the town. Their inheritance patterns are patrilineal, and the household pattern is patrilocal. Each of these cultural patterns defines the life-style of a *patzunero*. Deviations from the norm certainly occur, but the characteristic cultural pattern is adaptive to the environment of that area.

Environmental factors and disease

Disease is caused by varying sources in the inorganic and the organic environments and cultural patterns of behavior that affect susceptibility to and transmission of disease.

Inorganic factors. Among significant inorganic factors in the environment is climate. Climate affects the kinds of disease-causing agents that live in a given location and thus the kinds of diseases with which human beings living there will come in contact. Another example of the influence of climate on disease is the apparent improvement in arthritis in people moving to hot, dry climates.

Pathogens react differently under various physical conditions; for example, influenza viruses decay more rapidly under high humidity, while asthmatic attacks increase in similar environments. Yaws and elephantiasis are also diseases of particular ecological niches, which thrive in the tropics. In contrast, multiple sclerosis has its highest incidence in cool climates. Such genetically determined diseases as pernicious anemia and diabetes mellitus are seldom found outside the temperate zone (Sulman, 1976:81).

Popular interest in what effect atmospheric change has on psychological states is evidenced by numerous studies of the relationship between biological rhythms, atmospheric conditions, and various aggressive activities, such as accidents, suicides, and homicides (Licht, 1964; Lowry, 1970). Climatic changes also may bring health-related changes; for example, depressed persons are more prone to commit suicide when a weather front is moving in. An increase in thromboembolisms is associated with electrical storms because air ionization may provoke neural hormone changes that can precipitate a thromboembolism (Sulman, 1976:80).

Geography and geology are also factors that influence health. Clearly, a variety of natural disasters, such as floods, landslides, volcanoes, and earthquakes, are related to geological factors. Air pollution is a health hazard in most major U.S. cities and is frequently caused by an atmospheric inversion by which the cooler air is trapped by a heavy layer of warmer air. Thus the pollutants are maintained in the lower, cooler air and are prevented from dispersing into the upper atmosphere.

Inorganic factors, taken alone, influence the health of a population, but as part of a more complex interacting system in which the impact of organic and humanmade factors is also felt, they become even more powerful in influencing health in the contemporary world.

Organic factors. Organic factors include all living matter—flora and fauna, disease pathogens as well as human beings. All life on this planet is in some way related to or is part of the food chain. Neither human beings nor disease agents could exist without balance within the food chain. Physical factors, such as droughts and floods, affect this balance, while cultural features, such as level of technology, may increase food production. Major technical innovations in agricultural production, such as a mechanized plowing system or the development of new hybrids of grains and livestock, signify the importance of the interactions of the three major environmental factors (inorganic, organic, and cultural) in Subsystem I.

Another development demonstrating the critical relationships among the factors in the human ecosystem is the dramatic increase in world population by the year 2000 A.D. If the inorganic, organic, and humanmade variables cannot be manipulated in such a way as to ensure greater food production and to control population expansion, imbalance in the ecosystem may have disastrous results.

The very success of the human species in reproducing itself at a rate greater than the ecosystem can support is also fostering other problems that eventually influence health. Increased population density in cities, for example, has made the disposal of human waste and the ensuring of safe, adequate water supplies problems of grave concern. The demands of large populations for energy, especially in highly developed countries, has put these same societies at risk from the dangers stemming from energy production itself; the April 1979 accident at the Three Mile Island nuclear reactor in Pennsylvania was a graphic demonstration of these potential dangers.

Like human beings, disease pathogens also try to adapt and survive. Microorganisms compete with one another for resources and require a balance in their environments in order to survive. Their effects on human health are varied. Some pathogens have short life spans and reproduce rapidly, while others such as the one causing kuru, a disease found in New Guinea that affects the nervous system, have a long incubation period of about 2 years. The kuru virus is powerful, for after the incubation period the central nervous system is attacked and quickly degenerates. In contrast, other viral infections are not so virulent; for example, viruses causing colds and influenza usually have short-term effects and produce no long-lasting immunity to the diseases.

Other types of pathogens are bacteria, funguses, protozoas, and helminths. Bacterial organisms are classified by their various shapes, which are cocci (round), bacilli (rod shaped), and spirochete (spiral shaped). Funguses, usually attack the skin, and although they are not commonly a cause of death, they may result in severe damage to human mucous membranes (Alland, 1970:26). A third type of pathogen is the protozoa, or one-celled animal, which causes such human diseases as malaria, amebic dysentery, and African sleeping sickness. Helminths, or worms, are of various types and may be found affecting human populations in most parts of the world. They may have a severely debilitating effect on the host. Alland notes that the amount of blood lost each year in the United States because of hookworms is appalling but does not compare to loss in the population of Egypt where the infestation rate of schistosomiasis is about 95% of the peasant population (1970:181).

Other potentially harmful organic substances in our environment are associated with domestic animals. For example, dogs may be pets or sentinels, but they also may be menaces because they harbor a host of common infectious diseases. It is surprising that humans and domesticated dogs share sixty-five diseases (McNeill, 1976:51). Other domesticated animals that share infectious diseases with humans are: poultry (twenty-six), rats and mice (thirty-two), horses (thirty-five), pigs (forty-two), cattle (fifty), and sheep

and goats (forty-six) (McNeill, 1976:51). The benefits of domesticated animals are well-known, but knowledge about the liabilities of sharing infectious diseases is more recent. Also that liability may increase as human population density increases and there is more frequent interaction with domesticated animals.

Humanmade factors. The humanmade environment consists of the products of culture—the tools and methods by which human beings adapt to their environment (Bennett, 1976:234). All the varied ways of interacting—the rules and norms of a group—become the cultural pattern or, at the individual level, the blueprint for living. Culture is expressed through a variety of social institutions, such as kinship, religion, laws, education, economics, and medicine, as well as through such expressive systems as values, beliefs, language, play, art forms, myths, and folklore.

Cultural patterns alter the interaction between human beings and infectious pathogens. Eating, sleeping, and mating influence the transmission of disease. Settlement patterns, occupations, work roles and status are other culturally determined elements that significantly alter the incidence of various diseases. Cultural practices, such as religion, may be instrumental in curtailing or increasing diseases. For example, religious pilgrimages may increase disease prevalence by bringing together widely separated populations. Holidays, feasts, vacations, and trips may also affect the health status of groups and individuals. Finally, social institutions, such as schools and military service, where persons from widely dispersed environments are brought together, may act as breeding grounds for new diseases. Of equal importance to human health is the fact that, as is described in detail in Chapter 6, culture—in the form of belief systems and their related systems of curing disease—has a significant impact not only on how disease is acquired but also on how it is treated.

Macrolevel and microlevel analyses of the interaction of variables are important ways of how human populations through time have adapted to pathogens and other deleterious factors in the environment. Indeed the adaptive process is complex, for a disease does not merely result from an accumulation of environmental factors but rather from their multiple interactions. The response of human beings to this complex process depends in large part on individual adaptive capacity.

Subsystem II

The individual. The individual level of analysis in the model of the human ecosystem is an essential link in the chain of human evolution. From the time when our ancestors first began to walk upright to the moment when a human being first stepped onto the surface of the Earth's moon, the individual has been both the locus and the maker of change. It is within the individual that disease is most obviously manifested. For this reason, we must examine more closely the conditions that determine the state of health or disease in this smallest unit of analysis in the model of the human ecosystem.

Individual characteristics. A human being represents the union of inherited, species-specific characteristics and culturally determined traits. Although the influences of biology and culture are inseparable from one another in their action on individual adaptive capacity, we must first examine them independently in order to better understand their effect on the whole person.

Biological factors set certain adaptive limits to survival. For example, each physiological system has certain parameters for adequate functioning. Blood pressure, chemical and electrolyte balance, and other physiological functions have upper and lower limits that are similar in all human groups and under varying conditions. Another biological characteristic, blood type, appears in limited types (A, B, O, and AB), each of which is also shared by large human groups and has been linked to propensity for certain diseases. Brothwell (1971) describes some of these suspected associations as they have been found in samples of varying sizes (Table 1).

Other biological capacities may be affected by the cultural factors in an individual's environment; similarly, the biological base must be adequate for an individual to become a member of a culture. For example, in the event of severe mental retardation, a child may not become socialized into the norms of the culture; severe sensory deprivations, such as blindness, deafness, and the various syndromes that cause language impairment, also may influence the process of

Table 1. Some claimed (but by no means proven) associations between blood group phenotypes and disease*

Disease	Associated ABO or secretor phenotype
Bubonic plague	O
Smallpox	O, N
Syphilis	B and AB
Infantile diarrhoea	A
Influenza virus A_2	O
Bronchopneumonia	A or AB
Diabetes mellitus	A
Paralytic poliomyelitis	B (and excess of non-secretors)
Rheumatic fever	A, B (and non-secretors)
Pernicious anaemia	A
Duodenal ulcer	O
Cancer of stomach	A
Gastric ulcer	O
Salivary gland tumours	A
Tumours of the ovary	A
Cancer of the cervix	A
Pituitary adenoma	O
Cancer of the prostate	A
Cancer of the pancreas	A

*From Brothwell, D., 1971.

enculturation into a group's values and mores. Enculturation is a dynamic learning process, and it usually occurs within an individual's primary group, providing a guide to behavior that will be the most rewarding in that particular population.

Certainly cultural practices of individuals affect their biological selves. Such a cultural pattern as diet is a case in point. For example, quick service food outlets, common in modern urban centers in both developed and underdeveloped countries, influence the nutritional state of a population. Habits such as drinking and smoking also can engender biological stresses. Rest, relaxation, and psychological renewal are cultural patterns that affect the biological unit, as do learned patterns of behavior; for example, the high priority placed on speed and fast automobiles in many developed countries is linked with fatal automobile accidents.

Although human reproduction is similar throughout the world, cultural practices may influence the process. For example, Davis and Blake (1956) have developed a framework to study how sociocultural variables affect human reproduction. These variables include: age at first sexual union, postpartum abstinence, coital frequency, age of menarche, months of breast-feeding, the date at which menstruation is resumed postpartum, and use of modern contraceptives (such as the coil and the pill). For example, work roles are cultural patterns that may affect the frequency of intercourse. Even the manner in which the female transports her infant may influence the amount of work the female can do. In agricultural societies, where females engage in heavy physical labor requiring the use of both hands, a mother who carries an infant in a sling on her back is free to participate fully in the labor force. For example, a Cakchiquel mother carries the infant on her back while she engages in two-handed labor—embroidery work (Fig. 2-3). In con-

trast, Fig. 2-4 shows a Ladino mother and infant; the mother does not carry her infant on her back but rather in front. Consequently, the Ladino mother is not free to use both hands in work.

What differences do these culturally defined patterns have on fertility? Glittenberg (1976) found that the Cakchiquel mothers only partially breastfed their infants. Supplementary solid foods were introduced quite early into the infant's diet while the mother continued to do two-handed labor. In contrast, the Ladino mother did not engage in work while she was breastfeeding her infant. Although breastfeeding does not preclude conception, there is evidence that ovulation may be delayed (Perez, and others, 1971:491). The consequence of these two different breast-feeding patterns may result in

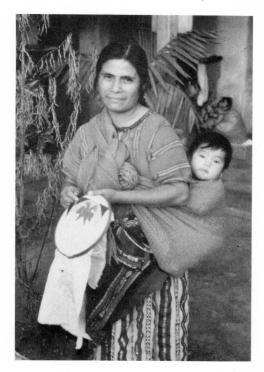

Fig. 2-3. Guatemalan mother carrying her infant on her back. (Photo by J. E. Glittenberg.)

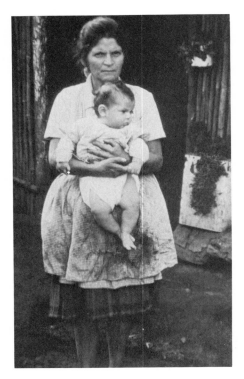

Fig. 2-4. Ladino mother holding infant in a typical manner. (Photo by J. E. Glittenberg.)

differences in the length of time before ovulation is resumed after giving birth (Glittenberg, 1976:90).

The adaptive capacity. The results of these two forces—the biological and the cultural—influence the whole person; it is the whole person who is either well or ill, not just the part of the organism that may be diagnosed as diseased. Adaptive capacity is also a result of a biocultural union; it is the capability of the whole person to adjust to changes in the environment, to cope with internal and external stress, and generally to maintain an equilibrium in all internal physiological and psychological systems. The stresses in the environment are innumerable, but they are not all stressful to every individual to the same degree. For example, a vacation flight to the island of Maui may be looked on by one person as a relaxing time, while to another individual the flight may be a horrendous experience. Each event is individually perceived as some point on a stress-relaxation continuum.

The adaptive capacities of some individuals are likewise greater than those of others; it is possible to demonstrate empirically that in some individuals, tolerance to stress is higher and coping behavior is more successful. Such persons are more frequently in a state of health than not. What are some of the factors that contribute to this success? Age is one, for as the individual grows older, adaptive capacity decreases; this relationship is described further in Chapter 5. Another time-related factor that influences the adaptive capacity is the number and the timing of stressful life events. Studies in recent years have identified how physical and psychological stresses are related to life events (see Chapter 5, pp. 00). Such events as death in the family, divorce, change of job or vocation, or a move to a new location all take their toll on the adaptive capacity of individuals. Such studies have been replicated cross-culturally and they are described in more detail in Chapter 5.

The proposition that life-style influences health is supported by some statistics on causes of death of males in the United States (see Table 2). The rates of death are based on the Hammond Report, a study of the life-styles of approximately half a million males in the United States. The figures indicate that, while there are differences in death rate patterns between whites and nonwhites, divorced males of either group are likely to die earlier than married males (Lynch, 1977: 41). Thus, the influence of life-style on health may entail the interaction of multiple factors, among them being marital state.

The adaptive capacity, in sum, is influ-

Table 2. Death rates of divorced and married men per 100,000 population, ages 15-64 in the United States, 1959-1961*

Cause of death	White males		Nonwhite males	
	Married	Divorced	Married	Divorced
Heart disease	176	362	142	298
Motor vehicle accidents	35	128	43	81
Cancer of respiratory system	28	65	29	75
Cancer of digestive system	27	48	42	88
Stroke	24	58	73	132
Suicide	17	73	10	21
Cirrhosis of liver	11	79	12	53
Hypertension	8	20	49	90
Pneumonia	6	44	22	69
Homicide	4	30	51	129
Tuberculosis	3	30	15	54

*From Lynch, James. *The Broken Heart.* New York: Basic Books, Inc., Publishers. 1977, p. 41.

enced by numerous factors, some of which are genetically inherited characteristics and others of which are developmental characteristics, such as the aging process and accumulated life events. Finally, the great variety of cultural patterns and social relationships also have a significant impact on an individual's adaptive capacity.

Health-sickness process. The health-sickness process is a dynamic continuum as it is represented in the model of the human ecosystem. Both health and sickness manifest themselves in degrees. The degrees of sickness may be related to a time factor; for example, a person may be suffering from an *acute* phase of a disease, or from a *chronic* condition that spans many years or a lifetime, such as cystic fibrosis. On the other hand, the degrees of sickness may be related to its physical extent. It may affect a single body part, such as a small wound in a finger; or it may involve a large portion of the body, such as an arm or even the total body, as is the case with septicemia or a systemic infection of the circulatory system. In the process, failure to cope with or repair the damage leads to increased sickness and, if the body fails to adapt, ultimately leads to

death. On the other hand, coping or repair of the body may lead to an augmented state of health or wellness. The result of the recovery process is thus a return to equilibrium, or health. Several indications, such as blood chemistry, healed wounds, and recovered feelings of alertness and relaxation, may be used to measure the outcome of coping and repair. The individual, while alive, is always at some point on the health-sickness continuum.

Death. Death is the result when the demands for coping and repair exceed the individual's adaptive capacity. This process may be gradual and predictable, or it may be sudden and its specific etiology unknown, such as occurs with sudden infant death syndrome or in deaths related to voodoo or severe fright. Other unexplained deaths may be associated with severe grieving and loss, such as may occur on an anniversary of a loved one's death or during special events related to severe loss. In the future these "unexplainable" deaths may be more thoroughly understood on the basis of physiological changes, but at this juncture their cause is not fully understood.

Death represents a failure to cope or to repair at the *organismic* level, and it removes an individual from active participation in the human ecosystem. However, the memory, the writings, and other artifacts of the individual may remain a part of the ecosystem for some time—several generations or longer for those individuals who leave a mark on human history. For the purposes of studying and explaining the dynamics of the ecosystem, however, the deceased individual can no longer be considered an active part of the system.

Behavioral feedback. As long as an individual is alive, the circumstances that engender health or sickness as well as the very state of being either well or sick evoke a behavioral response that feeds back not only into the organismic level of the ecosystem—that is, the individual—but also into the microlevel and macrolevel of Subsystem I. The behavioral response appears in many forms, some of which do not seem to have a direct relation to the health-sickness process. However, insofar as they express and reinforce an individual's attitude toward self and the world, these responses very definitely influence the individual's adaptive powers. Such responses may be expressive (for example, writing a poem about the struggle to survive or the joy of living), physical (such as planting a garden or digging a ditch), or cognitive (such as changing one's evaluation of the health care system). These behaviors may influence one or more of the Subsystem I environmental factors either directly or indirectly, either negatively or positively. For example, in the case of an individual's changing evaluation of the health care system, new forms of health care may result, or old forms may be destroyed or modified. Another behavioral response may be in the form of human reproduction; the biological condition of the parents will affect the progeny (as will be illustrated in the first case study in this chapter, related to high altitude), and deleterious genes may be maintained in Subsystem I through the transmission of genetic diseases. Thus at each level of analysis, the interaction of multiple variables directly or indirectly affects the whole human ecosystem. Consequently, when we address the issue of the biocultural basis of health, we incorporate in our hypotheses a holistic, dynamic view of human beings adapting in various degrees to and within a series of levels—the macrolevel, the microlevel, and the organismic.

We have now come full circle in describing the factors within Subsystems I and II, as well as discussing the value of dividing the systems into various levels of analysis. Using the two subsystems is a helpful way of separating the factors while still maintaining that human beings, and thus the human ecosystem, comprise a whole in which one part is not isolated from the others. The following three case studies illustrate the operation of Subsystems I and II by describing how individual adaptive capacities operate under three different sets of environmental stresses and so influence all levels of the human ecosystem.

CASE STUDY I: HUMAN ADAPTATION TO HIGH ALTITUDE

The study of human adaptation to high altitude provides a chance to view the relationship between human beings and their environment in a relatively simple fashion. As do the other case studies in this chapter, the example of high altitude provides the chance to see the operation of the human ecosystem in concrete terms. Characteristics of the physical, natural, and humanmade environment at high altitude are distinctive. Their effects on the individual and, in turn, the biological and cultural adaptive responses made can be shown to affect the health-sickness process in ways that are to some degree unique to high altitude. The most distinctive aspect of the high-altitude environment is the decreased oxygen supply. Because oxygen is vital to all biological processes and therefore to the survival of the individual, this case study emphasizes the importance of biological responses to features of the natural and physical environment, in comparison with the next two case studies, which focus on other major variables in the human ecosystem.

High-altitude regions comprise a small portion of Earth's habitable areas. Yet the value of studying high-altitude regions lies not only in understanding the conditions experienced by the persons living at high altitudes but also in the insight gained from recognizing the effects of limited oxygen supply on human health and disease. A large proportion of diseases that afflict humankind are diseases that affect oxygenation; these include heart, lung, circulatory, and hematological disorders that can interfere with one of several steps in the delivery of oxygen to the tissues—picking up oxygen in the lungs, transporting it through the body, and delivering it to the tissues. Such diseases are generally detectable only when their effects have become so severe as to limit normal physical functions. Individuals may then be diagnosed as having chronic obstructive lung disease, angina pectoris, arteriosclerosis, or anemia.

Characteristics of high altitude

High-altitude populations are found in the Andes of South America, the Rocky Mountains of North America, the Himalayas of Asia, and the East African Highlands (Fig. 2-5). In general, the term "high" altitude is reserved for those areas above 2500 m (8250 feet) (Fig. 2-6). Some 20 to 25 million people currently live at high altitudes (DeJong, 1970). Except in the North American areas, human populations have resided at high altitude for thousands of years, during which time genetic adaptations to high-altitude stress may have occurred in those groups.

The availability of oxygen decreases at high elevations as a result of the diminishing weight of the atmosphere (barometric pressure). At sea level, normal barometric pressure is 764 torr (or millimeters of mercury); at 3000 m, the barometric pressure is reduced to 530 torr. The proportion of oxygen in the air is 20.93% at all altitudes, but because of the decreased atmospheric pressure, the pressure exerted by oxygen (oxygen partial pressure, or Po_2) is lessened.

Decreased Po_2 is not the only effect of high altitude. Temperature drops by an average $0.5°$ C for every 100 m gain in elevation, but the drop varies in response to local conditions of humidity, season, and latitude. Increased ultraviolet radiation also occurs at high altitude, since the thinner atmosphere is less effective in screening out solar rays. The air is drier as a result of low rainfall, cool temperatures, and great diurnal temperature variation. Thus, a number of environmental characteristics accompany the drop in Po_2 at high altitude, but decreased oxygen availability, termed "hypoxia," is the universal and biologically most significant aspect of high altitude.

Process of high-altitude adaptation

A discussion of the possible components of high-altitude adaptation must necessarily take into account a broad range of factors. Aspects of the physical environment evoke biological and cultural responses that, in turn, can modify the effects of the environment. Fig. 2-7 diagrams some of the features of the high-altitude environment that could be considered.

If we consider the highland Andean Indian population as an example, we can see that features of this group's culture include a series of accommodations to the limited energy available in the environment, for the rigors of the climate and altitude decrease the productive capacities of plant and animal populations. In the altiplano area of southern Peru, cultural adjustments include: (1) spa-

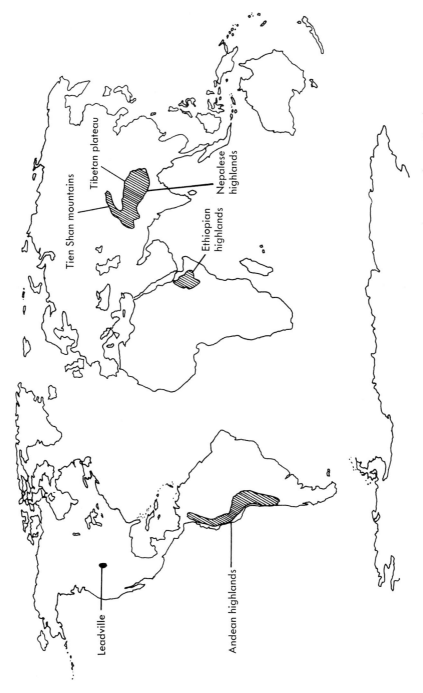

Fig. 2-5. The distribution of areas of the world over 2500 m. (From Pawson and Jest. In Baker, 1978:19.)

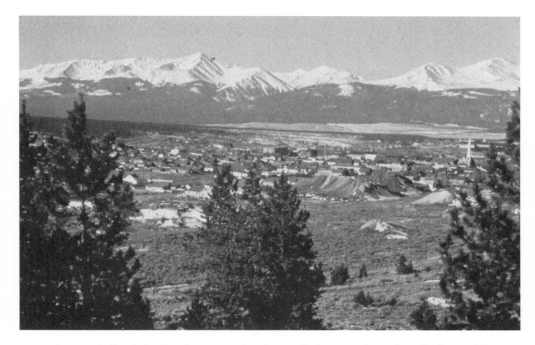

Fig. 2-6. Leadville, Colorado, elevation 10,200 feet, with Continental Divide in background (Courtesy R. F. Grover.)

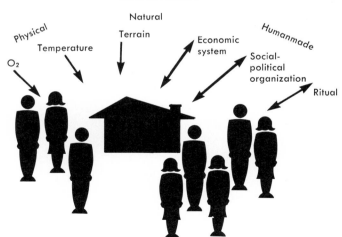

Fig. 2-7. Some components of adaptation to the high-altitude environment.

tially dispersed plant and animal resources, (2) exchange of food and other materials between climatic zones, (3) division of labor that relies on child participation, and (4) an activity pattern in which sedentary subsistence tasks occupy a large portion of the day (Thomas, 1976). The dispersion of resources is an attempt to match the climatic diversity over a small area with requirements for growth of particular plants and animals. Exchange between climatic zones permits products of animals adapted to the altiplano (llama, vicuna, alpaca) to be exchanged for high calorie resources of the lower altitudes. Children are an important economic asset to a household because their smaller size permits them to accomplish light or moderate work (for example, herding) at a lower energy expenditure than would be required of adults. Large family size (high fertility) is greatly valued, ensuring a large number of children for the household work force (Thomas, 1976). Apart from occasionally strenuous periods, adults and children commonly spend the majority of their time in sedentary activities that reduce energy expenditure.

Cultural responses appear primarily to be accommodations to the features of high altitude because the fundamental stress—low oxygen availability—cannot be changed by culture. Other environmental features such as the cold and low humidity can be modified by culture, but scarce vegetation and a paucity of heating fuels restrict their availability in Andean culture. To adapt to limited oxygen supply, high-altitude inhabitants must rely on biological responses.

Among the first biologic responses of the newcomer to the high altitude environment is an increase in pulmonary ventilation that serves to elevate the amount of oxygen (Po_2) in the blood. The barrel chest of the native Andean permits greater total lung capacity, which may increase the capacity for gas diffusion from the lungs to the capillaries and, therefore, help to maintain a higher Po_2 in the arterial blood during times of stress. Thus, for both native and newcomer, pulmonary adaptations serve to elevate oxygen tension and thereby reduce the level of hypoxia experienced. Hypoxia also stimulates the production of red blood cells with a resultant increase in the oxygen content of the blood. The net result of these pulmonary and hematological alterations is to permit a greater volume of oxygen to be carried from the lungs to the tissues. Biochemical adaptations inside the red blood cells also enable more of the oxygen carried by hemoglobin to be released. Finally, changes also may occur in the tissues to facilitate oxygen utilization.

These physiological responses to high altitude appear adaptive insofar as they effectively reduce the amount of tissue hypoxia; that is, oxygen availability is increased, which is comparable in effect to a reduction in altitude. Not all individuals appear equally able to make these adaptive responses. Surprisingly little is known about what is responsible for variation among individuals, but one factor would seem to be sex (Table 2). Higher arterial Po_2 is reported for female compared to male newcomers at high altitudes (Cudkowicz, Spielvogel, and Zubieta, 1972). At high altitude, female compared to male pigs have higher arterial oxygen tensions and less enlargement of the right ventricle of the heart; enlargement is commonly interpreted as a sign of impending right heart failure (McMurtry, Frith, and Will, 1973). Acute mountain sickness—a collection of symptoms experienced soon after ascent, including headache, nausea, and dizziness—appears to be less common and less severe in women. Too, chronic mountain sickness, as is discussed in this case study, is seen only rarely in females (Arias-Stella, 1971). Male mortality during infancy is commonly higher than female mortality at all altitudes, but the increase in male infant mortality compared to female infant mortality at high altitude is further accentuated (Spector, 1971). Thus, many of the clearest symptoms of failure to adapt are less common in women than in men. Physiologists over the past 70 years have noted an advantage for females in adjusting to high altitude:

I think on the whole that women suffer less than men.

T. H. Ravenhill, 1913

As a rule, females are supposed to suffer less than males.

F. F. Fitzmaurice, 1920

Chronic mountain sickness seen in La Paz favors predominantly males of a mixed or entirely European background.

J. Ergueta, H. Spielvogel, L. Cudkowicz, 1971

Results . . . establish the existence of cardio-pulmonary differences between the sexes, and suggest that females are better able to adjust to hypobaria than males.

I. F. McMurtry, C. H. Frith, D. H. Will, 1973

Available evidence suggests that sex hormones may play a role in accounting for differences observed between the sexes in adaptation to high altitude. Sex hormones influence variables that affect oxygenation. Progesterone increases ventilation at low and especially at high altitudes (Hasselbalch, 1912; Sutton, and others, 1975). In fact, progesterone is currently being used effectively as therapy for men suffering from chronic mountain sickness (Kryger, and others, 1978). At very high altitudes estrogen treatment prolongs survival in male rats (Davis and Jones, 1943). Testosterone stimulates the production of red blood cells and also enables more of the oxygen in the blood to be released to the tissues (Gorshein, and others, 1972). In a recent experiment by one of the authors, the effects of the sex hormones—progesterone, estrogen, and testosterone—on high-altitude adaptation were compared by treating rats with one of the hormones at either high or low altitude and comparing their cardiovascular and hematological responses. Contrary to expectation, the female hormones (progesterone and estrogen) had no protective effect on the physiological responses to high altitude that were measured. However, treatment with the male hormone, testosterone, appeared to adversely affect the animals by increasing the degree of enlargement of the right ventricle of the heart, thus increasing the propensity for right heart fail-

ure. These studies suggest that the advantage enjoyed by females in response to high altitude may not be caused, at least in the rat, by the presence of female hormones, but rather by the absence of testosterone (Moore, McMurty, and Reeves, 1978).

Sex hormones are also, of course, involved in the development and maintenance of reproductive ability. Is it mere coincidence that sex hormones affect both reproduction and physiological responses to high altitude? Pregnancy can be viewed as a link between the two insofar as pregnancy and high altitude both require modifications of oxygen transport. Not only do women fare better at high altitude, they also suffer less from diseases marked by chronic hypoxia and right heart failure, such as chronic obstructive lung disease (bronchitis, emphysema), sleep apneas and hypoventilation syndromes (disorders marked by a failure to breathe sufficiently, especially during sleep) (Webster, and others, 1968; Guilleminault, Tilkian, and Dement, 1976). Might the physiological effects of sex hormones have evolved in conjunction with the female's need for extra oxygen transport ability during pregnancy?

One of the difficulties encountered in adapting to high altitude concerns problems in reproduction that appear, at least in part, because of the growth-retarding effects of hypoxia during prenatal life. If some women are better able to supply oxygen to their fetuses than are others, their offspring would not show fetal growth retardation and thus would have a more favorable chance of survival. Limitations on the female's ability to respond to the combined effects of pregnancy and high altitude would then constitute a "bottleneck" for adaptation to high altitude.

This line of reasoning is being investigated in a study to examine the combined effects of pregnancy and high altitude on maternal oxygen transport in a nonnative (and thus theoretically more variable) population living in Leadville, Colorado (elevation 3300 m, or

10,200 feet). The question to be addressed is whether women producing growth-retarded infants are more hypoxic during pregnancy than mothers of infants with normal intrauterine growth. This study may shed light on whether the ability of women to respond to the combined effects of pregnancy and high altitude does indeed constitute a "bottleneck" for high-altitude adaptation.

Adaptive challenges of high altitudes

Early Spanish historians reported that the Spaniards colonizing Peru in the 1600s had great difficulty having children. Fifty-three years were said to have elapsed before a child survived in the city of Potosi at an elevation of 4500 m (14,900 feet); the child's survival was attributed to a miracle of Saint Nicholas of Tolentino (Monge, 1948). Spanish children born in the highlands were said not to survive unless they had some Indian admixture. Factors such as cold, poor nutrition, and economic deprivation are likely to have contributed to the Spaniards' inability to reproduce at high altitudes.

Pizarro moved the capital of Peru from the Incan city of Jauja at 3250 m (10,800 feet) to Lima at sea level in part because of reproductive difficulties experienced by the domestic animals brought to Peru by the Spaniards. The Act that founded Lima as the new capital of Peru pointed to the "great disadvantage and lack felt by the citizens who peopled this said city [Jauja], neither there nor in its surroundings nor anywhere in the upland could pigs, mares, fowls be raised because of the great cold and sterility of the land, and because we have seen by experience among the many mares that have dropped colts [that] their offspring usually die" (Monge, 1948:34-35). Confusion arises in these early accounts cited by Monge as to whether high altitude depressed fertility, increased mortality, or both.

More recent studies have not resolved whether or not fertility is depressed in high-land South America. The analysis of official birth records in Andean countries suggests that ferility is lower than in lowland regions (James, 1966). However, the records are likely to underestimate fertility, especially in highland areas where infant mortality is particularly high (Whitehead, 1969). Detailed studies of the high-altitude Indian community of Nuñoa in southern Peru show that completed fertility (that is, the number of children born to a woman during her reproductive years) averages 6.7. This is high by Western standards but low in comparison to other peasant societies and to the completed fertility of lowland populations. Further, migration to low altitude appeared to lead to an increase in fertility in persons coming from high altitudes when compared to the fertility of either high- or low-altitude natives or to migrants coming from other lowland areas (Hoff and Abelson, 1976).

Numerous experimental animal studies report diminished fertility at high altitude. Smaller litter sizes, ranging from 48% to 90% of those at sea level, have been observed in nonnative animals at altitudes above 3000 m. Higher proportions of unsuccessful matings have also been observed among native and nonnative animals at high altitude when compared to the same species at low altitude (Nelson and Srebnik, 1970). In addition, acute exposure to very high altitudes causes infertility, increased spontaneous abortions, abnormalities in the rat ovulatory cycle, and extensive fetal reabsorption in mice (Altland and Highman, 1968).

Thus, available evidence suggests that fertility is decreased at high altitude in both human beings and experimental animals, although the evidence is more clearcut in the case of nonhumans. Whatever the effect of high altitude on fertility, levels seen in Andean populations are well above requirements for population replacement and have proved sufficient to maintain human settlements in the Andes for 10,000 to 20,000 years.

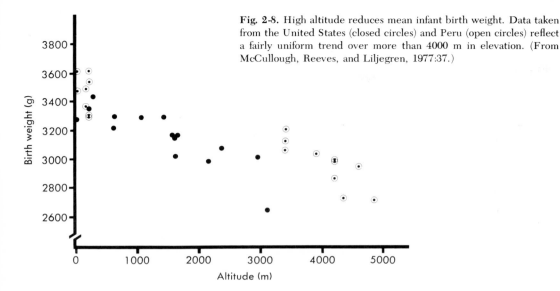

Fig. 2-8. High altitude reduces mean infant birth weight. Data taken from the United States (closed circles) and Peru (open circles) reflect a fairly uniform trend over more than 4000 m in elevation. (From McCullough, Reeves, and Liljegren, 1977:37.)

High altitude has consistently been shown to contribute to reduced infant birth weight. Data from South and North America show a uniform reduction in birth weight of infants in areas over 4000 m in altitude (Fig. 2-8). Normal gestational ages in the high-altitude samples point to fetal growth retardation rather than shortened gestation as the principal cause (McCullough, Reeves, and Liljegren, 1977). Placental size and weight are increased relative to the size of the infant at high altitude, possibly reflecting an adaptation to confer more nutrients to the developing fetus (McClung, 1969). In Andean communities, a greater reduction in infant birth weight occurs in Mestizo than in Indian residents at high altitude; this may indicate a genetic difference in adaptation between these two groups (Haas, 1976).

In all populations studied thus far, infants born at high altitudes are less likely to survive than are infants born at low altitudes. Mazess (1965) reported higher neonatal and infant mortality in highland than in lowland Peru. Perinatal mortality is also elevated in high-altitude regions of Ethiopia (Harrison,

and others, 1969). A recent study of vital statistics in Colorado indicates that while mortality for the state as a whole has declined, infant mortality in counties at elevations above 2740 m (9000 feet) is nearly twice that seen in lower-altitude portions of the state (McCullough, Reeves, and Liljegren, 1977). In Peru and Ethiopia, factors other than altitude in the highland and lowland communities make it difficult to detect the effect of altitude alone on infant survival. In comparison, the availability of good vital statistics records and comparable medical care in the high- and low-altitude settings in Colorado points to the likelihood that the higher altitude is responsible for increasing the infant death rate. Supporting this is the observation that the higher death rate results principally from the greater risk of preterm infants dying from respiratory disease (McCullough, Reeves, and Liljegren, 1977).

Postnatal growth (0 to 2 years) is also reduced at high altitude. Despite apparently adequate nutrition, high-altitude Andean Indians and Mestizo infants are lighter and shorter than their low-altitude counterparts (Haas, 1976). The same study indicates that growth retardation is more marked in males than in females, again reflecting the apparently greater effect of altitude on males than females. Growth continues to be reduced during the period from infancy through adolescence in the highland native. Both male and female residents of Nuñoa, Peru, evidence a late and poorly defined adolescent growth spurt and a prolonged period of growth when compared to sample populations in low-altitude Peru (Frisancho and Baker, 1970). The possibility exists that smaller body size at high altitude is adaptive, insofar as energy requirements are reduced. However, the degree of reduction in body size, especially at birth, must not be so great as to threaten survival.

High altitude affects the health-sickness process later in life as well as during prenatal and early infant stages. Newcomers commonly experience a collection of symptoms including headaches, nausea, and dizziness, together known as acute mountain sickness. High-altitude pulmonary edema may also develop on arrival; but it is a rare occurrence, and the causes are poorly understood. One hypothesis is that natives of a high altitude who have descended to a lower altitude for a brief stay are more susceptible to high altitude pulmonary edema on their return (Hurtado, 1960). Unless the victim of this condition returns to sea level or is given supplemental oxygen, the disease may be fatal.

Another condition, termed chronic mountain sickness, sometimes develops in residents of high altitude in whom acclimatization to high altitude is lost. The disease can be seen in both sexes and in all age groups, but it is more common in males over the age of 30 years and is only rarely seen in women. The hyperventilation normally seen at high altitude disappears; consequently, the amount of oxygen in the blood falls, and the individual becomes more hypoxic. The pressure of the blood flowing through the lungs rises (hypoxic pulmonary hypertension). Blood volume and, in particular, the number of red blood cells increase. The result, and most obvious symptom of the disease, is a hematocrit ranging from 60% to 80%. Elevated hematocrits result and are the most obvious symptom of the disease. The high blood viscosity caused by the increased hematocrit imposes a greater workload on the heart. The disease, in time, can result in a stroke or heart failure and can be fatal unless the hematocrit is lowered by repeated phlebotomy ("bleeding") or, as has recently proved successful, by the administration of progesterone.

An increase in respiratory disease and a decrease in cardiovascular disease have also been reported at high altitudes. Several studies in highland Peru have shown greater mortality from respiratory diseases throughout life when compared to lowland areas. Lower blood pressures and serum cholesterol levels, fewer signs of cardiovascular disease, and lower mortality from cardiovascular disease have also been observed at high altitudes in Peru (reviewed by Way, 1976). Death records from Colorado suggest that persons with emphysema at higher altitudes experience a higher mortality risk (Moore, Rohr, and Reeves, 1979). The analysis of deaths from coronary disease in Colorado did not reveal any altitude differences (Morton, Davids, and Lichty, 1964), but a report from New Mexico indicates a reduction in the number of deaths from cardiovascular disease in men living at higher altitudes (Mortimer, Monson, and MacMahon, 1977). Thus, while deaths from respiratory diseases appear more common at high altitude, protection from cardiovascular disease remains less clearly established.

Both reproduction and survival appear challenged by high altitude. Indications of lowered fertility, increased infant mortality, higher mortality from respiratory disease as well as the specific high-altitude disorders of chronic mountain sickness and high altitude pulmonary edema point to problems of human adaptation to high altitude. That populations have resided at high altitudes throughout the world for thousands of years is testimony to the ability of human beings to adapt to the high-altitude environment. Nevertheless, the health problems of recent migrants, such as the residents of Leadville, Colorado, and populations long resident at high altitudes elsewhere in the world point to the continuing challenge for adaptation.

Summary

This case study illustrates the effects of environment on the ability to live and reproduce at high altitude, in other words, to adapt. The high-altitude environment is distinctive insofar as a major feature—hypoxia—cannot be modified by culture. High altitude appears to challenge the adaptive capacities of human populations through possible reduction in fertility, increased infant mortality, and specific high-altitude diseases. Physiological responses that increase the amount of oxygen available to the tissues appear adaptive. Also, cultural adaptations serve as means of accommodating human activities within existing environmental constraints. Knowledge of the biological and cultural characteristics of high-altitude populations has increased in recent years, but there is a continuing need for more studies. The lack of genetic models for the inheritance of complex traits and the need for greater consideration of the interaction between biological and cultural modes of adaptation remain as limiting factors for building a comprehensive description of human adaptation to high altitude. Future studies, such as the investigation of maternal response to pregnancy at high altitude and its bearing on fetal growth, may provide information about the processes by which adaptation may occur. Expanding our knowledge about adaptation to high altitude can serve not only as a model of how adaptation to stresses of the natural physical environment occurs but also as a means of understanding the underlying processes that give rise to hypoxic diseases of the heart, lungs, circulatory system, and blood—disease that affect millions of Americans each year.

CASE STUDY II: HUMAN ADAPTATION TO NATURAL DISASTERS

This case study describes a population's response to a devastating earthquake and in so doing demonstrates the interrelationships of the three environmental factors in the model of the human ecosystem: the inorganic (the seismic activity along the Motagua fault in Guatemala), the organic (the death and injury toll of the inhabitants along the fault), and the humanmade (specifically, the maladapted house type introduced into the area by the Spanish conquistadores). As the previous case study emphasized the biological responses to the environment, this case study concentrates on the sociocultural responses to an environmental catastrophe. It points out that prevailing cultural practices may not necessarily be maximally adaptive because of conflicting demands. In particular, the study emphasizes that housing, a cultural trait, must be an asset rather than a liability to an individual's adaptive capacity and that when cultural practices are in fact liabilities, they must be modified to ensure the survival of the individuals in the population.

Disruptive effect of natural disasters

The tremendous annual toll natural disasters take on human life is sobering. The human suffering and economic disruption from such events are largely immeasurable. For example, more than a billion dollars is spent annually for disaster relief in the United States (Haas, Kates, Bowden, 1977: 25). Geological events in the United States cause damage to property in excess of 5 billion dollars a year (Cochrane, 1975). Hurricanes, cyclones, tornadoes, lightning, earthquakes, frost, tidal waves, drought, floods, wind storms, hail, and volcanoes are major catastrophes that occur annually around the globe. Their effects may be sudden, such as that of a hailstorm, or they may be long-term, such as the slow destruction from droughts. Only small areas may be damaged by lightning or tornadoes, while hurricanes, earthquakes, and floods may devastate broad and diverse geographical areas. The magnitude of some of these events may disrupt a whole nation, and their severity may be such that it will take many years for the stricken population to recover fully. In sparsely populated areas the impact receives less attention because the event directly affects fewer people. The disruption caused by the disaster may alter the equilibrium in each of the three subcategories (inorganic, organic, and humanmade) of Subsystem I of the human ecosystem. For example, flooding (inorganic) may alter the local food chain (organic), which in turn may alter the humanmade environment by changing dietary habits, food rituals, and perhaps folk myths and legends. The disruptive effect on the individual (Subsystem II) may be to reduce adaptive capacity or to inflict injury, illness, or death.

The effect of disasters thus involves the total human ecosystem through the disruption of the interdependent variables of the macrosystem, the direct costs of the disaster, and the pain of the dying and injured. The continuum of loss and injury has been depicted by Cochrane and associates (Fig. 2-9), indicating in a general way the types and degree of suffering that follow disaster. The diagram depicts the relationship between the direct effects of the event and the indirect responses of the larger population, the social and cultural factors. The total magnitude of loss is not merely the sum of the components; rather each loss has multiple ramifications. Thus, coping with natural disasters is a complex process of multiple and interrelated responses.

Coping with natural disasters

Human populations deal with these devastating situations through a number of strategies. They may attempt to avoid those disasters that can sometimes be anticipated; for example, settlements usually are not built on flood plains or in avalanche areas. Similarly, the good farmer will wisely avoid the risk of growing orange trees in a frost-prone area. Thus, caution against exceeding the system's adaptive capacity is one means of preventing disasters.

Another means of avoiding losses is through the prediction of disasters and, subsequently, the seeking of safety. Technical advances in weather prediction and monitoring other hazardous conditions, such as avalanches, protect many human lives (White and Haas, 1975:343). Steps have also been taken to prepare communities against possible catastrophes through precautions such as upgrading dams and drainage systems, constructing disaster-resistant houses, and improving warning systems. In densely populated coastal areas where hurricanes are a threat, evacuation plans are another means of adapting to a disaster and preventing overwhelming losses. Individual precautions for avoiding injury and death also may be part of the general knowledge of a society. Seeking underground shelter during tornadoes or avoiding open, high places during electrical storms are examples of precautions individuals learn in disaster-prone areas. Successful avoidance of injury may be linked to technological advances, such as radar warning sys-

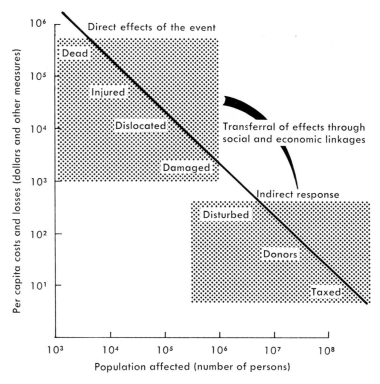

Fig. 2-9. Impact of disaster: a continuum of effects. (Adapted from Cochrane and others, 1975.)

tems, television and radio communication, and sturdy shelters. In underdeveloped countries these advances may not be present, and losses may be great. However, loss of human life and disrupted social systems also occur in densely populated urban centers of developed countries; for example, a tornado often does great damage to such areas but has comparatively little impact on the open plains. Although warning systems for impending disasters operate in the United States, the population frequently chooses to ignore the warnings and consequently, thousands of lives are needlessly lost each year.

Losses may be increased by poor judgment regarding living in a disaster-prone area. For example, a potential landslide area may have

great aesthetic value and so may lend a certain prestige to its purchase as a homesite. Or a building site may appear to be a bargain when its low price is hardly worth the risk of locating on a flood plain. It is obvious, then, that knowledge of the surroundings of one's dwelling is vital. Choosing an appropriate housing style is another factor in preventing loss from natural catastrophes, as this case study will demonstrate.

The Guatemala earthquake of 1976

Guatemala is the largest of the Central American countries, bordered on the north by Mexico and on the south by Honduras and El Salvador. It is a land of diverse physical splendor, of lush, green precipitous mountains, active volcanoes, and steaming jungles; however, it shares with the other Central American countries and parts of

Mexico the danger of being located on active, interlaced tectonic plates (Plakfer, 1976). Throughout history, seismic activity has been frequent as the tectonic plates continue to move. Scars of major earthquakes in Guatemala (1773 and 1918) are still apparent in the fallen cathedrals and denuded areas on the mountainsides from landslides caused by gigantic shifts in the earth's crust.

On February 4, 1976 at 3:02 A.M., Guatemala was struck again by a devastating earthquake that registered 7.5 on the Richter scale. Thousands of aftershocks occurred. The toll in life and injury was tremendous as more than 25,000 deaths occurred and approximately 75,000 people were injured (Bates, Farrell, and Glittenberg, 1979). More than a million people, or 20% of the population, were left homeless as their unreinforced adobe walls with heavy terracotta tile roofs gave way to the shaking earth. Lives were lost when the walls collapsed and the heavy tile roofs fell in on the sleeping victims. Many were crushed, while others suffocated in the thick adobe dust that surrounded them.

The earthquake extended along the Motagua fault that runs across the most heavily populated area of Guatemala. The impact was so tremendous that ground breakage from the disaster spread for more than 240 k along the fault. The epicenter of the main shock was about 115 km northeast of Guatemala City. In terms of lives lost, the disaster was the most severe in Guatemalan history, which has been marked by many other catastrophes such as floods, hurricanes, and volcanic eruptions. A major reason for the severity of this earthquake was the recent increased use of a house type that is maladaptive to that physical environment: the adobe brick house with tile roof. One of the authors (Glittenberg) is a co-principal investigator of a National Science Foundation research study of the longitudinal effects of this catastrophe. One of the goals of the study is to learn what features in the culture were the most vulnerable to destruction. A quasiexperimental research design was used. Twenty-six research sites were compared on the following dimensions: degree of damage, ethnicity, complexity of social organization, amount and type of relief agency aid received, and leadership styles within the communities. Control sites were also

used; they varied in ethnicity, complexity of social organization, and the degree to which they had suffered damage from this disaster. Three major types of data were collected. The first type was a 1400-household survey in the twenty-five research and control sites. The second was a survey of the leaders and a community inventory of each site. The last was a study of a sample of the more than a hundred relief and reconstruction agencies that provided aid to Guatemala after the disaster. The data are in the process of being analyzed. The findings from this study should help us to understand how individuals, families, small groups, and communities adapt to environmental threats such as earthquakes.

Housing: a social trait. Housing in any society reflects the value systems and technology of that society. Houses are more than mere pieces of construction; rather they are significant social objects with important cultural meanings. Houses are an important manifestation of a series of social processes that occur in response to the needs of a population and the environmental resources available. Their form and the methods and materials that are used to construct them are all features with significance to the social organization of the society, as well as to the life-styles of its members (Bates, Farrell, and Glittenberg, 1979). For example, in Guatemala house types reflect the different style of various sectors of the society: adobe with tile roof, cane with thatched roof, bajarique (cane-latticed walls filled with adobe mud), as well as modern cement block and brick houses.

Housing is a social trait and because it offers shelter against the severities of the physical environment, its form is evidence of human adaptability to a specific ecological niche. Thus study of the variation in house types is one means of studying the wide range of human needs for survival under varying environmental conditions. For example, elevated houses on stilts, such as those found in parts of the tropics, provide protection from predators as well as shelter from heavy precipitation and heat. Another example of an ecologically appropriate house type is the dome-shaped igloo, which is found in polar regions. The advantages of the igloo are: ease of construction, limited experience or training needed to construct it, availability of natural building materials, and its wind resistant and heat retentive qualities.

Both of these examples illustrate house types that are well adapted to their environments.

A house type may reflect not only the demands of the natural environment but also the technology and value systems of the society that has developed it. In Guatemala, the adobe brick and tile roof type of house was introduced by the Spanish conquistadors, who came from the plains of Spain in the mid-sixteenth century, bringing with them their ideal house type as it existed in their homeland. Tile roof and adobe brick walls surrounding a courtyard was the usual form of a Spanish house, adapted to the sunny plains of Spain. As the powerful Spaniards conquered the Mayan lands in Central America, the adobe house was adopted by the Ladino population (the ethnic group of mixed Spanish and Mayan Indian heritage), which eventually inhabited the urban centers of Guatemala City, Antigua, and Quezaltenango. Meanwhile, the rural people continued to live in the cane and straw thatched houses that they had inhabited for centuries. Even today the house type for the Mayan Indian in the rural areas is frequently of this type of construction.

However, cane walls offer little protection from heavy rains and cold nights, and they are not secure against intrusion. A cane and thatch house is easily broken into by thieves, while rodents nibble at the walls and other pests make their homes in the walls and roofs. Besides realizing these disadvantages, the Indians are aware of the low social value associated with living in a cane hut. The house type associated with the Ladino population is the adobe brick with tile roof, and Ladinos as a group have higher socioeconomic status than the Indians (Adams, 1970). They generally live in the urban centers, such as Guatemala City, or along the coastlands; they are better educated and have greater control over the economy, the church, the educational system, and the military. In contrast, the Indians control very little. They devote a greater part of their time to subsistence farming, with no accumulation of capital; they occupy less fertile land and own less of the land they work (Stavenhagen, 1970:238). To escape these restrictions, approximately 15,000 to 20,000 Indians become ladinoized each year (van den Berghe, 1968:522). Ladinoization is a complicated process involving several steps by which a person can become incorporated into lower levels of Ladino society. A visible indicator of ladinoization has been the diffusion of the adobe house type into the highland Indian areas.

During the past 50 years, the Ladino house type has spread out of the urban centers into the Indian rural hinterland. It is easily and inexpensively constructed, being made from the sun-dried clay that is quite accessible. New technological skills are needed to build an adobe house, but they are quickly learned. Consequently, over the past half century, densely populated Indian rural areas have begun to be filled with adobe houses. It is not known whether the Indians were aware of the danger of living in this house type in highly seismic areas.

The effects of socioeconomic and cultural forces leading Indians to become ladinoized and adopt an adobe house type are exemplified in Santa Maria Cauque, an Indian town about 20 km from Guatemala City. Fifty years ago, Santa Maria Cauque was a typical Indian town with only cane and thatched roofed houses. When the 1918 earthquake struck, no one from Santa Maria Cauque was injured or killed, whereas many were killed in nearby Guatemala City, where houses were built of adobe brick.

Possibly, in 1918 the Indians of Santa Maria Cauque were aware of the dangers of building adobe homes. However, their eagerness to gain the status and prestige associated with the adobe house may have outweighed their caution. The first adobe house was built in Santa Maria Cauque in 1925, and by 1971 more than 85% of the houses were of this type (Glass, and others, 1977).

Consequently when the 1976 earthquake struck, the physical stress on the adobe brick exceeded its tolerance threshold. Hundreds lost their lives, and many more were severely injured. Building materials were the most significant factor associated with death and serious injury. No deaths or injuries occurred in nonadobe houses in Santa Maria Cauque (Glass, and others, 1977), but the heavy, cheap adobe bricks became deadly projectiles in the adobe homes.

Changes in house type: an adaptation. Today Guatemalans who live in highly seismic areas do not build their houses only from adobe and tile. New ideas for earthquake-resistant houses have been introduced through the efforts of numerous aid agencies, such as the Red Cross, Salvation

Army, and Mennonite Disaster Relief. New construction materials, such as cement block and lamina tin roofs are being used, and safe building techniques are being taught. For example, the proper placement of doors and windows, the addition of cross beam supports, and the reinforcing of walls with steel rods are new means for ensuring a sturdy protective house (Figs. 2-10 and 2-11). In addition, a spontaneous return to the native housing materials of cane, mud, and thatch has occurred (Bates, Farrell, and Glittenberg, 1979).

Summary. This case study has illustrated how a feature of the humanmade environment—culture—may influence the choice of house type. The diffusion of a house type inappropriate to an area also illustrates the interaction between the three variables in Subsystem I of the human eco-

system. Thresholds for each of the variables—inorganic, organic, and humanmade—were exceeded, and the result was severe damage to all three elements on the macrolevel of analysis. Although the measures of impact on the microlevel are not as refined, we can identify at the community level—in the example of the Indian town of Santa Maria Cauque—that each of the three factors was also disrupted. Culture, the humanmade variable, showed the most rapid adjustment to the stress, as the natives rebuilt their houses with materials more resistant to earthquake damage, using new and traditional technologies. This example clearly demonstrates that populations can and do suffer from maladaptive living patterns. When a critical threshold is exceeded, the population either will resort to a more adaptive pattern or will not survive.

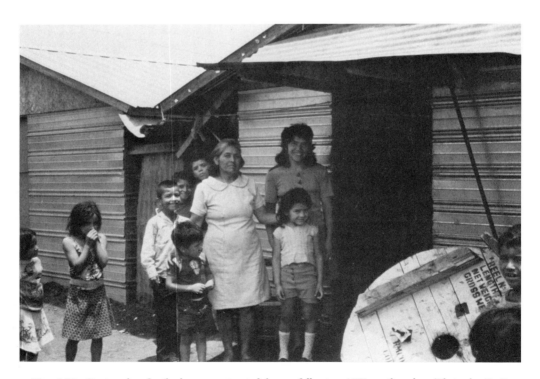

Fig. 2-10. Guatemalan family by reconstructed house following 1976 earthquake. (Photo by J. E. Glittenberg.)

CASE STUDY III: HUMAN ADAPTATIONS TO AN URBAN NEIGHBORHOOD

The two previous case studies described and analyzed biological and cultural adaptations to physical environmental factors: high altitude and natural disasters. In this case study we present two culturally varied groups, chicanos and Vietnamese, and their adaptations to a new environment, a Denver urban neighborhood. Specifically we examine their health beliefs and practices in order to discover the process by which human groups retain unity, support, and adaptive capacities when their previously held values are challenged in a new cultural environment. Because shared values and norms are vital to the survival of a group, we examine the process of acculturation that enables these two populations to adapt to a new environment.

The Chicanos

The term *chicano* is used here to refer collectively to the Spanish-surnamed residents of one of Denver's low-income housing projects known as Sun Valley. This housing project contains 419 units, consisting of 1-, 2-, or 3-bedroom multiplexes, each having a small front yard and a common rear area. A commercial and warehouse district is nearby, but no major traffic enters the development. A city-sponsored health center is located on one side and a grade school and recreation center on another (Afton, 1977). Some chicano families have lived in this immediate neighborhood for three generations. Effective links have long been established with other Spanish-speaking peoples of the city and state. Significant links (not all of which are judged to be effective) also have been established with non-chicano residents of Denver and with numerous agencies, community and educational organizations, and churches. Chicanos hold many of the positions of leadership in this portion of the city. They are in charge of many of the funded self-help

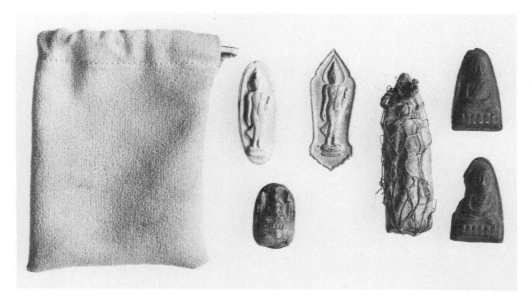

Fig. 2-11. A Vietnamese amulet bag, the contents having both medical and religious significance. (Courtesy K. Gengenbach.)

organizations such as the West Side Action Center, Brothers Redevelopment, and the Denver Inner City Parish. It was into this milieu that several hundred Vietnamese refugees began moving in mid-1975.

The Vietnamese

No exact agreement has been reached as to the number of Vietnamese war refugees entering the United States after the fall of the Thieu regime on April 30, 1975, but approximately 145,000 were resettled under the 1975 Indochina Migration and Refugee Assistance Act. Subsequent governmental authorization resulted in the admission of more than 35,000 more by mid-1978. Among these were many so-called "boat people" and other Indochinese who had spent weeks or months in southeast Asian resettlement camps before entering the United States. All totaled, it is probable that nearly 5,000 Indochinese came through Colorado between May of 1975 and December of 1978. As of Spring 1977, approximately 1500 Vietnamese had settled in the Denver metropolitan area; the number has risen slightly since that time (Van Arsdale and Latawiec, 1977:1-2).

Using socioeconomic and psychological criteria established by David (1970), we can classify most of the Vietnamese who moved to Sun Valley and other sections of Denver's west side as "involuntary migrants," whereas, most of the chicanos can be classified as "voluntary migrants." Sociologist Robert Marsh, who has completed numerous statistical studies on social, political, and economic correlates of change both here and abroad, stresses that a group's traditions are the key factors in current attempts at socioeconomic adjustment. Predictably, it has been found that the Vietnamese utilize a substantially different mode of adjustment to life in the Sun Valley Housing Project than do chicanos. This is reflected in demographic patterns and health practices.

The comparative study

In 1978 a demographic and health survey was administered to the Vietnamese and chicano residents to obtain comparable information on urban adjustment and adaptation. Information was obtained regarding geographical location, household income, and access to community or agency services. Determined qualitatively through partici-

pant observation and work with key informants, it was found that the greatest differences between the Vietnamese and chicanos lay in cultural background, length of residence in Sun Valley, and English-language fluency (chicanos being more fluent).

Vietnamese households. Demographically, one of the most important aspects of the refugee situation has been a migration adjustment process that for most Vietnamese can be broken down into four phases. Phase one consists of initial displacement and emigration from Vietnam to the United States. Phase two consists of processing through U.S. facilities and initial dispersion with sponsor aid to locations throughout the country. The third phase consists of resettlement, without sponsor aid, into still different neighborhoods or cities under the primary initiative of the Vietnamese themselves. Sociologically, at this point they properly no longer should be labeled "refugees." Historically, the label continues to apply. For many Vietnamese, phase three in Denver has consisted of moving from housing arranged by a sponsoring agency, such as Denver Catholic Community Services, to low-income city housing, such as Sun Valley, where rents are determined according to ability to pay. Phase four consists of moving from what might be termed "available rental units" to "more desirable rental units" or to one's own home (Van Arsdale and Latawiec, 1977).

As happens in similar cases, many Vietnamese tended to settle near their countrymen, resulting in enclaves of Vietnamese within the housing project. This enclave formation occurred primarily during phase three but was also seen to a lesser extent in phase four, especially among those who had achieved less English language fluency and economic mobility. At its peak, during mid-1977, the Vietnamese enclave in the Sun Valley Housing Project contained more than sixty families. Many had been attracted from other parts of the United States because of the presence of family members. As the Vietnamese refugees in Denver moved from phase three to phase four, the declining importance of the enclave was testified to by shrinking housing size. Based on a nonrandom sample of 41 Denver Vietnamese households, mid-1976 average household size was 6.2 persons (3.2 males and 3.0 females), with an average of 3.6 children per household (Van Arsdale and Latawiec, 1977:

4). A 1978 survey by the same researchers indicated a drop to 5.0 persons per household, with a range from one to ten persons per household. Some of the extended and joint families were separating into smaller nuclear families. For many, phase four, or moving into one's own home, was well underway.

Household size is important because at the microlevel it not only suggests trends in demographic variables, but also indicates the extent and possible strength of sociofamilial support networks. Changes in such networks, especially if they diminish in size relatively quickly, can indicate a trend toward more extensive integration into the wider urban environment.

Chicano households. A nonrandom sample survey found the average chicano household size in the Sun Valley Housing Project in 1978 to be 3.7. Households ranged in size from two to six people. These figures have remained relatively stable over the past few years, according to representatives of the housing project. Some of the households are comprised of single-parent families; few are extended families, in contrast to the Vietnamese. Births or pregnancies had occurred among eleven of the eighteen households surveyed during the past 3 years; an average of 0.8 births and pregnancies were reported per chicano household. By comparison, seven of the nineteen Vietnamese households surveyed reported births or pregnancies among their members (some of them occurring shortly before leaving Vietnam) during the same period of time. An average of 0.7 births and pregnancies were reported per Vietnamese household. Only one death had occurred among members of either group during the preceding 3 years.

Employment and occupational diversity

During the 3-year period of our study, income levels in the two groups were estimated to be approximately the same at the aggregate household level despite the differences in household size and individual earnings. As of early 1978, Vietnamese households had an average of 1.2 people employed per household, whereas chicano households had an average of 0.4. Because of the larger average size of Vietnamese households, the household work force was greater in the Vietnamese than in the chicano situations. However, an analysis of jobs by description and title suggests that employed chicanos earn more than employed Vietnamese. Thus, because both chicano and Vietnamese families traditionally have emphasized the sharing of resources among household members, aggregate household income totals for both groups were approximately the same.

Diversity among the Spanish-speaking population of the United States has been discussed; diversity among Vietnamese immigrants also needs to be recognized. Although almost all came from lowland areas of Vietnam, a wide range of social strata and occupations is represented throughout Denver. At the extreme are former South Vietnamese soldiers who were North Vietnamese prisoners of war. Overall, nearly half (48.7%) of the male household heads surveyed in 1976 had been in the military. Many of these were initially underemployed, especially during the end of phase two and beginning of phase three. Teachers and professionals are also represented, but in smaller proportions; most of these individuals did not move to the Sun Valley Housing Project. Former rural residents of Vietnam are even fewer in number.

In terms of years of education, among Vietnamese surveyed in 1978 belonging to the nineteen Sun Valley households, one person had the equivalent of a college or university education. Women had less education than men. Among all adults aged 18 years and over, the average number of years of education was 6.1, with nine having had no schooling. This compares to the chicano adults of Sun Valley, who had completed an average of 10.2 years of school each. One person had completed college. No adult surveyed had completed less than 5 years of schooling. In sum, the chicano adults surveyed were better educated than the Vietnamese.

Health care and its traditions

The chicano and Vietnamese in the Sun Valley Housing Project had distinctly different health care patterns, despite the fact that the same city facilities are used by both groups. The chicano pattern of interaction with the city health program and hospital facilities is one of "begrudging acceptance." At times there is vocal dissent. Complaints centered around a perceived lack of personal interest shown by physicians toward clients, inadequate time spent by physicians in making diagnoses, and (less frequently) incorrect diagnosis. For example, several clients were concerned that they had been given identical prescriptions for ailments they themselves judged to be very different. A number of people stated that it is difficult for "Anglo doctors" to acquire the cultural insights necessary to treat chicano ailments.

The traditions and methods of healing of Spanish-speaking people in the southwestern part of the United States are described elsewhere in this book and have been treated extensively in the literature (Kay, 1977; Kiev, 1968; Clark, 1959; Saunders, 1954; Klein, 1978; Hayes-Bautista, 1978). Numerous other articles written for more general audiences have also appeared (for example, Abril, 1975; Armijo, 1978). Dissatisfaction with the structure and function of the Anglo health network emerges, not surprisingly, as an important theme in several of these. But what ultimately is brought out in the present research is the culturally adaptive nature of responses of dissatisfaction, and the relatively minimal relationship of the urban "folk communication network" to population health maintenance.

Not surprisingly, Vietnamese health practices were found to differ considerably from those of the chicano residents, reflecting their unique Asian cultural background. Decades of French and subsequent Anglo-American influence in Vietnam had resulted in diffusion of some Western health practices into Vietnam. Similar influences of Western ideas on health care practices are also found in the urban chicano system after decades of Anglo-American influence: for example, extensive use of clinic and hospital facilities, reliance on Western prescription drugs, and confusion over the technical and bureaucratic aspects of Western health care services. Parallels in the diffusion and assimilation of these features can be traced to similarities in preexisting structural-adaptive arrangements in Vietnamese and chicano societies.

Residents of lowland Vietnam had a wide range of cures and healing modalities from which to choose. The influence of Buddhism, never an exclusive religious tradition of the country, was important. Paralleling Buddhist religious beliefs, which tend to incorporate competing modes of thought, was an integrative system of medicine that had grown to effectively accommodate Western, oriental, and tribal forms of health care. A sick person could visit a pharmacy offering Chinese herbal remedies or a clinic offering antibiotics. Because of close kinship networks and reliance on the knowledge possessed by members of the patrilineage, a cure was frequently initiated and often completed by attempting a self-help or home remedy (Fig. 2-11). Too, medical lore among the Vietnamese was thought to reflect the importance of human relationships. As with the lore of chicano healing traditions, its transmission through and among generations stressed familial and social responses to illness rather than the techniques of health care that are emphasized in Western traditions.

An example of this is the knowledge contained in Chinese medical texts, such as the eighteen volumes of the Nei-ching classic and the Shen Nung Ben Tsao materia medica, which diffused into Vietnam during the first millenium A.D. as sinification intensified. Chinese methods of irrigation and agricultural terracing were other important innovations introduced during this period. Yet the "little tradition" of folk remedies should not be dichotomized from the "great tradition" of the scholarly texts; as in China, they came to be united. A continuum existed that even the introduction of Western "miracle drugs" and the Vietnam war of the 1960s and 1970s could not shatter. This continuum of knowledge, belief, and practice reflects the belief that health is biocultural equilibrium; sickness is disequilibrium (Keyes, 1977: 181-257; Li, 1974:3-4; Topley, 1975:257-258; Silverman, 1977:29-33).

Certain of Vietnam's mountain tribes, such as the Mnong Gar described by Condominas (1977), cannot properly be viewed as reflecting this same cultural practice. Their shamanistic practices reflect an animistic, spiritual world view. Sorcery is thought to affect health as well. Chinese medical beliefs permeate this system only to a limited degree. However, only two Vietnamese families encountered in the Denver metropolitan region were found to adhere to an animistic belief system. A majority were Catholic; most others were Buddhist.

Chicano health care practices in the neighborhood. The medical and health knowledge available to the chicano population of Sun Valley is informal, heterogeneous, and in some ways contradictory. Available medical personnel and healers are varied—physicians, clinicians, social workers, dentists, *curanderas* (traditional folk healers), *brujas* (witches). Questions asked of the heads of the sample eighteen chicano households indicate that the clinic and its physicians are those from whom health information is obtained in most cases (78%), but that in a substantial number of cases (44%) neighbors or friends are consulted about an ailment before a physician's or *curandera's* advice

is sought. Several household heads (17%) stated they do not know from whom to seek health information, relying instead on their own knowledge. Although both interviewers who conducted the chicano portion of the survey (in Spanish, where needed) were themselves chicanos (one a resident of Sun Valley), it is possible that responses to questions concerning *curanderismo* were guarded (Fig. 2-12). Nonetheless, it is sig-

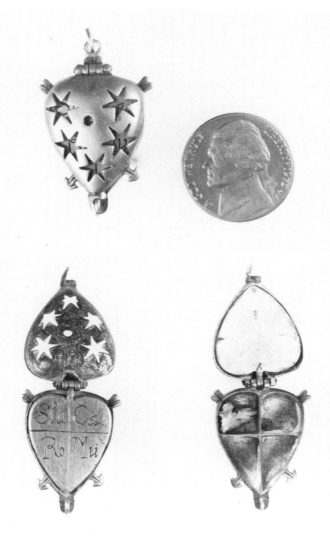

Fig. 2-12. A talisman, or locket, with four compartments for storage of medicinal herbs; also probably served as a protective charm for the wearer. Origin unknown; used by a contemporary Denver *curandera*. (Courtesy J. Afton.)

nificant that in two households they said they knew virtually nothing about these practices; one did not know what a *curandera* was. Kay reported similar findings in a small proportion of Hispanic populations she studied (1977:150-151).

When it comes to the actual receipt of health care services, almost all (89%) reported that the clinic and local city hospital are the primary sources. One-third (33%) also use the services of local *curanderas*. One *curandera* occasionally is consulted, although she is not a neighborhood resident, because she is well known throughout the region and holds the distinction of being certified as a mental health consultant by the state of Colorado. This *curandera* treats *enfermedades mentales* (mental illness). Another woman, a local person who is a self-proclaimed *bruja* offers herbal cures for a small proportion of Sun Valley's residents, but her curative powers are discounted by most. However, the director of a neighborhood action program reported his belief that hexes placed by her on community members may be effective. For example, one day the unoccupied automobiles of three chicanos hexed by the *bruja* were smashed by a fire engine that went out of control. An undercurrent of belief in *envidia* ("bad luck," often resulting from an episode of envy and the presumed actions of a *bruja*) was found to be widespread (Kiev, 1968:113-116).

Actual knowledge of diseases and remedies is found to vary widely among sample household respondents and among key informants. Two-thirds were able to name one or more diseases that they deemed important in each of the following four categories: among infants, children, adults, and the elderly. Virtually all responses elicited in this open-ended survey focused on temporary, passing, self-limiting diseases (*enfermedades temporales*), such as mumps, and on illnesses thought to be serious and in some instances incurable (*enfermedades graves*), such as heart attacks. To the degree that the questionnaire, as administered, was able to tap knowledge about other forms of illness such as *enfermedades mentales* that are known to be important to Spanish-speaking people of the United States, it was concluded that knowledge tends to be incomplete and fairly disparate among individuals. No support was found for the popular stereotype of widespread knowledge of folk illnesses and diseases among members of this ethnic minority.

Hayes-Bautista's (1978) paradigm is useful in understanding how medical knowledge is disseminated. Medical knowledge is usually unevenly distributed in a community, even among those from similar socioeconomic backgrounds. Furthermore, widespread dissatisfaction with the prevalent Anglo health network among chicano residents of Sun Valley may promote community unity in that the residents identify themselves as the "in group" and the Anglo network as the "out group." Even though actual medical knowledge varies widely among residents, stated shared beliefs as to the inadequacy of available care provide the functional means for the partial maintenance of internal group cohesiveness. At a somewhat broader level of analysis, such responses afford mechanisms for reducing stress brought about by disparities in resource availability between cultural groups and among urban neighborhoods (Press, 1978). The folk communication network, as manifested in Sun Valley and vicinity, while serving to spread medical and health-related knowledge to some extent, is far more important in the dissemination of information about problems in the functioning of the health system and its cultural subsystems. Feedback among residents serves to reinforce the image of dissatisfaction.

Vietnamese health practices in the neighborhood. Dissatisfaction with the available health services was also found among Vietnamese of Sun Valley. However, unlike in the situation with chicanos, the dissatisfaction did not emerge as a unifying, mutually reinforcing response of the group as a whole. Rather it was aimed primarily at individual physicians, pointing out that their lack of understanding of cross-cultural differences led to what were perceived to be incorrect diagnoses. Vietnamese informants also complained about the brevity of physician-patient interactions and about not seeing the same physician on subsequent visits. Visits to the hospital appeared to be more stressful than visits to the neighborhood clinic, although the requirement of rescreening patients on each visit to the clinic was found to be stressful. Concern was also expressed about the need for interpreters, although some had been provided (one was hired by the clinic, others by local community service agencies and a school). Severe problems were reported in the labeling and thus use of prescription drugs, not only because labels were in English, but also because instructions about dosages and their timing proved to be confusing. Even with the availability of refugee welfare assistance, the system of cash payment for health care proved baffling in many instances.

The Vietnamese also expressed displeasure that certain traditional rituals concerning health were unknowingly being violated by Western health practitioners. For example, mothers giving birth in Denver hospitals were being requested to shower or bathe immediately postpartum. Vietnamese believe that women having their first child should not bathe for 3 months, and women with several children should wait for 1 month. They also believe that ideally, after having given birth, a woman should remain in bed for a month or more. Sunshine should be avoided for

at least a month as well. In the extreme, it is thought that total disregard for these procedures will result in death. Another example is that in several instances the marks left on the back of a person because of the practice of coin-rubbing (to relieve "bad winds") were misinterpreted by Denver physicians as having resulted from abuse.

As was reported earlier for chicano residents, the medical and health knowledge available to the Vietnamese is also informal, heterogenous, and in some ways contradictory. Western health practitioners are utilized extensively, but the traditional Vietnamese curer also has a place. One person, aged 66, serves Sun Valley in this capacity. Catholic ritual is tied to the cures she offers. Some of the herbs used are purchased from Chinese sources in California; others are obtained from local sellers (Fig. 2-13). Responses to questions asked of the heads of the nineteen sample households (not all of whom responded on this topic) indicate that relatives, neighbors, friends, and

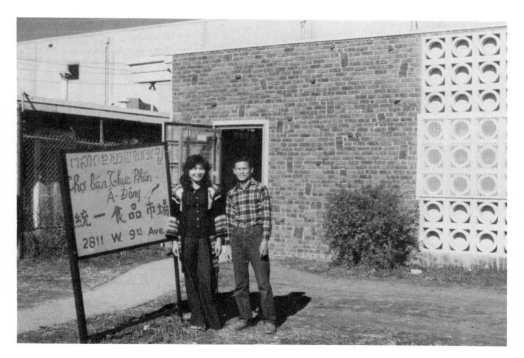

Fig. 2-13. A Vietnamese market owned and operated by immigrants to Sun Valley. Herbs, roots, and vegetables are sold here, as are certain curative ointments and powders. Most items are obtained from California suppliers. (Photo by P. Van Arsdale.)

American sponsors are those from whom basic health information is obtained in most cases (91%). Such persons are usually consulted about an ailment before advice is sought from a physician or traditional curer. One-third of the respondents stated that in Denver they did not rely on traditional curers.

In terms of actual receipt of health care services, most (88%) reported that the neighborhood clinic and city hospital were their primary sources. The data suggest a tendency for those who rely more heavily on city services to rely less on the traditional curers. One respondent stressed that she utilized the clinic "only as a last resort" because she perceived costs there to be prohibitive.

In comparison with the chicano respondents, actual knowledge of diseases and remedies was found to vary more widely among Vietnamese household respondents and key informants. Only one Vietnamese respondent was able to name one or more diseases that he deemed important for each of the four categories: infants, children, adults, and the elderly. However, this finding is misleading because non-elderly Vietnamese respondents tend to avoid answering when asked about ailments afflicting the elderly, presumably out of deference to them. In turn, one elderly respondent refused to answer about illnesses afflicting members of the other three categories. Half of the Vietnamese household heads responding were able to name diseases that they deemed important among infants, children, and adults. The knowledge of these individuals proved to be more extensive than that of most of the chicanos surveyed. Nearly all responses focused on self-limiting diseases, such as influenza, and on mild ailments, such as headaches. As with chicanos, mental illnesses were not mentioned here, in large part because they are conceptualized in a different way. Thus, it can be concluded that medical and health knowledge of the Vietnamese varies more widely than among chicanos, but that in comparing those who are knowledgeable (but do not serve as practitioners) in each group, Vietnamese tend to exhibit a wider range of knowledge and are also more adept at placing this knowledge into the context of tradition and ritual. Furthermore, more Vietnamese in Sun Valley rely on traditional curers than do chicanos.

The diversity among the Vietnamese health beliefs and practices results from their more recent migration into the United States and their familiarity with some aspects of the Western health care system. Nevertheless, the relationship of their health knowledge to the Western system can be classified as exhibiting "overlapping conflict." On the other hand, contact between the chicano health care system and the Western health care system may be interpreted as "overlapping congruity," except in certain illness episodes when the physician and client are not in agreement. The "overlapping congruity" of the chicano residents indicates that there is greater congruence between health care sought and health care received, while a Vietnamese resident frequently finds the health care received unacceptable; hence, the term "overlapping conflict." That conflicts have erupted between chicano and Vietnamese in this and other Denver housing projects—some of the events receiving national press coverage during the summer of 1979—merely serves to strengthen these interpretations.

Summary and conclusions

Health care must be placed in the context of adaptation. Specifically, as demonstrated by the analysis of data obtained in Sun Valley, urban health adaptation depends on cultural traditions, limiting factors of the immediate environment, and patterns of communication (as in Brownlee, 1978:123-126; Press, 1978). Seeking health care depends on rational decisions derived after evaluating available, and in this case competing, alternatives. Health-seeking decisions can be conceptualized as one subset within the larger set of decisions needed to cope with the migration process and initial adjustment to a new urban environment. For Vietnamese more than chicanos, the available information for making these decisions is less complete because of their more recent migration. Nonetheless, for both groups the decisions made are rational. Comparative studies of health care among different ethnic groups residing in a common urban environment, as Scott (1978) demonstrates, indicate that the ability to utilize multiple health resources is the ultimate key to eventual health adaptation for members of an enclave minority. Sun Valley's chicano population can be seen to have evolved a fairly stable pattern of enclave adaptation as is reflected in the analysis of health and communication variables. The Vietnamese have demonstrated a short-term pattern of adjustment which, for most of them, reflects their greater upward mobility and desire to assimilate into the wider urban milieu.

KEYS TO HEALTH

As these case studies demonstrate, the key to health and survival is the adaptation of the whole person to the environment. Thus, there is an obvious benefit in promoting a productive human ecosystem. One of the themes of this book is that health is best achieved by identifying factors at the macrolevel, the microlevel, and the organismic level that favor adaptation and ecological fitness. This philosophy runs counter to other approaches in medical anthropology that focus on disease and pathology and place greater emphasis on the curative aspect of medical systems. As Pelletier urges, "Researchers and clinicians need to consider healthy, well-functioning individuals from many realms of life in order to initiate a true profile of health and well-being" (1978:321). To this we would add that additional consideration be given to cross-cultural studies in order to learn about diverse ways of handling diseases under varying environments.

The macrolevel and microlevel

The species *Homo sapiens* has had obvious success in reproducing in varying environments. What is the key to this success? It lies in the fact that human beings have continued to modify the physical and natural environment in order to maximize their adaptive capacities. In the case study on high altitude, for example, the key is the biological accommodation to low oxygen levels. The earthquake case study illustrates how, at a microlevel, a cultural pattern—building adobe houses—can be rapidly altered with the introduction and acceptance of new building materials and house construction technology

and return to traditional modes. The last case study demonstrates the different patterns of adaptation affecting health in two cultural groups—chicano and Vietnamese—living in the same urban environment.

One way to understand societal keys to health at both the macrolevel and microlevel is to examine the social institutions for clues to mechanisms that encourage health. For example, a religious institution may intervene in times of overwhelming stress by uniting a population in a common belief. This institution might also provide expressive relief as well as plausible explanations for strange or mysterious occurrences. An example of this institutional function was the increased belief in cultural heroes after the 1976 Guatemalan earthquake. In three different areas, myths about legendary heroes arose. In an area called El Progreso a cultural hero, an "Old Man," supposedly had come begging house to house approximately a month before the disaster. Those who gave him gifts supposedly suffered less injury and loss, and those who did not act kindly toward the Old Man were punished accordingly. In another area, a revered saint, San Bernadino, supposedly made his appearance an hour before the earthquake in the Patzun town plaza where he was seen walking around the cathedral, apparently wanting to warn the people of the impending disaster. The last example is of a legendary saint and hero San Simon from the area of San Adres Iztapa. The shrine built to San Simon (called Maximon in the language of the Cakchiquel) was one of a few buildings left standing in this town after the large earthquake. Today the town is filled with miracle seekers from throughout Central America who visit the shrine of Maximon. These cultural heroes—the Old Man, San Bernadino and Maximon—continue to bring hope to the people that supernatural powers are available to forewarn and protect the population from impending danger. Thus these cultural heroes can be considered as examples of keys to health at the macro-level and microlevel in that belief in them reduces the fear and anxiety that the natives have of future disasters (Glittenberg, 1979).

Another social institution, the health care system, when it is responsive to the needs of the people, is a key to health. Chapter 1 describes the crisis in health care today. In it we note that the professional health care system is often unresponsive to the needs of the people, so much so that many are seeking new, alternative ways of meeting their health care needs. Alternative systems of curing can

also be considered adaptive social institutions, as is described more thoroughly in Chapter 6.

The educational system is another social institution that is vital in providing keys to health. Education can increase individual adaptive capacity through activities such as classes on health and fitness as well as by providing basic information on causes of sickness. In addition, courses on nonsmoking, weight reduction, and parenting are examples of the educational approach for improving the community's state of health that may have a long-term effect on increasing the adaptive capacities of a population.

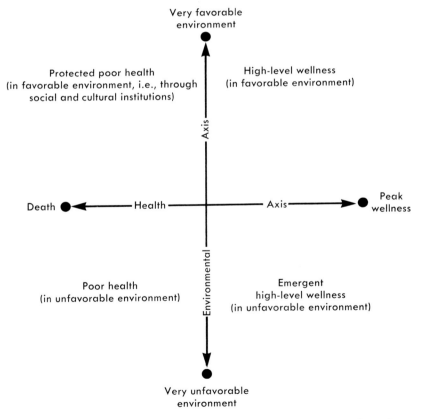

Fig. 2-14. The health grid, its axes and quadrants. (From U.S. Department of Health, Education and Welfare, Public Health Service, National Office of Vital Statistics, 1978.)

The organismic level

When we consider keys to health at the organismic level, we again must deal with the problem holistically. What factors in the environment promote health for the individual? A health grid prepared by the U.S. Department of Health, Education and Welfare is a useful guide in visualizing the continuum of peak wellness to death (Fig. 2-14). The key to optimal health would be to place or keep the individual functioning in the upper right quadrant of the grid. The grid provides a useful way of conceptualizing health and sickness, not as dichotomies but rather as states related to the environment. It supports our assertion that health is a balance between the individual and the environment. Such a balance may take on different meanings in different cultures. An imbalance, or disease, in one environment may not be considered an imbalance, or disease, in another. Some diseases can thus be considered "culture specific." For example in U.S. culture, the prevalence of stress-related diseases, such as vascular disease and cancer, is indeed alarming. Orthodox medical treatment seems often to come too late to place the individual back in a state of health. A number of accepted authorities on stress-related diseases have urged changes in life-style in order to reduce stress and maintain balance. Some techniques for reducing stress and establishing equilibrium are: biofeedback, autogenic training (relaxation), focusing, visualization, and meditation. The goal or key to health thus would be to reduce the conditions of extreme stress and reformulate life-styles to utilize energy for living rather than for combating disease (Pelletier, 1978:301).

Summary

The keys to health are the same for each level of the ecosystem. Whether at the macrolevel, microlevel, or the organismic level, health represents a balance in the system. Achievement of this balance takes time. At the macrolevel, it occurs through the process of species evolution over millions of years. At the microlevel, adaptation often occurs in societies in shorter spans of time—centuries or decades. Health at the organismic level is an outcome of processes affecting equilibrium at the macro- and microlevels as well as of factors determining individual adaptive capacity. The evolutionary processes giving rise to the macro-, micro-, and organismic levels of adaption seen today are described in the following chapter on evolution and the role of disease in human history.

REFERENCES

Abril, I. Mexican-American folk beliefs that affect health care. *Arizona Nurse*, 1975, *28*(3), 14-19.

Adams, R. *Crucifixion by Power. Essays on Guatemalan National Social Structure, 1944-1966.* Austin, Tex.: University of Texas Press, 1970.

Afton, J. Vietnamese in Denver: the development of the Sun Valley enclave. Paper presented at Rocky Mountain Psychological Association Meetings, Albuquerque, N.M., 1977.

Alland, A. *Adaptation in Cultural Evolution: an Approach to Medical Anthropology.* New York: Columbia University Press, 1970.

Altland, P., and Highman, B. Sex organ changes and breeding performance of male rats exposed to altitude. *Journal of Reproduction and Fertility*, 1968, *15*, 215-222.

Arias-Stella, J. Chronic mountain sickness: pathology and definition. In Porter, R., and Knight, J. (eds.). *High Altitude Physiology: Cardiac and Respiratory Aspects.* Edinburgh: Churchill Livingston, 1971, pp. 31-40.

Armijo, L. The curanderismo movement in the U.S. *La Luz*, 1978, *7*(3), 21.

Bates, F., Farrell, T., and Glittenberg, J. Housing changes following the 1976 Guatemalan earthquake. *Mass Emergencies*, 1979, *4*, 121-133.

Bennett, J. *The Ecological Transition.* Elmsford, N.Y.: Pergamon Press, Inc., 1976.

Brothwell, D. Disease, micro-evolution, and earlier populations: an important bridge between medical history and human biology. In Clarke, E. (ed.). *Modern Methods in the History of Medicine*, London: The Athlone Press, 1971.

Brownlee, A. T. *Community, Culture, and Care: A*

Cross-Cultural Guide for Health Workers. St. Louis: The C. V. Mosby Co., 1978.

Clark, M. *Health in the Mexican-American Culture.* Berkeley: University of California Press, 1959.

Chocrane, H. C. *Natural Hazards: Their Distribution Impacts.* Boulder, Colo.: University of Colorado Institute of Behavioral Science, 1975.

Condominas, G. *We Have Eaten the Forest: The Story of a Montagnard Village in the Central Highlands of Vietnam.* New York: Hill & Wang, 1977. (Translated by Adrienne Foulke.)

Cudkowicz, L., Spielvogel, H., and Zubieta, G. Respiratory studies in women at high altitude (3,500 m or 12,200 ft. and 5,200 m or 17,200 ft.). *Respiration*, 1972, *29*, 393-426.

David, H. P. Involuntary international migration: adaptation of refugees. In Brody, E. B. (ed.). *Behavior in New Environments: Adaptation of Migrant Populations.* Beverly Hills, Calif.: Sage Publications, Inc., 1970.

Davis, K., and Blake, J. Social structure and fertility: an analytic framework. *Economic and Cultural Change*, 1956, *4*, 211-235.

Davis, B. D., and Jones, B. F. Beneficial effect of estrogens on altitude tolerance in rats. *Endocrinology*, 1943, *33*, 23-31.

DeJong, G. Demography and research with high altitude populations. *Social Biology*, 1970, *17*, 114-119.

Ergueta, J., Spielvogel, H., and Cudkowicz, L., Cardiorespiratory studies in chronic mountain sickness. *Respiration*, 1971, *28*, 485-551.

Farge, E. J. Medical orientation among a Mexican-American population: an old and a new model reviewed. *Social Science & Medicine*, 1978, *12*, 277-282.

Fitzmaurice, F. E. Mountain sickness in the Andes. *Journal of the Royal Naval Medical Service*, 1920, *6*, 403-407.

Frisancho, A. R., and Baker, P. T. Altitude and growth: a study of the patterns of physical growth of a high altitude Peruvian Quechua population. *American Journal of Physical Anthropology*, 1970, *32*, 279-292.

Glass, R., Urruita, J., Sebony, S., and others. Earthquake injuries related to housing in a Guatemalan village. *Science*, 1977, *197*, 638-643.

Glittenberg, J. A comparative study of fertility in highland Guatemala: an Indian and Ladino town. Unpublished doctoral dissertation, University of Colorado, Boulder, Colo., 1976, p. 84.

Glittenberg, J. Cultural heroes aid in coping. Unpublished paper presented at the Pscyhiatric Nurse Clinician Symposium, Denver, Colo., April 18, 1979.

Gorshein, D., Delivoria-Papadopoulos, M., Oski, F., and others. The effect of androgen administration on erythrocyte 2, 3-diphosphoglycerate level and hemoglobin oxygen affinity in primates. *Clinical Research*, 1972, *20*, 487.

Guilleminault, C., Tilkian, A., and Dement, W. C. The sleep apnea syndromes. *Annual Review of Medicine*, 1976, *27*, 465-484.

Haas, J. D. Prenatal and infant growth and development. In Baker, P. T., and Little, M. A. (eds.). *Man in the Andes.* Stroudsburg, Pa.: Dowden, Hutchinson, & Ross, Inc., 1976, pp. 161-179.

Haas, J. E., Kates, R. W., and Bowden, M. J. (eds.). *Reconstruction Following Disaster.* Cambridge, Mass.: MIT Press, 1977.

Harrison, C. F., Kuchemann, M. A., Moore, S., and others. The effects of altitude variation in Ethiopian populations. *Philosophical Transaction of the Royal Society of London*, 1969, *256*, 147-182.

Hasselbalch, K. *Skandinavian Archives of Physiology*, 1912, *27*, 1-12.

Hayes-Bautista, D. E. Chicano patients and medical practitioners: a sociology of knowledge paradigm of lay-professional interaction. *Social Science & Medicine*, 1978, *12*, 83-90.

Hoff, C. J., and Abelson, A. E. Fertility. In Baker, P. T., and Little, M. A. (eds.). *Man in the Andes.* Stroudsburg, Pa.: Dowden, Hutchinson, and Ross, Inc., 1976, pp. 128-146.

Hurtado, A. Some clinical aspects of life at high altitudes, *Annals of Internal Medicine*, 1960, *53*, 247-256.

James, W. The effect of altitude on fertility in Andean countries. *Population Studies*, 1966, *16*, 97-101.

Kay, M. A. Health and illness in a Mexican American barrio. In Spicer, E. H. (ed.). *Ethnic Medicine in the Southwest.* Tucson: University of Arizona Press, 1977.

Keyes, C. F. *The Golden Peninsula: Culture and Adaptation in Mainland Southeast Asia.* New York: The Macmillan Co., 1977.

Kiev, A. *Curanderismo: Mexican-American Folk Psychiatry.* New York: The Free Press, 1968.

Klein, J. *Susto:* the anthropological study of diseases of adaptation. *Social Science & Medicine*, 1978, *12*, 23-28.

Kleinman, A. Social, cultural and historical themes in the study of medicine in Chinese societies: problems and prospects for the comparative study of medicine and psychiatry. In Kleinman, A., and others (eds.). *Medicine in Chinese Cultures: Comparative Studies of Health Care in Chinese and Other Societies.* Washington, D.C.: DHEW Publication No. (NIH) 75-653, 1975.

Kryger, M., McCullough, R. E., Collins, D., and others. Treatment of excessive polycythemia of high altitude with respiratory stimulant drugs. *American Review of Respiratory Disease*, 1978, *117*, 455-464.

Li, C. P. *Chinese Herbal Medicine.* Washington, D.C.: DHEW Publication No. (NIH) 75-732, 1974.

Licht, S. *Medical Climatology.* New Haven, Conn.: Licht, E., 1964.

Lowry, W. P. *Weather and Life: an Introduction to Biometeorology.* New York: Academic Press, Inc., 1970.

Lynch, J. J. *The Broken Heart.* New York: Basic Books, Inc., Publishers, 1977.

McNeill, W. H. *Plagues and People.* Garden City, N.Y.: Anchor Books, 1976.

Mazess, R. Neonatal mortality and altitude in Peru. *American Journal of Physical Anthropology,* 1965, *23,* 209-213.

McClung, J. *Effects of High Altitude on Human Birth.* Cambridge, Mass.: Harvard University Press, 1969.

McCullough, R. D., Reeves, J. T., and Liljegren, R. L. Fetal growth retardation and increased infant mortality at high altitude. *Archives of Environmental Health,* 1977, *32,* 36-39.

McMurtry, I. F., Frith, C. H., and Will, D. H. Cardiopulmonary responses of male and female swine to simulated high altitude. *Journal of Applied Physiology,* 1973, *34,* 459-462.

Monge, C. *Acclimatization in the Andes.* Baltimore: The Johns Hopkins University Press, 1948.

Moore, L. G., McMurtry, I. F., and Reeves, J. T. Effects of sex hormones on cardiovascular and hematologic responses to chronic hypoxia in rats. *Proceedings of the Society for Experimental Biology and Medicine,* 1978, *158,* 658-662.

Moore, L. G., Rohr, A. L., and Reeves, J. T. Emphysema mortality at high altitude. Unpublished observations, 1979.

Mortimer, E. A., Monson, R. R., and MacMahon, B. Reduction in mortality from coronary heart disease in men residing at high altitude. *New England Journal of Medicine,* 1977, *296,* 581-585.

Morton, W. E., Davids, D. J., and Lichty, J. A. Mortality from heart disease at high altitude. *Archives of Environmental Health,* 1964, *9,* 21-24.

Nelson, M., and Srebnik, H. Comparison of the reproductive performance of rats at high altitude and at sea level. *International Journal of Biometeorology,* 1970, *14,* 187-193.

Olson, R. The Guatemalan earthquake on 4 February 1976: social science observation and research suggestions. *Mass Emergencies,* 1977, *2,* 69-81.

Pawson, I. G., and Jest, C. The high altitude areas of the world—their cultures. In Baker, P. T. (ed.) *The Biology of High-Altitude Peoples.* New York: Cambridge University Press, 1978, pp. 17-45.

Pelletier, K. R. *Mind as Healer, Mind as Slayer.* New York: Delta, 1977.

Perez, A., and others. Resuming ovulation and menstruation after childbirth. *Population Studies, 25,* 491-503.

Plafker, G. Tectonic aspects of the Guatemalan earthquake of 4 February 1976. *Science,* 1976, *193,* 1201-1208.

Press, I. Urban folk medicine: a functional overview. *American Anthropologist,* 1978, *80*(1), 71-84.

Ravenhill, T. H. Some experiences of mountain sickness in the Andes. *Journal of Tropical Medicine and Hygeine,* 1913, *16,* 313-320.

Saunders, L. *Cultural differences and medical care: the case of the Spanish-speaking people of the Southwest.* New York: Russell Sage Foundation, 1954.

Sayers, R. and Weaver, T. Explanations and theories of migration. In Weaver, T. and Downing, T. (eds.). *Mexican Migration.* Tucson: Bureau of Ethnic Research, University of Arizona, 1976.

Scott, C. S. Health and healing practices among five ethnic groups in Miami, Florida. In Bauwens, E. E. (ed.). *The Anthropology of Health.* St. Louis: The C. V. Mosby Co., 1978.

Silverman, M. L. United States health care in crosscultural perspective: the Vietnamese in Denver. Unpublished masters thesis, University of Denver, 1977, Denver, Colo.

Spector, R. M. Mortality characteristics of a high altitude Peruvian population. Unpublished masters thesis, Pennsylvania State University, University Park, Pa., 1971. (Quoted by Hoff, C. J., and Abelson, A. E.)

Stavenhagen, R. Classes, colonialism, and acculturation. In Horowitz, I. L. (ed.). *Masses in Latin America.* New York: Oxford University Press, 1970.

Sulman, F. G. *Health, Weather, and Climate.* Basel: S. Karger AG, 1976.

Sutton, F. D., Zwillich, C. W., Creagh, C. E., and others. Progesterone for outpatient treatment of Pickwickian syndrome. *Annals of Internal Medicine,* 1975, *83,* 476-479.

Thomas, R. B. Energy flow at high altitude. In Baker, P. T., and Little, M. A. (eds.). *Man in the Andes.* Stroudsburg, Pa.: Dowden, Hutchinson & Ross, Inc., 1976, pp. 379-404.

Topley, M. Chinese and Western medicine in Hong-Kong: some social and cultural determinants of variation, interaction and change. In Kleinman, A., and others (eds.). *Medicine in Chinese Cultures: Comparative Studies of Health Care in Chinese and Other Societies.* Washington, D.C.: DHEW Publication No. (NIH) 75-653, 1975.

Van Arsdale, P. W., and Latawiec, J. A. Vietnamese in Denver: research strategies and population dynamics. Paper presented at Rocky Mountain Psychological Association Meetings, Albuquerque, N.M., 1977.

van den Berghe, P. L. Ethnic membership and cultural

change in Guatemala. *Social Forces*, 1968, *46*, 514-522.

Way, A. B. Morbidity and postneonatal mortality. In Baker, P. T., and Little, M. A. (eds.). *Man in the Andes*. Stroudsburg, Pa.: Dowden, Hutchinson and Ross, Inc., 1976, pp. 147-160.

Webster, J. R., and others. Chronic obstructive lung disease: a comparison between men and women. *American Review of Respiratory Disease*, 1968, *90*, 1021-1026.

White, G. F., and Haas, J. E. *Assessment of Research on Natural Hazards*. Cambridge, Mass.: MIT press, 1975.

Whitehead, L. Altitude, fertility, and mortality in Andean countries. *Population Studies*, 1969, *22*, 335-346.

Yee, B. and Van Arsdale, P. W. Breakdowns in traditional culture and the effects of learned helplessness among Vietnamese elderly. Paper presented at Society for Applied Anthropology Meetings, Merida, Yucatan, Mexico, 1978.

CHAPTER 3

Human adaptation: the evolutionary and historical record

As the model of the human ecosystem (see Fig. 2-1) clearly implies, contemporary humankind's state of health has its biocultural basis in the processes of human biocultural evolution. Millenia of interactions among biological, cultural, and environmental variables have resulted in a present-day condition of general human health that, at the organismic level, is exemplified by the ability of some to survive for as long as 100 years or more and, at the species level, is exemplified by the expansion of the human population throughout the world. However, rather than referring to the condition of health as a concept that is necessarily "good" for an individual, group, or species, it is more appropriate to view health as an ongoing process wherein the organism's functions—biological, psychological, and sociological—are in equilibrium with its environment. Illness and disease conversely imply that such functions are in disequilibrium. Health can be understood from the viewpoint of ecology, where adaptive interactions among biocultural and environmental variables are assessed.

PERSPECTIVES ON EVOLUTION AND ADAPTATION

The terms health, disease, and illness have numerous connotations, apart from the definitions presented above and in Chapter 1. From the view of medical anthropology,

most are attributable to labels associated with concepts that have arisen in the West. Thus, problems can arise when cross-cultural comparisons are attempted; for example, the health of a Navajo shaman in a trance-induced state might be labeled incorrectly as psychotic by an outside observer unfamiliar with this practice. Such labeling problems can be minimized by referring instead to health-related processes of adjustment and adaptation that contribute differentially to human well-being and survival. Cohen (1968) has provided a useful definition for the anthropological use of these terms: adaptation is a long-term change process (or complex of processes) that affects a group's relationship to its environment. Dobzhansky defines adaptation as "a feature of structure, function, or behavior of the organism which is instrumental in [enabling it] to live and to reproduce in a given environment" (1968: 111). Through adaptation, chances of survival are enhanced. One example of adaptation is the development of complex economies, relying on the domestication of plants and, later, animals, in the Middle East some 10,000 years ago. An adjustment, on the other hand, is a short-term response made by the organism to an environmental stimulus. The introduction of a new "wonder drug" provides one such example, although its continued use raises the possibility that it will later become ineffective against an infectious organism that evolves into a drug-resistant strain.

In summary, adaptation refers to an ongoing phenomenon that is broader in scope than is adjustment. Short-term adjustments may contribute to long-term adaptations. Health is one product of both these processes. Witnessing the broad range of conditions in which human beings successfully reproduce points to the adaptability of our species. Yet such recent technological successes as the development of nuclear power may have potentially disastrous effects on the future of the species. Hence, adaptations of the present may have maladaptive consequences in the future.

Mechanisms for achieving adaptation

Adaptation can be achieved by biological (genetic and developmental) and cultural mechanisms. While potentially independent, each functions as part of a biological-behavioral continuum by which adaptation is ultimately achieved.

Genes, as components of chromosomes, are the transmitters of heredity. It has been estimated that a set of forty-six chromosomes, the normal human complement, contains in excess of 100,000 genes. Together these determine the genotype of an individual. Genes act to produce polypeptide chains that function as enzymes or structural proteins. The role of enzymes is to catalyze a reaction between chemical substances in the body so as to decrease the time required for the reaction to take place. Reactions are linked in biochemical pathways through the specificity of enzymes for substrates, which are the raw materials for enzyme reactions. Biochemical pathways serve to supply three essential needs: (1) the appropriate substances for the individual organism's maintenance and growth, (2) the chemical energy required for the conversion of substances into usable forms, and (3) the energy released as heat to maintain constant body temperature.

If the form of a particular gene varies as a result of mutation, the characteristics of the enzyme or structural proteins produced also will vary. The resultant changes in enzymes or proteins may be harmful, beneficial, or neutral in terms of affecting the ability of the organism to function. As discussed in Chapter 1, the presence of a genetic variant of hemoglobin, hemoglobin S, along with normal hemoglobin in an individual, confers resistance to malaria. Another example concerns the forms of proteins that reside on the surface of red blood cells—antigens—which have been shown to vary and to give rise to different blood types (for example, A, B, AB, or O; Rh+ or Rh−). The work of Baruch Blumberg and his colleagues at the University of Pennsylvania (Blumberg, 1977) has revealed the existence of variation in another red blood cell antigen, the Australia antigen. They discovered that patients who had hepatitis B shared this otherwise rare antigen. Further study revealed that the virus causing hepatitis B contained the Australia antigen on its surface (surface antigen, HBsAg) as well as another antigen in its core (core antigen, HBcAg). People varied in their ability to respond to the presence of either or both of these antigens through the production of antibodies (substances able to neutralize the particular antigen). An individual may develop hepatitis followed by complete recovery, during which time HBsAg and antibodies to HBsAg and HBcAg appeared. Acute hepatitis may be followed by chronic hepatitis in which HBsAg and antibodies to HBcAg persisted. People with HBsAg and antibody to HBcAg may develop chronic liver disease or, alternatively, may be free of chronic hepatitis but may develop liver abnormalities. Finally, some people with chronic liver disease may develop panhepatic cell carcinoma, a cancer of the liver particularly common in middle-aged males in Africa and Asia. The transmission of the hepatitis virus has been shown by the Blumberg group to occur both "horizontally," from person to person, and "vertically," from parent to offspring. A maternal effect has been suggested in which transmission to offspring may occur during labor and delivery or during early mother-child interactions. Insects such as bedbugs can transmit the virus in societies where mother and child share the same bed. Thus, features of structure (antigens), function (recovery from hepatitis), and behavior (mother-child interactions) may all be involved in as yet incompletely understood adaptive processes that confer protection against a chain of diseases that include acute hepatitis, chronic hepatitis, chronic liver disease, and panhepatic cell carcinoma.

Over time, bioculturally patterned forms of behavior have developed that provide additional mechanisms for achieving adaptation. According to an outline provided by Svejda (1978), key elements in the evolution of mother-infant interaction systems illustrate this. Maternal behavior can be conceptualized as an organized set of activities that the mother carries out for her child to ensure its survival. Certain maternal behaviors have been selected for through evolution (and modified to some degree cross-culturally) because of their tendency to increase the probability of survival. Successful care-giving behaviors should not be interpreted so much as short-term adjustments to current technologies but rather as long-term adaptive responses to emergent biocultural processes (for example, among hominids, minimizing the threat of predation). Some of the maternal behaviors that contribute to infant survival are:

1. Carrying, since the infant has limited means of locomotion, and its grasp is not such that it can cling to the mother's body
2. Touching, which helps to bind the infant to the mother via skin-to-skin contact and which has a quieting effect on the infant.

3. Breast feeding, which helps ensure that the mother will have the baby in a protected position in relation to her body, with the content of the milk and colostrum contributing to nutrition and the provisioning of protective antibodies against disease.
4. Maintaining temperature through skin-to-skin contact by which the infant's body temperature can be kept at or near normal
5. Positioning, since an upright position quiets and alerts the infant and allows for maternal odor to be transmitted
6. Responding to infant signals, since immediately after birth infants begin to provide cues as to their needs. Different types of crying inform the parents whether the infant is angry or hungry and thus present information upon which they can act in a culturally patterned manner. (For example, among Anglo parents of the United States, attempts are made to encourage the infant to terminate angry crying, whereas among the Asmat of New Guinea no such termination is usually sought.) Visual cues also are transmitted, especially when the infant is held 20 to 30 cm from the parent's face. Carrying, visual cues, and touching contribute to the overall timing of activities that relate to the infant's state and needs and bring the infant into synchronization with parental caregiving activities
7. Maintaining the infant's physical condition, since at the most general level, the parents provide food and care (such as protection and cleanliness) and can place the infant in contact with appropriate health providers or curers

Fitness, fertility, and mortality

Adaptation, as we have illustrated, can stem from a range of biological and behavioral process, all of which affect our ability to live and to produce viable offspring. Adaptations influence fertility and mortality. Differential fertility refers to variation among individuals in their chances of reproducing;

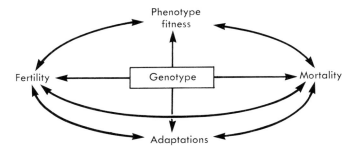

Fig. 3-1. Adaptations act through the genotype to produce phenotype fitness according to their net effects on fertility and mortality.

differential mortality refers to variation in their chances of survival.

The relationships among adaptation, fertility, and mortality are diagrammed in Fig. 3-1. The net effects of adaptations that affect fertility and mortality, in conjunction with an individual's genetic attributes (genotype), determine observable or phenotypic fitness. Fitness can be defined as the relative survival of the genotype, or, as Dobzhansky has written, "the differential perpetuation of genotypes or of genetic systems" (1968:115). Fitness is an outcome of factors that determine relative survival. It is critical to recognize genotypic and phenotypic levels of fitness. Genotypic fitness can be approached by viewing changes over time in genotypic proportions or gene frequencies. Stimulus for this change is the operation of selective forces. The outcome is a change in fitness where some genotypes have increased and others have decreased in number; the process contributes to the evolution of the species. The phenotype comprises the observable attributes of the genotype along with the independent effects of the environment, and effects of the environment in interaction with genetic effects. In most instances, researchers have been limited to assessing effects of adaptations on phenotypic, not genotypic, fitness.

Adaptation and fitness are not equivalent concepts since the same adaptation may have opposite effects on fertility and mortality. Slobodkin (1964:53) points out the relative independence of fitness and adaptation by means of a theoretical example in which an adaptation could result in a high reproduction rate (high fertility) and a low tolerance to food shortage (high mortality). The organism has a low fitness overall because of opposing adaptations. Dobzhansky (1968:115) shows that fitness and adaptability are not equivalent since it is possible for an organism to have a genotype with zero fitness relative to other genotypes and yet to be viable and fertile and thus to qualify for adaptation.

To summarize, an adaptation is specific either to mortality or to fertility effects, whereas fitness pertains to a genotype and is measurable relative to other genotypes. The sum of differential mortality and differential fertility, each a function of adaptations plus chance factors, constitutes fitness. In turn, changes in fitness constitute evolution. Organisms with increased fitness contribute more offspring to subsequent generations. Their genes, therefore, will predominate in future populations to the extent that their heritable adaptations continue to evidence increased relative fitness.

Clearly, only genetic attributes can be transmitted directly from parent to offspring. However, given the importance of physiological and cultural mechanisms of human adaptation and the possibility that genes influence complex behavioral as well as biologic traits (for example, "heritable diseases," such as diabetes mellitus), we need not limit our attention to the role of genetic factors in the evolution of health. Physiological and cultural adaptations are equally important. As the model of the human ecosystem (Fig. 2-1) suggests, these different but related types of adaptations contribute through time to a system of biocultural integration, an issue that will be discussed in more depth later in this chapter.

Evolutionary interpretations

Pre-Darwinian evolutionists. Any theory of evolution provides an interpretation of the relationship between ourselves and our surroundings. Contrary to popular opinion, the concept of evolution did not begin with Charles Darwin's formulations in the mid-1800s. There is no indication of when or where the recognition of relationships between things in the environment first appeared. Archeological testimony such as that evidenced at Stonehenge, the Big Medicine Wheel in Wyoming, and the observatory at Chichen Itzá suggests widespread and remote origins of interest of human populations in the relationship among things in the environment.

Views of evolution in the eighteenth and early nineteenth centuries in Europe accorded a noncentral position for the Earth in the universe, in line with Copernicus' teachings, but retained a central position for human beings among all living things. A literal interpretation of creation as told in the Bible's Book of Genesis prevailed. According to this view, humankind was created last and in God's image and, thus, justifiably, was given dominion over all other living and nonliving things. The task of scientists was perceived of as learning more about the wisdom of the Creator. Thus, Linnaeus undertook the classification of all living things in order

to better understand the Creator's plan. Agassiz believed that the task of the naturalist was "complete as soon as we have proved His existence" (as quoted in Mayr, 1972:983). The view of evolution during this time emphasized steady change toward the attainment of perfection. The "ladder of perfection" linked "lower" and "higher" forms in a progression from the simple to the more perfect; evolution as such neatly fit God's plan (Mayr, 1972).

The literal interpretation of creation was threatened in the early nineteenth century by the discovery of the great age of the Earth and the large number of extinct forms of life in the fossil record. Previous to these findings, creation was considered a recent event that had produced the world in its contemporary state. Analysis of the number of generations cited in the Bible provided a date for creation of 4004 B.C. In one variant of pre-Darwinian evolutionary theory, the extinction of certain species could be accommodated by the story of Noah's flood. Since multiple extinctions were evident, however, multiple floods and, subsequently, multiple creations were advanced. The replacement of the idea of a single creation with that of multiple creations led to the formulation of a second variant of pre-Darwinian evolutionary theory: catastrophism. In this interpretation the idea of multiple creations modified the view of creation as stated in the Bible but reaffirmed the view in which humankind retained a special, superior place in the natural order.

The Darwinian era and beyond. Darwin's formulation of evolution as published in 1859 departed so radically from the creationist and catastrophist conceptions that it has been described as the Darwinian revolution. Not only were the particular tenets of creationism and catastrophism opposed, but also refuted were the ideas of an anthropocentric, essentialist picture of the relationship among living things (Mayr, 1972). Charles Darwin and, simultaneously, Alfred Russell Wallace proposed that the world was not created in its present form, rather that species evolved through the operation of natural selection acting on naturally existing variation. Change was not a function of creation and extinction. Rather, it was the continual result of the natural forces of variation and natural selection.

In its present form, Darwinian evolutionary theory is recognized as a process of change that (1) is initiated by effects of mutation that supply new genetic variation, (2) produces either a decrease or increase in fitness, and (3) is given direction by natural selection, acting to preserve variants that increase fitness. Mutation is interpreted as generally harmful to the organism (decreasing fitness) but, under some circumstances, may confer increased adaptive capacity. Other factors capable of affecting the genetic composition of a given population—genetic drift and gene flow—operate in a nondirectional (random) fashion. The emphasis on natural selection as a directional force results in Darwinian theorists at times being referred to as "selectionists."

Darwinian evolutionary theory continues to prevail in interpretations of human adaptation and human evolution. Variation and change are seen as results of selective processes, possibly leading to the emergence of a species adapted to a new set of environmental circumstances. Recently, however, the primacy of Darwinian evolution has come under question by proponents of an opposing or non-Darwinian interpretation (as in King and Jukes, 1970; Lewontin, 1974).

In the non-Darwinian view, mutations do not necessarily produce an increase or decrease in fitness as is assumed in Darwinian theory. The mutation may be neutral; in other words it may have no effect on fitness. Mutations that do not change the amino acid

sequence coded for by a particular gene (that is, those resulting in an alternate code for the same amino acid) are, by definition, neutral, but non-Darwinian theorists propose that mutations that change the amino acid sequence also may be neutral. The concept of neutral mutation permits a large number of genes to be polymorphic (a case where there are two or more variants of a gene, each with a frequency in a population greater than 5%). In Darwinian formulations, the amount of genetic variation is expected to be small; mutations that decrease fitness would be eliminated, and the amount of variation that could be maintained would be limited by the "genetic load," a concept advanced as the cost to the population of having some less fit genetic variants. The observation in the late 1960s (Lewontin, 1967; Lewontin and Hubby, 1966) that genetic variation was much more common than previously expected thus challenged the Darwinian concept and contributed to the formulation of non-Darwinian theory.

Non-Darwinian evolution opposes the premise that natural selection is the guiding force in evolution by contending that random, or stochastic, forces have had a major role. The elimination of one genetic variant and the resultant fixation of the other variant by genetic drift (that is, random change in a gene pool reflecting the fact that some variants are not transmitted to the next generation due to small population size) is a possible mechanism for evolutionary change of this type. Critics have referred to this view as evolution by "random walk." In the non-Darwinian scenario, the random fixation of neutral genes becomes a driving force for evolution that yields a constant rate of evolutionary change over time. Thus, it is possible to calculate evolutionary distance between species and, once a calibration factor has been established, to compute an estimate of the amount of time that was required for the evolutionary divergence observed (Sarich and Wilson, 1969).

In summary, evolutionary theory provides a means of interpreting the relationships among living things. Early evolutionary thinking accorded human beings a privileged place in the natural world consistent with Western religious interpretations. Darwin sparked a controversy that continues into present times with the view that humankind did not occupy a special position but was subject to the same natural laws and processes that affected other forms of life. In the latest phase of the controversies surrounding evolution, non-Darwinian evolutionists have pointed to the possibility that evolution results from random forces operating on neutral genetic variation. Both the Darwinian and non-Darwinian evolutionary theories emphasize that human beings exist as a part of, not apart from, their environments. The perspective on humankind as just another part of the environment is carried even further in the non-Darwinian view by raising the possibility that evolution operates without sole reference to natural selection.

Biocultural evolution: the hominid pattern. The complexity of the issues raised by evolutionary theories is compounded further by some apparently simple questions, as posed by Dobzhansky (1971:45), "What is man, whence came he, and whither is he going?" He suggests that as humans transmit their "two heredities"—biological and cultural—consciousness and self-awareness must be taken into account. These originated at some later stage in the evolutionary process and, in conjunction with the emergence of culture, have enabled a transcendence beyond humankind's purely biological form and function to occur. Following Dobzhansky, we would agree that such transcendence does not imply the injection of some novel kind of energy, fundamentally different from that found in other living organisms. How-

ever, it does imply an interactive, biocultural distinctiveness that sets human beings apart from other species.

Attempts to analyze this distinctiveness have been complicated by the necessity for unravelling philosophical as well as biocultural variables. Darwin, not the first to attempt such analysis, encountered similar difficulties. His conceptualization limited the validity of parts of his work, because, as Harris (1968:121) points out, like his contemporaries, Darwin did not "separate changes in a group's learned repertory from hereditary modifications." Harris (1968:121) illustrates this with a longer version of the following passage from Darwin's *Descent of Man:*

At the present day civilized nations are everywhere supplanting barbarious nations, excepting where the climate opposes a deadly barrier; and they succeed mainly, though not exclusively, through their arts, which are the products of the intellect. It is, therefore, highly probable that with mankind the intellectual faculties have been gradually perfected through natural selection.

In contrast to this view of differential intellectual capacity, which in part reflects a nineteenth century philosophical stance, we now know that the mean and variance of brain size and general intellectual capability are approximately the same among all human populations. This is a result of uniform "progressive evolution" but not in the sense of "improvement." There was an overall trend toward increasing size and complexity of the human brain that occurred in all populations over the past million years. The progression was a function of adaptive successes modulated through environmental and cultural feedback as tool use, language, and social skills developed. Dobzhansky (1971:49-50) believes that the feedback concept neatly illustrates the integration of biological and cultural processes. Looking toward the future, however, he stresses the dilemma that we do not yet know exactly how this relationship operates, nor where it is taking us as a species.

PATTERNS OF ADAPTATION IN HUMAN EVOLUTION
Our place in nature

Understanding the place of the human species in the natural world requires a knowledge of how humankind is related to other living things and how humankind evolved to its present position. Health, disease, and illness are part of this evolutionary process.

One description of our place in nature is afforded by the taxonomic chart in Fig. 3-2. In keeping with the rules laid down by Linnaeus during the eighteenth century, all life forms can be classified into an array of progressively narrower, more restricted categories. A human being is thus classified as an animal, a chordate, a eutherian mammal, an ungulate, and a primate. Included among the chordates are all animals that have a tubular nerve cord running down the spinal or dorsal surface and have gill slits at some stage of the life cycle. Mammals are animals that produce milk from the mammary glands, maintain constant body temperature, have hair, and have a single bone in

the lower jaw. Eutherian mammals are a group of mammals that develop placentas for nourishing the fetus during gestation instead of laying eggs (like protheria) or giving birth at an early stage of fetal development and maintaining the young in an external organ (as do marsupials). Ungulates are those eutherian mammals that have nails instead of claws and have four limbs. The order to which human beings belong was named "first order," or primates, by Linnaeus, reflecting the philosophical stance of both the classifier and others of his century. Primates are a group of mammals with a high degree of dexterity, a large brain, and in many cases, more generalized means of adaptation.

Within the primate order, human beings can be further classified as anthropoid, hominoid, hominid, *Homo*, and *sapiens* (Fig. 3-3). The Anthropoidea are a suborder of primates with juvenile and adult sets of dentition and hemochorial placenta. Hominoidea are anthropoid primates that have no tails and include those who subsequently have developed arboreal brachiation (Pongidae) and terrestrial bipedalism as forms of locomotion. The Hominidae—hominids—are hominoids that have become specialized for bipedal locomotion. Finally, hominids that make tools

Kingdom: Animalia

Phylum: Chordata

Class: Mammalia

Infraclass: Eutheria

Cohort: Unguiculata

Order: Primates

Suborder: Anthropoidea

Infraorder: Catarrhinae

Superfamily: Hominoidea

Family: Hominidae

Genus: Homo

Species: Sapiens

Fig. 3-2. The taxonomic position of humankind.

and rely on culture are members of the genus *Homo*. Those with brains approximately as large as those of living human beings have the species designation *sapiens*.

Two groups with which human beings have great affinity stand out in the classification scheme: mammals and primates. Mammals, as judged from their numbers and distribution, are very successful animals. Internal fertilization and gestation ensure a relatively predictable survival for offspring who have demonstrably greater complexity than do other forms of life. Our mammalian heritage includes the presence of four limbs and five digits (pentadactility) on each extremity. Both of these characteristics are old,

adaptive traits that are generalized and conservative in nature, that is, their adaptive value has been retained in the face of other more specialized alternatives. Most primates share these generalized mammalian features. Primates also all have opposable thumbs and/or great toes; stereoscopic, color vision; eyes situated on the same frontal plane of the head; enclosed bony eye orbits; a large brain relative to body size; and three kinds of teeth (incisor, premolar, molar). These primate features can be seen as reflections of adaptation to an arboreal way of life in which manual dexterity, three-dimensional color vision, and a large brain emphasizing visual (as opposed to olfactory) centers are advantageous.

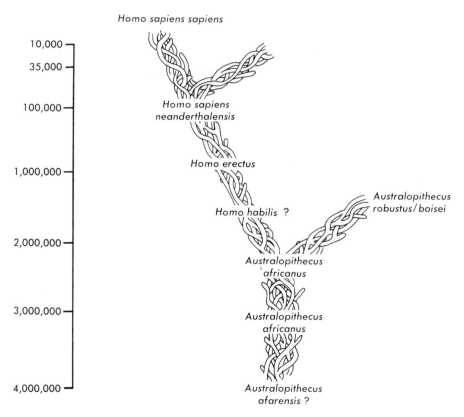

Fig. 3-3. The human evolutionary "tree," expressed in years. Multiple lines, reflecting the existence of numerous populations and species, are likely to have characterized the human evolutionary record.

Bipedalism

The taxonomic family to which human beings belong is distinguished from other primate families by our habitual form of posture—bipedalism. Bipedalism entails a number of anatomical modifications in the structure and function of the spinal column, hips, lower limbs, and feet. Body weight is delicately cantilevered from the spine and is balanced over the hips and the two supporting limbs (see Schultz, 1950).

The appearance of bipedalism altered the relationship of hominids to their environments. A major benefit was that it freed the hands from locomotor functions. In an already dextrous, visually oriented primate, freeing the hands for tool use and manufacture is likely to have operated in a feedback relationship with bipedalism in which each reinforced the emergence and perpetuation of the other. This interpretation has recently been challenged by Johanson and White (1979) who suggest, based on analysis of skeletal fragments of a hominid species christened *Australopithecus afarensis,* that full bipedalism preceded early tool use.

In either case, environmental change is also thought to have been a factor in the emergence of bipedalism. During the Miocene epoch, the previously unbroken expanse of tropical forest stretching across what is now Africa, the Middle East, and Asia began to be divided by open grasslands. A new ecological niche opened for the primates that, in the course of adaptation to terrestrial life, aided the emergence of the hominids. A bipedal primate living on the ground at least part of the time is likely to have been vulnerable to attack from other animals. A biped is not very fleet footed compared to quadrapeds. The trees may have continued to offer refuge but were not a place wholly out of reach of other animals. Thus, increasing reliance on extracorporeal means of defense (and offense)—tools—was a likely, eventual accompaniment of bipedalism.

Another possibility recently proposed by Owen Lovejoy (quoted in Kolata, 1977) concerns the advantage afforded early hominids by the shortened time interval between births. *Homo sapiens,* compared to other living primates, has a short birth interval. Assuming that the shortening occurred in the past, Lovejoy suggests that the increase in reproduction and number of offspring permitted would have been pressures for increased bipedalism and social cooperation to facilitate caring for the larger number of dependents produced.

The precise origins of bipedalism in the paleontological record are unclear. Some assume a late Miocene origin, approximately 20 to 12 million years ago; others suggest Pliocene origins. *Ramapithecus,* known from teeth and jaw fragments found in India and Africa, is the Miocene primate most frequently proposed as the first hominid. Given the paucity of fossil remains and difficulties in interpreting them, however, the hominid status of *Ramapithecus* is far from established (Frayer, 1974).

Bipedalism was established by the late Pliocene or early Pleistocene epoch. *Australopithecus,* the hominid genus first identified by Raymond Dart in 1924, was clearly bipedal. Low, broad illiac blades, an S-shaped spinal column, a centrally-positioned foramen magnum, and lower limb bones adapted for bearing weight attest to this. Numerous subsequent discoveries of Pliocene/Pleistocene hominids have resulted in the identification of several species in two proposed genera, *Australopithecus* and *Homo.* These include *Australopithecus africanus, Australopithecus robustus, Australopithecus boisei,* the newly designated *Australopithecus afarensis,* and *Homo habilis.* It is unclear which among these eventually

People of the Lake

The people of the lake should not properly be called "people" at all, if the latter term is meant to be equated with the term "human." Yet they exhibited many humanlike characteristics and may well have been some of our forebearers. As described by Leakey and Lewin (1978) in their book *People of the Lake,* these hominids lived 2.5 million years ago on the eastern shores of what is now known as Lake Turkana in Kenya. Crocodiles could be seen nearby. Hippopotamuses wallowed in the mud, while pelicans crowded the air. The savannah-covered hills not far from the shores were interspersed with forested valleys. Fig trees and acacias lined some of the streams leading into the lake. Animals resembling pigs, colobus monkeys, and mangabeys would have been but a few of the animals seen as these Pliocene/Pleistocene creatures traversed the denser forest regions.

The economy was a mixed one. Both plants and animals were consumed, plants most likely taking precedence. Roots, shrubs, buds, and leaves probably were preferred. When available, insects, lizards, and birds' eggs likely were eaten as well. Leakey and Lewin suggest that these hominids already may have begun to develop a sexual division of labor. Given the requirements of nursing and general child care, combined with the demands made on bipedal females to carry their offspring as a function of a mobile existence, females may have done more of the gathering (as is seen among contemporary human bands) and males more of the hunting and scavenging. It is unlikely that these early hunters were reliant on stone weapons—Leakey's finds indicate an origin of simple stone tools in this part of Africa of about 2 million years B.P.—but rather on their hands or wooden implements to catch immature small game or lame animals. The scavenging of leftover meat from the carcasses of animals killed by lions, leopards, and other carnivores may have served as an important source of protein. Unlike other primates whose food-getting is primarily individualistic even though other of their activities are intensely social, early hominids such as those of Lake Turkana may have developed an unusual adaptive strategy: food sharing. Males and females returning to temporary encampments sharing mixed food resources would have had an advantage over other animal species.

If the remarkable find by Donald Johanson of the fossilized partial remains of ten or more hominids in a single site in Ethiopia is an accurate indication of group size, it can be concluded that the hominids dwelling near Lake Turkana lived in small, flexible bands. Inferences derived by Leakey in his study of late Pliocene encampments suggest that certain bands may have been as large as twenty-five individuals. It is unlikely that matri- or patri-lineality, or other more rigid forms of social organization, had yet emerged. But if these researchers are correct, one very important social characteristic had appeared: cooperation. Ecological and economic considerations indicate that cooperative behavior in many social interactions is an outgrowth of food-sharing activity. Other anthropological investigations suggest that complex language did not develop until the era of *Homo sapiens,* some 2 million years later, and so it must be presumed that call systems and social interactions were sufficient to transmit basic information regarding cooperative activities. No clues exist as to whether such cooperation included care of those individuals who were sick or injured. However, Leakey and Lewin do conclude with the assertion that cooperation was a key to what eventually made humans distinct from other animals, not warfare, as others have stressed.

became extinct, but at this point it is most likely that *Homo habilis, Australopithecus africanus,* or both evolved into later Pleistocene hominids. Evidence indicates that all of the species in both hominid genera were bipedal (see People of the Lake, p. 63).

Little direct evidence exists as to the diseases that may have prevailed during the late Pliocene and early Pleistocene epoch. A style of life dependent on foraging, the eating of carrion, and irregular hunting in a savannah environment would likely have been associated with two types of infectious disease: parasitic and zoonotic. Parasites that had become adapted to prehominid populations of the Miocene epoch, such as the dryopithecines, would be expected to infest subsequent lineages. Head lice, body lice, and pinworms are examples of such parasites (Armelagos, 1978:102). The intestinal protozoa found in *Homo sapiens sapiens* today are shared in large part with apes and monkeys, suggesting ancient origins. Small population size, low population density, and lack of a sedentary life-style would have limited the prevalence of infectious diseases (Dunn, 1968; Cockburn, 1971). Livingstone (1958) has suggested that malarial infections would not have been prevalent in early hominids. A savannah orientation combined with the mobile life-style of small bands would have inhibited the spread of malaria. The second type of disease—zoonoses—consists of those parasites that have adapted to other hosts and are transmitted via bites, wounds, or the consumption of infected meat. Diseases such as sleeping sickness, tetanus, and schistosomiasis (bilharzia) follow this mode of transmission (Armelagos, 1978:103).

Geographic expansion

Darwin speculated that human origins would be found in Africa. Early paleontologists, such as Eugene Dubois who searched for the "missing link" and discovered *Pithecanthropus erectus* (now renamed *Homo erectus*) in Java, ignored Darwin's advice. The recent discoveries by the Leakey family and other investigators in eastern and southern Africa attest to the importance of this continent in the evolution of early humankind. However, whether hominid origins were confined to Africa remains in question, since fossil remains found in Asia (that is, *Meganthropus palaeojavanicus,* dated at 1.9 million years B.P.) suggest that the early hominids were more widely distributed.

In any event, *Homo erectus* remains from Africa and Asia and evidence of occupation sites in Europe attest to the widespread distribution of hominid groups during the middle Pleistocene epoch. Besides Dubois' discoveries in Java, Von Koenigswald also found several specimens in Java. There are also extensive remains at Choukoutien in China and in eastern Africa. Skeletal fragments indicate that *Homo erectus* was a medium-sized biped with increased cranial capacity and decreased jaw size compared to the australopithecines. *Homo erectus* lived from approximately 1 million to one-third of a million years ago. In keeping with its considerable antiquity, *Homo erectus* was distinguished from subsequent human ancestors by the absence of a forehead, by a smaller cranial capacity, and by the presence of comparatively robust cranial features.

Homo erectus pursued the animals and presumably also the plants that comprised its diet with greater intensity and in a more systematic fashion than did earlier hominids. Among the prey at middle Pleistocene sites appear large animals, including gazelle, oxenlike herbivores, and rhinoceroses. At Torralba and Ambrona in Spain, elephant remains have been found with flake tools between the animal's ribs. Charcoal fragments indicate that fire may have served as a means of guiding the animals to sites where killing could more easily be accomplished. The stone tool technology of the middle Pleistocene epoch includes a variety of heavy-duty multifacial and bifacial tools that could have been used to dismember game animals but that would not seem well-suited as weapons for killing large prey. This evidence leads us to conclude that full-fledged hunting and gathering as a systematic, patterned hominid way of life can be said to have begun with *Homo erectus* (see People of the Plateau, below).

People of the Plateau

The adjacent sites of Torralba and Ambrona on a plateau in north-central Spain have yielded some of the most extensive evidence of late *Homo erectus* populations. Dated at approximately 400,000 B.P., Torralba was first discovered in 1888 by workers digging a ditch for a water main. An amateur Spanish archeologist subsequently excavated it more thoroughly in the early 1900s. Clark Howell (1966) and his associates resumed the effort more systematically in the 1960s, excavating more than 20,000 square feet of earth to a depth of 8 feet. Their efforts revealed abattoirs, places for butchering animals and processing the meat, and remains of human habitation sites.

Elephants were prominent in the fossilized remains. They may have been killed by *Homo erectus* after being driven into swamps, there to be clubbed, speared, or stoned to death. Other important fauna included horses, red deer, wild oxen, and rhinoceroses. Cleavers and other bifacial stone tools were used in the butchering. Charcoal remains give evidence of hearths and, in certain widely scattered locations nearby, indication that grass fires were purposefully set in order to drive game into the swamps (Pfeiffer, 1978:110).

Hominids were now occupying temperate zones. Certain patterns of local and occasionally long-distance migration probably were well established. Thus new and different parasites would have been present if compared with those of the Pliocene/Pleistocene epoch. Since some food was being cooked, certain parasites would have been killed in the process (Armelagos, 1978:103).

Humans of this era are likely to have developed fairly sophisticated types of social and economic organization (Fig. 3-4). Seasonal encampments were situated such that game trails could be monitored. The ability for people to effectively organize can be attributed to a tradition of cooperation, to the evolving ability to plan for the future, and to what may have been a complex form of gestures and sound communication. It is unlikely, however, that true speech had yet emerged (Hewes, 1973).

Some remains suggest ritual practices among the people of the plateau. The orderly alignment of elephant bones in one location suggests a purposeful human activity in which there may have been some significance attached to the order of the bones. Examination of the cranial vault of an elephant skull indicates that it had been purposefully smashed open. The brain was probably extracted and eaten. Fossil human skulls from Choukoutien in China indicate that the basal opening of the skull had been enlarged, perhaps for the extraction of the brain. Among subsequent *Homo sapiens sapiens,* ritual cannibalism became an important way of life for some cultures; perhaps *Homo erectus* also engaged in such rituals.

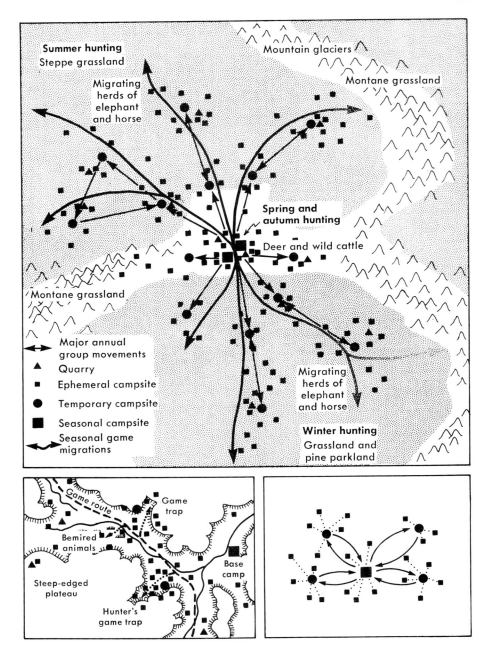

Fig. 3-4. A seasonal mobility model for Acheulian hunters and gatherers in mid-Pleistocene Spain, based in part on information from Torralba and Ambrona. During spring and autumn, the hunters preyed systematically on migrating herds forced to pass through the mountain routes (see detail, lower left), while during winter and summer, the hunters subdivided into smaller groups and fanned out into a succession of temporary sites. The mobility model is abstracted in the lower right. (From Butzer, K. Environment, culture, and human evolution. *American Scientist*, September 1977.)

The beginnings of culture

The evolution of culture cannot be separated from the evolution of humankind. Viewed in contemporary perspective, human beings are human because they have culture; in paleontological perspective, the genus *Homo* emerged as reliance on culture increased.

Culture is comprised of such extrasomatic adaptations as tools, shelter, fire, and social relationships. Clearly, such inventions bypass the lengthy biological adaptations that are required to fell game or to protect against cold temperatures. Culture, especially in its early manifestations, is made, at least in part, with the hands. Thus, the change to a bipedal posture that freed the hands for other activities was a critical event in the evolution of culture. Likewise, by increasing the range of environments and potential for control over environmental challenges, culture contributed to forces pressuring for cranial expansion and subsequent human evolution.

The continuing expansion of brain size

People of the Cave

Beginning about 100,000 years ago, *Homo sapiens neanderthalensis* first began to occupy a large cave in a remote mountainside in northern Iraq. Even today families of modern Kurd people live there. Shanidar Cave, as it is called, has shed light on the origins of modern humans. It also has revealed evidence of Neanderthal ritual practices dating back to 60,000 B.P.

At the back of Shanidar Cave, in a layer estimated to be 60,000 years old, Ralph Solecki in 1960 unearthed the grave of a hunter with a severely crushed skull. This was one of nine individuals whose remains were found in the cave. The skeleton was fairly complete and was found lying on its side. It faced to the west with the head to the south. Unbeknown to the investigators until soil analysis had been initiated at the Musée de l'Homme in France was the presence of extensive amounts of pollen of various flower species (Leroi-Gourhan, 1975). The several pollen types in the soil surrounding the grave supported the idea that bunches of flowers had been placed there. Bright flowers had been chosen, such as hyacinths, daisies, and hollyhocks. Certain of the plants were herbs that are presently used as medicinals by tribes in the area. Very small pieces of wood were found that may also have had ritual significance.

Shanidar IV, as this hunter's remains have been labeled, likely met his death during a rockfall within the cave. Other of the excavated individuals seem to have met a similar demise. Analysis of their remains indicates amputation of an arm of one and the presence of numerous microfractures in some ribs (Kerley, 1971:136, 141). It is likely that the cave's inhabitants lived in and among the rockfall areas. "Their household debris and accumulated soil gradually filled in the areas between the stones, leveling the rough parts of the cave floor until another ceiling collapse started the whole process all over again" (Solecki, 1971:213). It can be inferred that human culture had evolved to a point where more abstract notions of life and death had emerged. Perhaps disease was coming to be understood and medicinals were being used. Furthermore, not only do there seem to have been burial rituals but associated funeral feasts as well. Split and broken mammal bones concentrated around another of the Shanidar burials indicate that a feast of this sort may have occurred.

during the middle Pleistocene epoch reflects the increasing complexity and challenge of *Homo erectus'* world. During the middle Pleistocene epoch, average body height increased from 4½ to 5½ feet, but average cranial capacity changed from 600 cc to 1000 cc. Thus, the relative expansion of cranial capacity exceeded the increase in body size by a factor of 3 (22% increase in body size in comparison to 66% increase in cranial capacity). The occupation of environments from cave sites in Choukoutien to lake shores in Tanzania, along with charcoal fragments and the presence of hearths, attests to *Homo erectus'* growing control over the environment.

In the late Pleistocene epoch hominids existed who had cranial capacities within the range of modern human beings. These were the much-maligned Neanderthals, classified as *Homo sapiens neanderthalensis* or as a predecessor subspecies of the living human species. While the Neanderthals were distinguished by larger and more robust dimensions of the face than modern humans, the average cranial capacity of Neanderthal specimens actually exceeds the modern average. The initial Neanderthal find was of a skullcap, which was discovered in 1856 in the valley *(thal)* of Neander in Germany; hence, it was termed Neanderthal. It is noteworthy that this discovery coincided closely with the publication of Darwin's views on evolution. Among the reactions to Darwinian views was the response that "fossil man did not exist"— a response that relegated the Neanderthal specimen to being the remains of a diseased or deformed individual. Subsequent discovery of many remains at various sites helped establish that "fossil man" indeed did exist. The Neanderthal specimens reveal great variation in cranial vaulting, brow ridge, jaw size, and tooth size features, but consistently had modern postcranial skeletons.

Cultural remains at Neanderthal sites evidence increasing sophistication of stone tools. Several stone tool traditions become apparent in Europe, Africa, and Asia, perhaps as a response to varying environmental and cultural traditions. Burials have been found at several sites, indicating that special treatment was extended to the dead, perhaps as preparation for an afterlife (see People of the Cave, p. 67).

DISEASE EVIDENCE IN PAST HUMAN POPULATIONS
Paleopathology

In 1914 Sir Marc Armand Ruffer defined paleopathology as "the science of the diseases which can be demonstrated in human and animal remains of ancient times" (Janssens, 1970:1), and this definition has persisted. The objectives of paleopathology in light of medical anthropology are threefold: (1) to analyze and describe the evolution of diseases that afflict humans, (2) to illuminate the cultural circumstances of the populations involved, and (3) to provide understanding of the processes of human adaptation. Nonhuman, reptilian evidence of disease dates at least to the Permian period some 250,000,000 years ago (Janssens, 1970:25). As applied to medical anthropology, paleopathology primarily deals with prehistoric and nonliterate societies. However, whether in humans or nonhumans, the evidence of disease or injury usually is inferred from physical remains. Such remains most often consist of skeletal materials, but in certain instances, such as mummies and "bog people" (see p. 69), soft tissue remains have been preserved. When available, written records also may be used.

Paleopathology provides information to aid in the understanding of paleoecology, the study of the former habitats of living organisms. As in the study of ecology, the focus is on organism-environment interrelationships and the ways in which adaptive or maladaptive modifications occur through time.

The Bog People of Iron-Age Denmark

Well-preserved remains of human corpses, containing both soft tissue and bone, have been found intermittently over the centuries in certain of Denmark's peat bogs (Glob, 1969). During the past 200 years alone, more than 150 men, women, and children have been uncovered. The constant action of moderately acidic bog water is the key to preservations of this sort. The two discoveries that most dramatically served to bring the "bog people" a share of international anthropological acclaim and detailed paleopathological analysis took place within 2 years of one another in the early 1950s.

First to come to light was the so-called "Tollund man," named for the bog in which peat diggers uncovered his remains. He lived during the Iron Age, approximately 2000 years ago. His flesh (particularly that of the face, abdominal region, and feet) was preserved so well that minute wrinkles and pores could be seen. The stubble of a beard was found on his chin. His hair was approximately 2 inches in length but was not dressed in any way. It was hidden under a cap made from pieces of leather that had been sewn together. Of particular interest was the plaited skin rope found tied in a slip-knot around his neck. Clearly visible rope marks were found on the skin under the chin and along the sides of the neck. Although the neck vertebrae did not appear to be damaged, a team of medical, and anthropological experts concluded that he had died by hanging. Without the preservation of the soft tissue, no such determination could have been made.

The second find was that of the "Grauballe man." He was uncovered near the village of Grauballe just 11 miles east of the Tollund find. Again most of the flesh and bones were remarkably well-preserved. Perfect finger prints were obtained from the right hand. A combination of dating techniques led to a determination that the man was of late Iron Age origin, having lived some time between 200 and 400 A.D. Analysis of bone materials indicated that the left femur and tibia had been fractured, probably on burial rather than before death. The Grauballe man also had been killed, but not in the manner of the Tollund man. His neck had been cut from ear to ear. The wound was so deep that the gullet was severed completely. The skin revealed the evidence of more than one stroke of the cutting implement.

Combining the paleopathological evidence with that derived from the studies of paleoecologists and historians, a fairly complete picture of the life of Jutland's Iron Age population has been reconstructed. An ancient highway, later used by pilgrims traveling from Iceland to Rome, passed through the region. Peat was used for fuel 20 centuries ago just as it is today. Although meat played a role in the diet, analysis of the intestinal remains of the two individuals described here indicates that wild grasses, weeds, and cultivated grains were prominent. Between 12 and 24 hours before he was hanged, the Tollund man had consumed his last meal. It consisted of a gruel made primarily from barley, linseed, "gold-of-pleasure," and knotweed, as well as other sorts of weeds that grow on ploughed land. Apparently the Grauballe man had eaten his last meal immediately before death. He had likewise consumed a gruel, but of even more mixed variety: sixty-three different types of grain, grass, and weed were represented. In addition to those species mentioned for the Tollund man, clover, rye, goosefoot, and buttercup were found during intestinal analysis. Brothwell (1978:131) notes that the intestinal remains of the fungus *ergot sclerotica* were also isolated. Paleoecological analysis indicates that small fields of barley and rye were tended in the open areas near Jutland's bogs. Weeds were allowed to grow among the grains. Uncultivated land was covered with scrub vegetation that included birch, willow, and mountain ash. Cranberries were commonplace in the bog areas themselves, particularly in spots where peat had not been cut for some time.

Disease processes and the response of human populations contribute to these modifications.

Within the sphere of Western science, the earliest known observations of pathological fossil bones were published by Johann Friedrich Esper in 1774. His publication dealt with "sarcoma"—actually a fracture indicating healing callus—in a cave bear (Campbell, 1976:59; Ackerknecht, 1977:72). As the field of paleopathology emerged, first with emphasis being placed on animal remains and then only more recently with attention turning toward humans, problems of misinterpretation were frequent. The classic case involved French paleontologist Marcellin Boule. He did not recognize that the skeleton of a Neanderthal male discovered at La Chapelle-aux-Saints bore signs of extensive arthritic processes and tooth decay. Boule's 1911 to 1913 reconstruction mistakenly referred to the effects of these diseases (for example, stooped posture, bowed legs) as attributes of Neanderthals in general, a reconstruction that served for decades as the presumed model for western European populations.

Such misinterpretations of fossil material can arise through improper analysis of the cause or the reconstruction of skeletal attributes. After normal inhumation, bones can be affected by soil conditions, percolating water, mineral deposition, invading insects, bacteria, or plant roots. Dripping water can create a hole in a skull bone which may be confused with an unhealed wound inflicted during the individual's lifetime. Rodents and carnivores leave gnaw marks on bones, as exemplified by osteological remains uncovered from the Belgian cave of Furfooz, that can be misinterpreted as being caused by disease in the living individual or cannibalism of the deceased (Janssens, 1970:20, 21). An indentation caused by trauma, such as a blow to the head, can be misinterpreted as resulting from disease *per se* (see Wells,

1964:21). Even the shovel of an errant excavator can leave a mark that, if bone patina is not examined closely, might be misconstrued.

Paleopathological evidence, when interpreted in the strictest sense, tells of a disease's existence but not of its prevalence (the number of cases in a population) nor its incidence (the number of new cases during a specified interval, usually a year). Once the existence of a disease has been established, which can be done by one incontestable case, inferences can be made about associated ecological and cultural circumstances. Biocultural factors thus can be elucidated through paleopathological investigations. For example, occupational diseases can serve to clarify patterns of biocultural adaptation. It can be inferred that Neolithic miners from Spiennes and Obourg, Belgium, using staghorn pickaxes to hack flint out of limestone, might have suffered from the lung disorder silicosis (Janssens, 1970:4). Miner's elbow may also have been a problem. Were osteological remains of certain contemporary Americans to be uncovered some centuries from now, evidence of tennis elbow could be seen. If interpreted correctly, a greater understanding of the general life-style of the population (or, at least, a portion of it) could then be derived. However, the exact incidence of the ailment and the proportion of those engaged in such behavior would probably remain unknown.

Varieties of paleopathological evidence

Bone growths. Neoplasms ("new growths") can be either benign or malignant. Both may leave evidence on bones that can in turn tell the paleopathologist or medical anthropologist something about the conditions that affected individuals at a particular time and place. However, in many instances little more than the immediate cause can be accurately determined.

Simple osteoma is one type of neoplasm that is extremely common and is usually benign in nature. As Wells (1964:70-71) indicates, it has been found on the skeletal remains of numerous peoples during the course of excavating ancient cemeteries throughout the world. Osteomas usually resemble small, hard knobs on the surface of bones. One unusual example that was found in a French skull dated to the Middle Ages was an interior osteoma large enough to occupy a sizable portion of the cranial cavity.

Exostoses are much like osteomas in appearance. However, they are not primary growths but osteological reactions to trauma. One of the most well-known in the anthropological records is the protruding knob on the *Homo erectus* femur discovered by Dubois in Java in 1891 (Campbell, 1976:207). Exostoses are common, but unless the type of traumatic injury is known, they shed little light on the health of ancient populations. In most cases, therefore, patterns of such population's behavior do not emerge from the paleopathological record, and it must be assumed that the exostosis resulted from a sudden blow or fall or a prolonged irritation. The results of the latter have been found among populations whose members squat for prolonged periods of time, so that exostoses develop on the third facet of the ventral side of the ankle joint (Janssens, 1970:4).

In comparison to such benign neoplasms, malignant bone growths are of more importance to health because of the greater probability that disability or death will result. Such growths are subject to a wider range of interpretations than are simple osteomas. Sarcoma and carcinoma are the two most common types of skeletal cancers. Unlike growths of the body's soft tissue, sarcomas and carcinomas survive inhumation well. Some of the earliest sarcomas yet found are those on the femurs and humeri of fifth dynasty Egyptians living about 2750 B.C.

(Wells, 1964:73; Janssens, 1970:68); some pre-Columbian skulls found in Peru also exhibit them (Ackerknecht, 1977:76).

Sarcomas begin in osseous (bone) tissue and subsequently spread into surrounding organs. By contrast, carcinomas usually originate in a gland, mucous membrane, or organ and later may spread to bone; they begin as soft tissue neoplasms. Carcinomas tend to be found in elderly persons. Hence, they are not common in the skeletal remains of ancient populations in which comparatively few individuals reached old age. Only two or three carcinomas have been located in the thousands of Egyptian mummies studied to date (Wells, 1964:74). Thus, while carcinomatic etiologies are not thoroughly understood, this form of cancer can perhaps be thought of as a "disease of civilization." That is, populations that exhibit greater life expectancies—inhabiting areas sometimes referred to as "the civilized world"—also tend to have a greater prevalence of carcinomas.

Arthritis. Osteoarthritis attacks the joints, especially those of the limbs and vertebrae, resulting in the deterioration of the cartilage that covers opposing surfaces of bone. This can lead to alterations in the bones themselves. The causes of osteoarthritis remain unknown. Famed medical historian and paleopathologist Henry Sigerist suggested an infectious etiology for arthritic diseases, but other paleopathologists are not ready to support this assertion fully. Endocrine and metabolic considerations, as well as repeated trauma, all have been suggested as playing a role (Wells, 1964:59-60; Janssens, 1970:75-77).

Evidence of various forms of chronic arthritic disease is widespread in the human and nonhuman fossil record. Dinosaurs and early reptiles exhibited it (Janssens, 1970:82). Pliocene/Pleistocene hominid remains show evidence of spinal arthritis (Johanson, 1977). Osteoarthritis seems to have been relatively widespread among Neanderthal populations, being evidenced in individuals from the sites of Krapina, La Ferrassie, La Quina, and La Chapelle-aux-Saints. The jaw is especially affected in these cases and at an early age. "We can assume that they fed on a tough, perhaps uncooked, diet and put their jaws to vigorous use gnawing bones, cracking nuts and chomping roots" (Wells, 1964:62). Among populations of *Homo sapiens sapiens*, the ancient Nubians, living in what is now southern Egypt and northern Sudan, frequently exhibited osteoarthritis of neck vertebrae. Various explanations have been offered. It could have arisen through the compression induced by carrying water vessels on the head (causing repeated instances of minor trauma). It could have resulted secondarily from an oral-dental infection (as discussed in Armelagos, 1977). Early twentieth century paleopathologist Roy Moodie and others before him had suggested the relationship, in both New and Old World osteological remains, of oral infection and spinal change (Wells, 1964:64). The understanding of osteoarthritis and associated behavior patterns is enhanced if one considers the results of Pales' research (reported in Janssens, 1970:84). Focusing on mandibulo-temporal osteoarthritis, he found no evidence of it in modern Peruvians or Egyptians, but a prevalence of 26.4% among inhabitants of Melanesia's Loyalty Islands. High prevalence was found among other inhabitants of Melanesia as well. This suggests that prolonged chewing of tough, fibrous plant substances leads to wearing out articulating bone surfaces. The type of resources used, therefore, can play an important role in the proliferation of certain diseases; consequently, disease prevalence is frequently related to patterns of group behavior.

Fractures. Fractures of the limbs are among the most common injuries found in osteological remains. Among the numerous kinds that have been described, the "parry fracture" of the ulna is remarkable for the in-

formation it sheds on human behavior. Janssens investigated it in several different contexts (1970:18, 32) and concluded that it results from a blow inflicted as warriors battle one another. Such injuries usually occur in the middle of the forearm. In contrast, other types of forearm breaks (such as those resulting from a fall) usually occur near the wrist. Healed parry fractures have been identified in the Neolithic populations of Furfooz and Sclaigneaux and in a late Roman skeleton from the fourth century A.D.

Fractures of the skull are also commonplace (Fig. 3-5). The paleopathological record reveals instances of partial crushing (as in the Grauballe man) and of skull fracture (as in the Obourg man). In the latter case, the injury, brought about by the caving in of a flint mine during Belgium's Neolithic period, resulted in death (Janssens, 1970:31). A very different type of skull fracture is found among certain early inhabitants of Peru. It consists of a double or triple depression of the parietal bone, inflicted in battle by means of a mace shaped like a six-pointed star (Wells, 1964: 49). Other wounds of the skull, commonly in the form of circular or rectangular holes, are the result of the practice of trephination. This was a form of surgery in which recovery of the patient was intended. Among some peoples of Neolithic western Europe and pre-Columbian South America, it is likely that this practice had magical or ritual connotations (Bandelier, 1904). Clearly, primitive surgeons demonstrated a high degree of sophistication in certain of the techniques they employed.

There is some disagreement among paleopathologists as to the measures that earlier populations of *Homo sapiens sapiens* may have taken to aid the healing of bone fractures. It is likely that many limbs healed without the aid of splints; even in a sample of gibbons,* 30% showed evidence of

---

*An arboreal anthropoid ape of the genus *Hylobates*.

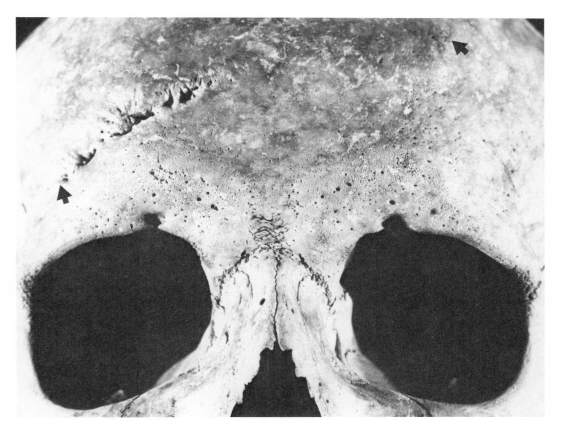

Fig. 3-5. This skull comes from a pioneer grave found in the eroding banks of the Little Muddy River near Fort Bridger, Wyoming, by Dr. George W. Gill of the University of Wyoming. Analysis of the bone materials revealed that the individual was a male Caucasian, approximately 35 years of age who had suffered a blow to the forehead sometime prior to death. A 100 mm scar extends between the two arrows. (Courtesy G. W. Gill.)

healed fractures (Armelagos, 1979). However, among certain peoples such as the Mayans, bone-setting became a well-developed specialty (Paul, 1976).

Infectious diseases. Paleopathological evidence for infectious diseases has been uncovered in tissue remains (see, for example, Allison, 1979) and more frequently from bone lesions. In both cases, clues occasionally can be obtained as to the approximate antiquity of certain diseases in human populations. For example, it would appear that tuberculosis has had a very long history, but lepromatous leprosy a short one, spanning only the past 1500 years (Black, 1975:515). As was emphasized earlier in this chapter, infectious disease transmission depends on population size. Small, isolated hunter-gatherer bands and incipient horticulturalists of the Paleolithic, Mesolithic, and Neolithic eras could not have provided a pool of individuals large enough to have sustained measles, influenza, smallpox, or poliomyelitis. Humankind's adaptation to these diseases has probably covered a span of less than 200 generations (Black, 1975:518).

Infectious and parasitic disease rates, both in terms of prevalence and incidence, are related to ecosystem diversity and complexity and to patterns of human geographic dispersal. A tropical rain forest (in which human technology has not yet appreciably reduced species diversity) represents a complex ecosystem. We would expect that occupants of such prehistoric ecosystems were exposed to many species of parasitic and other infectious organisms, with many potential vectors present, but that any given infection resulted in only low to moderate mortality. Occupants of simple ecosystems, such as the early desert bands in central Australia, were exposed to few infectious species, with few potential vectors present, but a given infection might result in high mortality (Dunn, 1968).

A recent landmark study in the area of infectious disease in early human populations is that of Cockburn (1971). He skirted the more traditional data of paleopathology (for example, evidence of bone lesions) in order to develop a model that is evolutionary in scope. Since infectious diseases do not often leave osteological or even soft-tissue traces, other types of information are needed. Cockburn's approach focuses on both human and nonhuman primates and makes extensive use of analogy and ecological principles that exemplify processes of socioeconomic adaptation.

Cockburn notes the importance of settlement patterns in understanding changes in certain disease patterns. The advent of agriculture in the post-Pleistocene epoch correlates with semisedentary and eventually sedentary settlements of increasing size and complexity. The loss of mobility meant that various parasites could establish themselves through infection and reinfection within the host population. Hookworms are one such example (1971:48); malaria is another and is described later in this chapter.

The transmission of infectious diseases has been aided by indiscriminate deposition of human feces by sedentary villagers. Continual, albeit accidental, contact with these materials permits reinfection within relatively immobile populations. In other cases, such as in China, the use of excreta as fertilizer has brought about infection by intestinal flukes. As with the well-known schistosome liver flukes of Africa (Nelson, 1960), snails were involved in this cycle of disease transmission in China. The development of fish and water-plant cultivation over the past few millenia in the orient transformed this initially incidental infection into one of severe proportions (Cockburn, 1971:49).

Kunitz and Euler (1972) have followed a similar vein of ecological analysis in their assessment of paleopathological conditions in the pre-Columbian Americas. Their focus is on paleoepidemiology and the impact of infectious diseases on demographic and resource variables. For example, they suggest that *oroya* fever played an important role in certain areas of the Andes. This geographically restricted bacteriological infection can lead to the acute involvement of as much as 90% of the body's red blood cells. *Oroya* fever is likely to have caused numerous deadly epidemics; if a population remains untreated, mortality can reach 40%. In endemic areas of the Andes, 5% to 10% of the population could have been carriers. Several species of sandfly serve as vectors among humans.

The cyclical change in disease vectors and human population size illustrates, in sum that ". . . infectious disease represents an imbalance between parasite and host and is part of a process of continuing mutual adaptation" (Kunitz and Euler, 1972:13). In the pre-Columbian era, *oroya* fever seems to have been a disease with which native populations learned to adapt. Outbreaks were probably more severe when carrier populations came into contact with neighboring native groups. Spaniards arriving in the region also suffered considerably from the disease (Kunitz and Euler, 1972:17-19). (A detailed treatment of the cross-cultural implications of transmission of infectious disease during the colonial era appears later in this chapter.)

DEMOGRAPHIC PROFILES AND RECONSTRUCTIONS

Demography is the study of population dynamics as related to biocultural factors. The combining of methods of inquiry devised by archaeologists, paleontologists, biological and cultural anthropologists, and demographers within the past 15 years has led to a greater understanding of the population dynamics of both prehistoric and historic peoples. This is of particular importance where ecological and evolutionary considerations weigh heavily. Demographic analysis provides medical anthropologists with a more inclusive way of looking at cultures, as well as a set of specific methodological tools by which to assess the multiple factors that influence health. Analysis of the age-sex structure of a population by peer group (that is, "cohort") can provide information on the differential impact of a disease. This in turn can shed light on patterns of adjustment and adaptation. Birth, death, and migration rates serve to place a population in the statistical context necessary to make cross-cultural comparisons; this is of particular importance for the medical anthropologist attempting to generalize about health and illness among, for example, a number of tribal societies or among the inhabitants of similar ecological zones. Demographic analysis ultimately can provide information useful in the understanding of genetic and biocultural mechanisms of adaptation in both stable and transitional populations.

The analysis of demographic, resource, and disease variables is central to the understanding of long-term population growth. Malthusians would claim that significant world population growth during the past 6000 to 8000 years resulted from innovations in the domestication of plant and animal species, as well as changes in disease patterns; others (Boserup, 1965; Binford, 1968) suggest that population growth pressures served as an impetus to agricultural innovations and, eventually, to dramatic changes in patterns of health. Whichever view is accepted, the exponential increase in the size of the human population during the post-Pleistocene epoch has been accompanied by significant changes in social structure, resource utilization, and health in most societies.

Demographic studies of contemporary band and tribal populations—groups that have preserved evolutionarily older subsistence patterns—can serve to clarify patterns of adaptation and disease of prehistoric cultures (as discussed in Lee and DeVore, 1968). Methodologically, such comparisons across time rely on the premise that ethnological and ecological analogies can be extended from the analysis of contemporary hunters and gatherers to preexisting cultures with similar subsistence activities. The theory of uniformitarianism states that processes observable in the present also occurred in the past, justifying such a method (Sarma, 1977:2). For example, if archaeological and paleoecological remains suggest a close similarity between settlement pattern and resource availability in a southwestern United States, pre-Columbian pueblo and those of a contemporary group, ethnological and ecological comparisons may be made in an attempt to better understand demographic and other biocultural processes not evidenced directly in material remains (Longacre, 1975). The Asmat case study found later in this chapter (see p. 79) exemplifies certain of the comparative premises.

A caveat must be interjected. Even for contemporary band and tribal populations, specific demographic information is inadequate, and ethnographic and ecological analogies must be used with caution. Leading the American anthropological effort to provide appropriate, rigorous methodologies have been Kenneth Weiss, James Neel, B. J. Williams, George Armelagos, Alan Swedlund, and Nancy Howell; who have relied on the slightly earlier biocultural and demographic work of Moni Nag, Steven Polgar, Richard Lee, Peter Kunstadter, G. A. Harrison, and others. They have employed analogy only in conjunction with ecological, paleoecological, archeological, and derivative statistical data (where available) to infer demographic processes among prehistoric and contemporary societies. The work of Weiss (1973) stands out in this regard, providing methodological insights and information of importance to the understanding of adaptation processes.

Age-sex distribution. An age-sex distribution, or "pyramid" is a data-based graphic representation of the numbers and proportions of persons by age cohort and sex in a society. Age-sex distributions are central to demographic analysis where data are based on rigorous population-wide censuses, such as those conducted in the United States or in instances where data are derived from tribal populations using census or sampling techniques. This pertains whether or not written records (such as birth and death certificates) are available. Age cohorts usually are analyzed in units that cover 5-year intervals (0-4.9, 5.0-9.9, and so on). From such representations can be derived other important demographic statistics, such as life expectancy at birth (E[0]) and at age 15 when the reproductive years begin (E[15]).

Age-sex distribution can be calculated for those prehistoric populations where sufficient numbers of skeletal and/or mummified remains are available, and for contemporary preliterate bands and tribes where demographic data have been systematically collected. Computer-generated models have

been used by Weiss (1973) to help generalize from the data available and to simulate the survivorship experience of those cohorts where data are incomplete. For example, in this way skeletal series that yield exceptionally low life expectancies—those thought to be in error because of underrepresentation in certain cohorts—can be corrected. Still remaining to be discovered is the determination of more specific cause-effect relationships between disease and mortality for most of the populations analyzed by Weiss and others. Results of Weiss' work (1973) are seen in Tables 3 and 4. Table 3 summarizes the estimates of life expectancy at age 15—E(15)—for most of the populations analyzed, including calculations of average error. Table 4 combines the calculations of life expectancy at birth and at age 15—E(0) and E(15)—derived from the pioneering work of Acsádi and Nemeskéri as well as those of Weiss. Clearly, life expectancies have shown a tendency to increase throughout the Pleistocene epoch, but little difference is found on comparison of E(15); for example, among preindustrial Europeans and living primitive populations. Significant increases in life expectancy have only been achieved within the past century, as sanitation, nutrition, and medicine have interacted to reduce infant and childhood mortality.

Allison (1979) provides an example of the importance of demographic data for reconstructing the health and disease profiles of past cultures. Among pre-Columbian peoples of the Ica region of Peru, analysis of numerous mummified remains indicates that 27% of the people lived past the age of 40 years, and that 50% of all children died before the age of 10 years. However, in part because of hardships endured under Spanish rule, including diseases such as miner's silicosis, only 12% of the native population lived beyond age 40 during the early colonial era. A study of children in the Ica region suggests

Table 3. Life expectancy data for selected populations*

Population	E(15)	Average absolute % error	Average years in error	Population	E(15)	Average absolute % error	Average years in error
Living groups				**Skeletal series**—cont'd			
Baker Lake Eskimos	27.7	3.3	1.0	*Preurban*—cont'd			
Angmagssalik Greenland	19.2	5.6	1.4	Chalcolithic Turkey	21.8	1.3	0.7
East Greenlanders	23.5	15.4	4.6	Iran	18.3	5.4	1.0
San Luis Obispo	23.4	9.0	2.0	Bronze Age Austria	23.4	0.0	0.0
Guarani	26.1	15.0	4.6	Eneolithic East Spain	18.4	5.8	0.7
Caingang	25.1	8.5	2.5	Eneolithic France	24.5	6.7	1.2
Yanomamö	21.4	7.1	1.8	Neolithic Greece	14.6	5.9	1.0
Birhor	24.0	6.5	1.6	Neolithic Denmark	16.6	18.3	3.0
Tikopia	27.0	10.5	3.1	Neolithic North Africa	14.9	12.2	2.2
Tsembaga	28.0	9.8	3.5	Norton Mound Michigan	25.7	6.2	1.5
Australians, North Terr.	34.0	8.2	3.4	Hiwassee Island Tenn.	15.5	13.1	1.5
Australians, Groote Eyl.	23.3	4.5	1.6	Occaneechi Virginia	16.5	16.7	3.2
Tiwi	33.1	6.7	3.0	Neolithic Switzerland	28.7	1.5	0.7
Boni	32.9	2.5	1.2	Illinois Middle Miss.	19.0	11.7	2.6
				Illinois Hopewell	22.9	9.5	2.7
Skeletal series				Illinois archaic	24.3	11.1	2.4
Preurban				Texas aboriginals	23.1	10.3	4.0
Japan Jomon (hunters)	14.4	5.3	0.8	Pecos Pueblo	21.5	12.1	3.2
Western African Tribes	18.4	5.7	0.6				
Protohistoric Saharans	19.1	10.3	2.0	**Urban and medieval**			
Upper Paleolithic	16.9	7.2	1.2	Classic Athens	19.3	17.5	4.3
Ibero-Maurusians	15.5	15.9	2.5	Ancient Greece	22.4	6.9	1.7
Australopithecines†	12.7	11.5	1.6	Roman period Egypt	21.9	1.3	0.3
Japan Edo period	27.0	3.4	1.1	Westerhus Sweden	16.9	6.7	1.5
Karatas, Turkey bronze	13.2	7.3	2.0	Ptuj Yugoslavia	31.2	3.3	0.7
Macedonia Neolithic	12.3	20.7	2.8	Scarborough England	24.0	12.2	2.8
Neolithic Turkey	13.8	21.1	2.5	Hungary	32.0	1.7	0.4
Anatolia Copper Age	21.2	4.3	1.0	Danube Basin	34.6	0.0	0.0

*From Weiss, 1973:21-22.
†Australopithecines included for comparison with human groups.

that those who were healthiest lived with their families on the coast, benefitting from a high-protein diet of fish and shellfish. In contrast, mountain-dwelling farm families had less protein in their diet. Their closer living quarters, which probably posed some sanitation problems, also suggest that infectious diseases would have spread more rapidly than among those residing on the coast.

Demography and warfare of primitive populations. Building on the information already presented, and on the Asmat case study (pp. 79-81), several points of more gen-

eral applicability stand out. While population growth rates have been low over the long term—the average over centuries having been less than 0.01% annually (Petersen, 1975)—there may have been periodic fluctuations among earlier groups of *Homo sapiens sapiens*. Variations were attributable to changes in the food supply, the differential impact of diseases through time, stochastic changes in fertility and mortality, the effects of warfare, and environmental changes.

It has been suggested that, even in the precontact era, warfare-related deaths did

Table 4. Human life expectancy*

Cultural group	N†	Mean E(0)	Mean E(15)	E(15) range
From Acsádi and Nemeskéri‡				
Paleolithic	4	19.9	20.6	15.0-26.9
Mesolithic	4	31.4	26.9	15.0-34.8
Neolithic	8	26.9	19.1	15.0-24.3
Copper Age	5	28.4	22.2	15.2-28.4
Bronze Age	6	32.1	23.7	20.4-27.0
Iron Age	3	27.3	23.4	15.0-34.5
Classical Period	19	27.2	24.7	18.0-32.4
Medieval Europe	23	28.1	25.3	18.0-20.9
From Weiss				
Australopithecines	1	—	12.7	—
Neanderthals§	1	—	17.5	—
Hunter-gatherer averages	4	—	16.5	15.0-19.1
Proto-agricultural averages	22	—	19.8	15.0-28.7
Urban agricultural averages	8	—	25.3	16.9-34.6
Living primitive averages	14	—	26.3	19.2-34.0

*From Weiss, 1973:49.
†N in this table refers to the number of populations in each case.
‡As adapted by Weiss.
§Data from Vallois 1960, smoothed by Gompertz graduation. Minimum E(15) value set at 15 years.

not contribute to significant episodic mortality patterns among the Asmat of New Guinea. Averaged out, such effects were usually smaller and more processual instead. This is in contrast to findings obtained by researchers in the New Guinea highlands (Vayda, 1976; Heider, 1970; Meggitt, 1977; Rappaport, 1968; Koch, 1974). The most important feature of warfare there was that it was a persistent, large-scale, institutionalized process that served as part of a larger ritual system to help adjust human populations and their activities to changing ecological conditions. Because ecological changes vary in type and magnitude through time, warfare (as a response to such changes) varied in its form and in its effects on highland peoples. A group's perception of such changes also must be taken into account, in that perceptions differed among groups regarding "acceptable" ratios of human beings to horticultural land and natural resources.

Thus, while population pressures in New

Guinea were primary factors behind intensive warfare in many cases, the actual number of people per unit of land required to initiate armed conflict has varied widely through time and among groups. Large numbers of people were occasionally killed in a single battle or an intense series of battles (for example, 150 out of 2000 among a group of Dani in 1966 [Heider, 1970:131]). This can be correlated with greater population pressures and more intensive cultivation practices as compared with traditional Asmat society. This was not, however, a simple cause-effect relationship. Ritual cycles involving pig raising and slaughter functioned as key intervening variables in the system. Through ritual, perceptions of change can be translated into action. Similarly, through healing rituals responses to disease can be translated into action.

The relationships among population pressure, warfare, and ecological conditions such as described for traditional New Guinea

The Asmat of New Guinea

Demographic analysis techniques were recently used by Van Arsdale (1978b) to aid in the interpretation of health information obtained in 1973 and 1974 among the Asmat tribe of southwestern Irian Jaya (Indonesian New Guinea), and to place health and disease information in longitudinal perspective. The Asmat are a scattered, relatively sedentary group of more than 40,000 hunting, fishing, and sago-gathering Papuans who inhabit a portion of the coastal lowland swamp and rain forest. They have been in continuous contact with outside change agents only since 1953 when the first permanent mission, Dutch government post, and trade operations were established. During the 1950s warfare, headhunting and cannibalism were largely suppressed by these agents introducing new programs in religious, economic, educational, and political spheres. As these events have transpired, health care has been altered; nonindigenous diseases have been introduced, while inroads have been made in the eradication of others. The population growth rate has increased.

A complete explanation for the demographic patterns of the Asmat during the pre- and postcontact eras is lacking, but strong inferences can be drawn despite a lack of adequate written records. Based in part on an analysis of oral history, it was determined that during the latter half of the nineteenth and first half of the twentieth centuries, the Bismam area of Asmat, where change agents have since made the greatest impact, was experiencing a strong atypical surge in growth, indicating that the area was well below "carrying capacity" (admittedly a controversial concept in itself). Food resources can be presumed to have been relatively abundant throughout this time period. Traditionally, warfare-related deaths usually occurred in small numbers, and during this period can be treated demographically as having ongoing processual (that is, gradual) rather than episodic (that is, "battlefield decimation") effects. Indigenous diseases likewise were hypothesized to have contributed processual rather than epidemic effects for the most part. Three village-level migrations that occurred, the effects of two large battles, and an average annual growth rate of 1% account for the increase from a presumed population in about 1850 of 750 Bismam Asmat to a population of 2300 by 1952— the end of the precontact era. As with population growth during the contact era, it is assumed for demographic purposes that the Asmat represented a stable population. They presumably were characterized by little in or outmigration, relatively constant birth and death rates, and relatively constant age-sex distribution, and a relatively constant rate of growth.

An analysis of the age and sex structure of the Bismam Asmat was developed from data collected from 1973 to 1974. The data indicate a relatively young population—42.3% are in the 0 to 14.9 years age range and 13.3% are in the 0 to 4.9 years cohort. As calculated using equations presented by Weiss (1973), Asmat life expectancy at birth, $E(0)$, is approximately 25 years as of 1974. By comparison, in the United States in 1975, $E(0)$ was over 72 years. For those surviving the prereproductive years (0 to 14.9), Asmat life expectancy at age 15 years was found to be 27 years more. The average 15-year-old therefore could be expected to nearly reach "old age"—thought by the Asmat to begin at about 45. These figures, especially that for $E(15)$, accord very closely with averages derived for other living primitive populations, such as the !Kung of Botswana (Howell, 1976:34-35). The $E(0)$ of 25 is lower than that for numerous contemporary societies of Papua New Guinea (van de Kaa, 1970, 1971), a situation largely attributable to high Asmat infant mortality. During the contact era the death rate frequently has exceeded 300 per 1000 live births. Furthermore, although reduced owing to pressure applied by missionaries and the present Indonesian regime, infanticide still continues.

Continued.

The Asmat of New Guinea—cont'd

Based on an analysis of census materials compiled by Catholic missionaries during the contact era, and on a comparative analysis of scattered data on birth and death rates collected by Van Amelsvoort (1964) and Van Arsdale (1978b), it has been determined that the population growth rate has averaged about 1.5% annually during the past 25 years. This growth rate, while significant, is less than that for other comparable areas of Melanesia. Other peoples have recently experienced rates as high as 2.3% to 2.8% annually (van de Kaa, 1971; Stanhope, 1970:36-37). The Asmat crude birth rate (CBR) for 1973 was fifty-six; in other words, there were fifty-six live births for every 1000 persons. By comparison, the state of Colorado in 1975 had a CBR of fifteen. Although the CBR has fluctuated widely during the contact era, dipping as low as twenty-eight in one large village in 1961 (Van Amelsvoort, 1964:196), an estimate encompassing the past 25 years suggests that an average yearly crude birth rate of fifty-five would be conservative. A summary of similar scattered statistics available as to the crude death rate (CDR) since 1953 suggests that it has averaged about thirty-five to forty per 1000. In 1973 it was thirty-seven per 1000 persons. By contrast, in Colorado in 1975, the CDR was seven per 1000.

Primary causes of death among adults since 1953 have been malaria, complications surrounding yaws, filariasis and its associated disease elephantiasis (Fig. 3-6), pneumonia, intestinal disorders, and diseases not indigenous to the Asmat region, such as smallpox, cholera, whooping cough, and influenza. Although not causing death, venereal disease (not

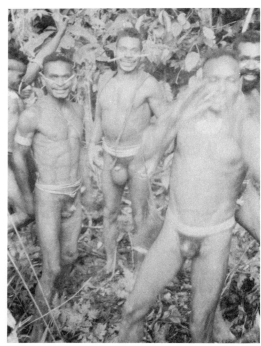

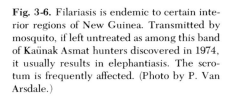

Fig. 3-6. Filariasis is endemic to certain interior regions of New Guinea. Transmitted by mosquito, if left untreated as among this band of Kaünak Asmat hunters discovered in 1974, it usually results in elephantiasis. The scrotum is frequently affected. (Photo by P. Van Arsdale.)

indigenous) has reached endemic proportions in some villages. The main factors associated with infant and child mortality during the contact era seem to have been pneumonia, malaria, diarrhea, birth complications, and occasional epidemics of nonindigenous diseases, such as smallpox and cholera. The Dutch experienced moderate success in the treatment of some of these diseases. Under their regime clinic stations were established, outpatient programs were begun, and systematic immunization campaigns were mounted. The yaws eradication program was very successful, for example. Furthermore, intricacies in the interaction of traditional Asmat belief patterns and Western health practices were recognized early on by Dutch medical personnel and their Papuan assistants during the 1950s. Attempts were made to preserve traditional cultural norms; for example, while maternal and child outpatient health-care programs were being initiated.

Little sensitivity to traditional beliefs has been demonstrated by Indonesian officials and health personnel. In addition, immunization and clinic programs have not been systematic. In part because of these reasons and in part because neither Dutch nor Indonesian personnel have been able to minimize death from epidemics (for example, a cholera epidemic from 1961 to 1962 killed over 600 Asmatters), the demographic pattern during the contact era encompasses what might be termed a "disease-mortality cancelling effect." For Asmatters under the impact of nontraditional health and medical regimes there have been about as many negative as positive effects on acute disease–related mortality.

How then can an average annual population growth rate of 1.5% be explained? It is suggested that the key, in part, lies in the high annual birth rate of approximately fifty-five live births per 1000 inhabitants. It is probable that this rate has climbed during the contact era. This is not in accord with the theory of demographic transition (which suggests that the populations of developing areas experience first death rate and then birth rate declines), but is in accord with other more specific hypotheses. As measured in 1973 among a sample of Asmat women, the total fertility rate was 6.9. This falls within the upper range for human societies and lends support to a hypothesis of an increase in fertility since 1953. It may be the case that, while disease-related care has not improved, nutrition-related health has. Slight reductions in the birth intervals may indicate that a few young women are undergoing physiological changes that in turn are contributing to increasing fecundity (see Frisch and McArthur, 1974). Newly introduced foods, such as garden crops and rice, may be improving nutritional status, which will in turn translate into future increases in infant survival rates (see Katz, 1972:357-358). Although highly speculative, it is possible that decreased birth intervals are related to physiological changes accompanying the Bismam Asmat transition to a somewhat more sedentary life-style (see Kolata, 1974:934). Also, the Bismam woman's workload, as demonstrated elsewhere (Van Arsdale, 1978a), has been shown not to be excessive, a factor that may be contributing to increased fertility (see, for example, Dahlberg, 1974).

It is also possible that mortality compensation (greater number of births per woman owing to a desire to offset high infant mortality), falling on the heels of externally introduced epidemics, is partially responsible for the postulated increase in fertility among some of the younger Asmat women. To be sure, warfare-related deaths—even during the precontact era—have not made the impact on population size that has been suggested for other New Guinea societies (see, for example, Vayda, 1976). Research about the Asmat thus indicates that cultural and biological factors can interact fairly rapidly to produce new modes of adaptation to a changing environment. That population size is increasing without degradation of the environment is, according to Alland (1970:180), "the proper measure of adaptation."

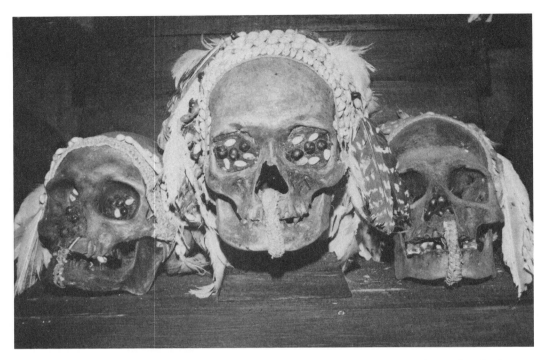

Fig. 3-7. Certain skulls of ancestors and enemies alike were decorated with "Job's tears" and other colorful items for ritual purposes by the Asmat of coastal New Guinea. Left to hang from the rafters of houses, most enemy skulls remained undecorated, however. Warfare traditionally resulted in relatively few deaths, the loss per year usually being less than 2% of the total population. (Photo by P. Van Arsdale.)

highland societies, were likely atypical compared with most other societies of prehistoric and protohistoric humans. Evidence indicates that most other groups had not developed intensive horticultural practices, nor populations of the density found in the highlands (see, for example, Lee and Devore, 1968). Demographic fluctuations undoubtedly also occurred, but like warfare, they were less dramatic.

Certain parallels, therefore, can be drawn between the demographic and ecological factors that influenced primitive populations of the pre- and postcolonial eras. Patterns of warfare and ritual indicate that biocultural processes of adaptation were affected significantly by human intervention and that a vari-

ety of systems control mechanisms existed. In many cases, patterns that had represented successful modes of adaptation were disrupted by change agents from Europe, often with disastrous effects. Nevertheless, as the data on contemporary tribes of New Guinea indicate, such groups have frequently demonstrated a great deal of adaptive resilience.

COLONIALISM: ADAPTATION IN LATER HISTORY

Few examples in human history provide as clear an opportunity for studying biocultural adaptation as does the phenomenon of colonialism. Both to the colonized and the colonizers, the sudden and frequently imposed contact between two cultures produced effects that reached far beyond the colonizers' simple expectations of wealth and power. From our current vantage point in history and by using the research tools now available to the medical anthropologist, we can trace the routes of colonizers to new territories and so can witness the impact of diseases imposed on new populations and eventually on the course of history.

Early European exploration and expansionism

Euro-American colonialism had its seeds in a milieu of complex changes that arose during the Middle Ages. The Renaissance and Enlightenment periods were accompanied by some improvements in medical knowledge, hygiene, and precision of technique, but more pervasively by patterns of internal sociopolitical and demographic changes and by externally oriented processes of exploration and discovery. International trade linkages extending beyond Europe had been established prior to this time (such as with the Middle East), but extensive colonial contacts had not been made. A desire on the part of such emergent sea powers as Italy, Portugal, and Holland to increase their resource bases and trading capabilities led to an extension of oceanic routes to the Indies and the Far East. Persian and Arabic traders had pioneered certain of these routes, just as their countrymen had pioneered certain medical innovations that were later adopted by Europeans. The Far East, by the 1500s, was also being brought into the Western sphere of influence. As mentioned in Chapter 1, such explorations brought recognition of the existence of "very dangerous diseases" (Van Amelsvoort, 1964:9) stimulated, perhaps, by externally visible maladies, such as yaws, in the indigenous populations.

The search for spices such as cinnamon and cloves was not the sole impetus for early colonial penetration into the Far East. The political and economic climate in Europe, combined with improved navigational techniques and instruments (like the astrolabe) and recognition that territorial acquisition was assured by superior European naval technology, led to complex expansionist programs.

Yet, to the eye of the general public and the seafarer alike, the lure of the Spice Islands (the Moluccas), was indeed powerful. These islands symbolically represented the wealth of the Far East as well as the gateway to China and the Pacific. According to the Catalan Atlas, presented to Charles VI of France on his coronation in 1381, there were thought to be more than 7500 islands in the Indian Ocean. In addition to spices, it was said that gold, silver and precious stones were abundant. The island of "Trapobana" was described as "the last island of the Indies," perhaps a gateway to still greater riches further east (Sanders, 1978:3ff).

It was, of course, partially in extending the search for riches, which were presumed to be beyond Trapobana, that Columbus and others pursued alternative oceanic routes. If indeed the world were round, the discovery of an east-to-west route from Europe to the Indies would obviate the need to sail around Africa and India. And it was in the furthering of contacts with native American and Caribbean populations, discovered in the pursuit of these routes from 1492 onward, that resulted in dramatic cross-cultural and intracultural transformations and adaptations.

Details of the processes of colonization and induced culture change that transpired during this era are of interest here to the extent that they can be related to longitudinal changes in health. As exemplified again by the Moluccas, the staple part of their diet had been low in protein and fat (and thus in vitamin B), owing to a reliance on the starchy pith of the sago palm. However, the diet had traditionally been supplemented with caterpillars, worms, maggots, and other species, effectively supplying much of the needed protein and fat. As May (1977:723) points out, a correlate of contact with Western civilization was an eventual abandonment of such foods from the Moluccan diet, and a resultant increase in beriberi, pellagra, and bladder stones. All of these can be related to protein–vitamin B deficiencies.

Policy and disease in the Americas before 1900

Patterns of disease and health care have played a major role in shaping the events that have transpired in the Americas during the past 500 years. As McNeill (1976:1) stresses, in the analysis of post-Columbian events, disease factors must be given tremendous importance.

As everyone knows, Hernando Cortez, starting off with fewer than six hundred men, conquered the Aztec empire, whose subjects numbered millions. How could such a tiny handful prevail? . . . (Certain) undeniable technical superiorities the Spaniards had at their command do not seem enough to explain wholesale apostasy from older Indian patterns of life and belief. Why, for instance, did the old religions of Mexico and Peru disappear so utterly?

He believes that most historians have neglected the impact of disease in shaping world events. For instance an epidemic of smallpox was raging in the Aztec capital of Tenochtitlan at the time when these native Americans might otherwise have succeeded in driving out Cortez and his troops. McNeill believes that historians also have neglected consideration of the psychological implications that a disease such as smallpox can have on a population showing no prior immunity. This latter theme was raised years earlier, in 1957, by William Langer, during his presidential address to the American Historical Association, when he stressed the need for what is now known as psychohistorical analy-

sis, specifically as it might be applied to a disease's impact on society. Citing research suggesting that even the ancient Etruscan civilization may have owed much of its collapse to epidemics of malaria and that Europe's black death dramatically changed the course of events on that continent as well, Langer (1958:292-294) queries: what could inferential analysis tell us of the psychological impacts on these populations? In the context of present-day anthropological research, Lea (1973) addresses essentially the same issue: how does disease contribute to psychological stress in a population undergoing induced culture change?

Los Indios was the name Columbus gave to the Caribbean people he encountered on what is now known as the island of Hispaniola. *Los indios*, the Indians, initially were thought to be just that, inhabitants of the Indies. Thus began in the Americas what has proved to be a seemingly endless series of misconceptions and stereotypes applied to the indigenous inhabitants. Nowhere is this more clear than in some of the early writings concerning the health of *los indios*. Quoting from Simpson, McNickle (1972:77) notes that Ovando, first governor of the Indies, included this statement in one of his orders in the year 1501: The Indians "are not to bathe as frequently as hitherto, as we are informed that it does them much harm." From Vespucci's *Mundus Novus* (published in 1504 or 1505), the following extract has been taken: "They live one hundred and fifty years, and rarely fall ill, and if they do fall victims to any disease, they cure themselves with certain roots and herbs" (quoted in Berkhofer, 1978:9).

Racism is manifested in many of the earliest writings as well, further contributing to the emergence of a negative stereotype:

These folke lyven lyke bestes without any resonablenes and the wymen be also as comon . . . they hange also the bodyes or persons fleeshe in the smoke/as men do with swynes fleshe. And that lande is ryght full of folke/for they lyve commonly [300] yere and more as with sykeness they dye nat . . . (quoted in Berkhofer, 1978:9-10)

The above quote, taken directly from an English version of a Dutch pamphlet published between 1511 and 1522, clearly indicates not only the ethnocentric bias of the colonists and their countrymen, but also the paucity of information then available to Europeans on primitive peoples' biological and cultural conditions. Such attitudes severely limited the positive effects of those few contributions (such as soap) that Europeans could offer native Americans. This was especially true during epidemics of nonindigenous diseases, which, in the manner of smallpox in Tenochtitlan, continued to influence the course of history in the Americas. Rosen (1973:238) puts this kind of situation in a still broader historical-cultural perspective: ". . . whether a given society emphasizes a particular stage of biological development in relation to health depends on social and cultural factors acting over a period of time."

Health of the native people. Neither conqueror nor colonist seemed greatly interested in the health of the indigenous people. The Spanish did, however, introduce a vaccination program (Smith, 1974) and showed some interest in the high-altitude adaptation of Peru's Andean natives (Monge, 1948:4). Epidemics were feared because Europeans had had experience with contagious diseases, such as the black death (bubonic plague) (Amundsen, 1977:403-404). The very frailty of the native people seemed in part to justify their conquest. As Berkhofer notes, "In so far as Native Americans like other alien peoples figured in the history of European expansion over the world, their conquest seemed to justify to Europeans their understanding of history as progressive and their superiority to other peoples" (1978:44). It was thought that in primitive people were

seen cultural and even biological images of the ancient ancestors of Europeans, a stage through which Europeans had long since passed. Progress through colonialism was seen as one way to further separate civilized people from their savage brethren (McNickle, 1972:83). Native Americans were being decimated by diseases; this seemed to serve as further evidence of the Indians' less developed state of being.

For example, in Virginia the powerful Powhatan Confederacy had been a force to reckon with in the early seventeenth century. This Confederacy may have had as many as 10,000 members. After years of peaceful coexistence, the Confederacy mounted an attack in 1622 that succeeded in killing approximately 350 English colonists. However, these Native Americans were already suffering the effects of such diseases as measles, smallpox, and typhoid, and (much like the Aztecs a century earlier) they were not able to follow through after their initial victory. Within 75 years, only a few Indians remained in Virginia east of the Blue Ridge Mountains (Jones, 1976:250-251). Although frequently devastating to colonists as well, disease surely was an ally of the "progressive" Europeans.

Emergent colonialist policies, all in the name of progress, thus focused on reducing the "threat from below," while at the same time maximizing resource (including land) availability. This can be conceptualized as a situation in which initially different systems interlock through time, as a result of occupying the same territory and competing for the same scarce resources. Brookfield (1972:1-2) uses a similar approach in presenting a comprehensive definition of colonialism:

[It is a] thoroughgoing, comprehensive and deliberate penetration of a local or "residentiary" system by the agents of an external system, who aim to restructure the patterns of organization, resource use, circulation and outlook so as to bring these into a linked relationship with their own system. The objective is an externally wrought or guided transformation of the residentiary system, revolutionary in the sense that it involves termination or diversion of former evolutionary trends.

Early U.S. policies were aimed at broad patterns of social, political, and especially economic control. By the nineteenth century the United States was not advocating total elimination of Native Americans, but was engaged in a systematic diversion of what had been their resources to suit settlers' needs. Indians were being forced to become increasingly responsive to external motivation and control.

Changes in the indigenous systems of land use and tenure were crucial to colonists. In some instances, this meant a change in Indian subsistence patterns; in others, removal and relocation. As May (1977) stresses, geographic factors are important determinants of disease patterns. Relocation can contribute to problems of short-term adjustment, long-term adaptation, and increased incidence of disease. Whereas the Royal Proclamation of October 7, 1763 had at least recognized certain of the mutual interests of native Americans and colonists, President Andrew Jackson's Second Annual Message in 1830 left no doubt as to the course future U.S. policy would take:

Humanity has often wept over the fate of the aborigines of this country, and Philanthropy has been long busily employed in devising means to avert it, but its progress has never for a moment been arrested . . . But true Philanthropy could not wish to see this continent restored to the condition in which it was found by our forefathers. What good man would prefer a country covered with forests and ranged by a few thousand savages to our extensive Republic . . . (quoted in McNickle, 1972:84)

The Removal Act of 1830 bore out the President's intent. Native Americans were forced to move from east to west. Large numbers died from disease in the process, as has been documented from the "trail of tears."

The impact of malaria on colonialism. Given this background on colonialist policy and its effects on health in the Americas, it is instructive to investigate more fully the impact of a single disease—malaria. Its effect on colonial and postcolonial America was profound. During the eighteenth and nineteenth centuries, its impact was felt on both coasts and in much of the interior as well. It was, along with other deadly nonindigenous diseases (such as smallpox), implicitly responsible for the way in which much of colonial and frontier life unfolded. Malaria at times served to structure the nature of many of the sociopolitical relationships between colonists and native Americans.

The common form of malaria in human population is transmitted by *Plasmodium falciparum* via an intermediate agent, or vector. Most infectious diseases that are transmitted via vectors utilize arthropods, and malaria is no exception. Species of anopheline mosquitoes serve as the malarial intermediaries. As May (1977:717) points out, anophelines vary greatly in their habits. Some bite at dusk, others at dawn. In some areas one human population will be "favored"; in other areas, another.

Climate and environment affect this disease cycle in significant ways, but in almost all cases the potential for anopheline survival and infestation is enhanced where a human population alters a forest environment to the extent that standing or stagnant water accumulates. Breeding takes place in water of this sort. Slash-and-burn horticulture and colonial logging and agriculture, with the removal of forest cover, have been conducive to the breeding of anophelines. The soil, alternately moistened by rain and dried by the sun, becomes hard and virtually impervious to water. Puddles of water form readily

(Laderman, 1975:590). As human population density increases with the advent of villages and towns, the potential for the presence of endemic malaria is further enhanced.

Falciparum malaria probably was introduced to the eastern seaboard colonies via slaves brought in from Africa. Anophelines, which had not previously served as vectors owing to the presumed prior absence of the disease in the New World, became efficient transmitters. Jones (1976:255) suggests that by the mid-1700s there was significant mortality from malaria among Virginian colonists and Native Americans alike. By the late 1700s and early 1800s, fevers that can, in retrospect, probably be attributed to this disease were endemic throughout most of the area east of the Mississippi River (Anonymous, 1976:248).

West coast settlers and Native Americans in particular, also began to fall victim to malaria in the early nineteenth century. S. F. Cook (1972), one of the leading authorities on the interpretation of disease patterns through ethnohistorical and historical reconstruction, has argued convincingly that the deadly "fever and ague" epidemics of 1830 to 1833 in California and Oregon were indeed malaria. Despite the incidence of malaria east of the Mississippi River, Cook infers that these epidemics found their beginnings in parasites brought to the west coast via traders traveling from Hawaii and other Pacific islands. This conclusion is based on the finding that the first malarial outbreak was at Ft. Vancouver, not inland nor along an interior trading route. People hit hardest in 1830 seem to have been those along the lower Columbia River, and by 1833 those in the Sacramento and San Joaquin valleys. As was the case along the eastern seaboard, anophelines that had not previously served as vectors were rapidly incorporated into the disease cycle. Hudson Bay Company trappers and others traveling from north to south near the coast probably served as carriers from Oregon to California. Cook estimates that nine out of ten such persons had a chance to be carriers.

White settlers were severely affected by what was rapidly becoming endemic malaria, but Native American populations in some cases were being also totally eradicated. Travelers reported seeing so many dead Native Americans that, by virtue of not having enough survivors to bury them, their corpses were left (according to one account) "unburied and festering in the sun" (Cook, 1972:183). Writing in 1846, Samuel Parker said:

Since the year 1829, probably seven-eighths . . . have been swept away by disease, principally by fever and ague . . . This great mortality extended not only from the vicinity of the Cascades to the shores of the Pacific but far north and south; it is said as far south as California. The fever and ague was never known in this country before the year 1829 . . . (quoted in Cook, 1972:174)

Cook concludes that, while many travelers' reports were undoubtedly exaggerated as to the extent of malarial mortality, among certain Indian populations a 75% death rate probably was reached. Sociopolitical relationships were, concomitantly, dramatically affected, and resources were rapidly expropriated to the detriment of the once numerous indigenous inhabitants.

Disease continued to influence the course of intercultural relations in the Americas well into the twentieth century. For example, in 1903 the Caypao tribe of interior Brazil accepted a single missionary priest into their midst. Despite what is described as his "every effort to safeguard his flock from the evils and dangers of civilization," a tribe that had counted at least 6000 members in 1903 had only 500 by 1918, twenty-seven by 1927, and two descendants by 1950 (McNeill, 1976: 204).

Colonialism and disease in Oceania

Colonialism brings together two radically different cultures. The outbreak of disease in both populations, as was evidenced in the settling on New World soil by Europeans, indicates some preexisting patterns of biocultural adaptation. The colonization of the Pacific islands, Oceania, indicates a different response to the impact of nonindigenous diseases. A comparison of the two colonialization processes—America and Oceania—may be useful in understanding variation in the colonizers as well as in the colonized.

Early explorations, such as that by Magellan of the Micronesian atolls in 1521, others of New Guinea in 1526, and Tahiti by Europeans in 1767, indicate the length of time over which the indigenous peoples had contact with nonnative diseases. Pirie (1972) notes that records of single, deadly epidemics invading previously isolated populations are found from the eighteenth century onward. Other such epidemics in the previous 200 years may have gone unrecorded. Not unexpectedly, many areas of Oceania experienced long periods of population decline. Newbury (1972:145) reports eastern Polynesian depopulation from initial European contact through the middle of the nineteenth century. In the Marquesa Islands it continued disastrously until about 1925. In addition to sporadic epidemics, including strains of venereal disease occasionally fatal to native inhabitants, prolonged trade, mission, and colonial contacts with the Western world seem to have raised the overall incidence of disease as well.

In contrast to the general incidence of disease and depopulation, research on Nukuoro Atoll, a Polynesian outlier in the Trust Territory of the Pacific Islands, presents a contrasting view. For Nukuoro, ethnohistorical, historical, and demographic reconstruction indicates that nonindigenous diseases that may have reached the atoll did not produce high mortality during the past 150 years (Carroll,

1975). Gonorrhea was present, however, and may have accounted for reduced fertility in the last half of the nineteenth century.

Carroll suggests that during the nineteenth century, and presumably prior to that, Nukuoro had low rates of fertility and mortality. The precontact population appears to have remained at a size far below that of the atoll's "carrying capacity" without constant recourse to abortion and infanticide. Carroll suggests that this was accomplished, in part, by appropriate recognition of resource availability and proper use thereof, and also through recognition and maintenance of atoll ethnic identity, population boundaries, and relative isolation. "Their cults were devoted to keeping certain things *away* from the island—natural catastrophes, epidemic sicknesses, and people" (Carroll, 1975:366). The colonial impact was not thwarted, but it was altered to some degree. Community leadership at times played a role in this process.

Carroll presents a model that places Nukuoro in an ecosystem context, which resembles somewhat that postulated in the model of the human ecosystem (Fig. 2-1). The atoll represents a subsystem whose self-regulatory controls have been interfered with by input from the larger colonial system, but which nonetheless has retained a degree of self-regulation. Nonindigenous disease can be considered as an input, one that has at times caused short-term disequilibrium, but not devastation. Colonial policies at times also have contributed to disequilibrium (Maddocks, 1975). To the extent that Western medicine has been able to offset certain of the recent ill-effects of Western intervention, the Nukuoro subsystem has benefitted adaptively.

Among the Asmat of Irian Jaya (western New Guinea), the introduction of nonindigenous diseases has not resulted in overall depopulation either (see the insert on the Asmat, p. 80). Since permanent contact with these tribes was first established in 1953, a kind of "disease standoff" has developed; the overall disease-related mortality does not seem to be appreciably different from that in the immediate precontact era.

The great range of responses demonstrated by colonized peoples to the biological and cultural influences imposed by their various colonizers serves to reaffirm our contention that health and disease are products of multiple, complex interactions. The devastation among the Aztecs of post-contact Mexico and among Native Americans was not reproduced among the populations of Oceania because the many individual factors that contributed to the final result in each of the meetings between two cultures were never quite the same. Nevertheless, where similarities occurred among influencing factors, so also were there degrees of similarity in outcome. It is impossible to speculate whether a recognition of this delicate balance among macro- and microlevel subsystems would have averted some of the disasters that followed colonial expansion. However, our retrospective view of these relationships should help us to prevent comparable efforts that promise to further unbalance the human ecosystem, whether it be in the response of one culture to another or of an individual to a biocultural environment.

REFERENCES

Ackerknecht, E. H. Paleopathology. In Landy, D. (ed.). *Culture, Disease, and Healing: Studies in Medical Anthropology.* New York: The Macmillan Co., 1977.

Alland, A., Jr. *Adaptation in Cultural Evolution: An Approach to Medical Anthropology.* New York: Columbia University Press, 1970.

Allison, A. Polymorphism and natural selection in human populations. *Cold Springs Harbor Symposium on Quantitative Biology,* 1954, *20,* 137-149.

Allison, M. J. Paleopathology in Peru. *Natural History,* 1979, *88*(2), 74-82.

Amundsen, D. W. Medical deontology and pestilential disease in the late middle ages. *Journal of the History of Medicine and Allied Sciences,* 1977, *32*(4), 403-421.

Anonymous. Two hundred years of medicine in the United States. *Journal of the History of Medicine and Allied Sciences,* 1976, *31*(3), 247-249.

Armelagos, G. J. Disease in ancient Nubia. In Landy, D. (ed.). *Culture, Disease, and Healing: Studies in Medical Anthropology.* New York: The Macmillan Co., 1977.

Armelagos, G. J. Personal communication, 1979.

Armelagos, G. J., and Dewey, J. R., Evolutionary response to human infectious diseases. In Logan, M. H., and Hunt, E. E., Jr. (eds.). *Health and the Human Condition: Perspectives on Medical Anthropology.* North Scituate, Mass.: Duxbury Press, 1978.

Bandelier, A. F. Aboriginal trephining in Bolivia. *American Anthropologist,* 1904, *6,* 440-446.

Bennett, J. W. *The Ecological Transition: Cultural Anthropology and Human Adaptation.* New York: Pergamon Press, Inc., 1976.

Berkhofer, R. F., Jr. *The White Man's Indian: Images of the American Indian from Columbus to the Present.* New York: Alfred A. Knopf, Inc., 1978.

Binford, L. R. Post-Pleistocene adaptations. In Binford, S. R., and Binford, L. R. (eds.). *New Perspectives in Archeology.* Chicago: Aldine-Atherton, Inc., 1968.

Black, F. L. Infectious diseases in primitive societies. *Science,* 1975, *187,* 515-518.

Blumberg, B. S. Australia antigen and the biology of hepatitis B. *Science,* 1977, *197,* 17-26.

Boserup, E. *The Conditions of Agricultural Growth.* Chicago: Aldine-Atherton, Inc., 1965.

Bowers, N. Demographic problems in montane New Guinea. In Polgar, S. (ed.). *Culture and Population: A Collection of Current Studies.* Chapel Hill, N.C.: Carolina Population Center, 1971.

Brookfield, H. C. *Colonialism, Development and Independence: The Case of the Melanesian Islands in the South Pacific.* Cambridge: Cambridge University Press, 1972.

Brothwell, D. The question of pollution in earlier and less developed societies. In Logan, M. H., and Hunt, E. E., Jr. (eds.). *Health and the Human Condition: Perspectives on Medical Anthropology.* North Scituate, Mass.: Duxbury Press, 1978.

Butzer, K. W. Environment, culture, and human evolution. *American Scientist,* 1977, *65*(5), 572-584.

Campbell, B. G. *Humankind Emerging.* Boston: Little, Brown, and Co., 1976.

Carroll, V. The population of Nukuoro in historical perspective. In Carroll, V. (ed.). *Pacific Atoll Populations.* Honolulu: The University Press of Hawaii, 1975.

Cockburn, T. A. Infectious diseases in ancient populations. *Current Anthropology,* 1971, *12*(1), 45-62.

Cohen, Y. A. Culture as adaptation. In Cohen, Y. A. (ed.). *Man in Adaptation: The Cultural Present.* Chicago: Aldine-Atherton, Inc., 1968.

Cook, S. F. The epidemic of 1830-1833 in California

and Oregon. In Walker, D. E., Jr. (ed.). *The Emergent Native Americans: A Reader in Culture Contact.* Boston: Little, Brown and Co., 1972.

Dahlberg, F. M. Women's workload and fertility. Paper presented at the annual meeting of the American Anthropological Association, Mexico City, Mexico, 1974.

Dobzhansky, T. Adaptedness and fitness. In Lewontin, R. C. (ed.) *Population Biology and Evolution.* Syracuse, N.Y.: Syracuse University Press, 1968.

Dobzhansky, T. Evolution—organic and superorganic. In Bleibtreu, H. K., and Downs, J. F. (eds.). *Human Variation: Readings in Physical Anthropology.* Beverly Hills, Calif.: Glencoe Press, 1971.

Dunn, F. L. Epidemiological factors: health and disease in hunter gatherers. In Lee, R. B., and Devore, I. (eds.). *Man the Hunter.* Chicago: Aldine-Atherton, Inc., 1968.

Frayer, D. W. A reappraisal of Ramapithecus. *Yearbook of Physical Anthropology,* 1974, *17,* 19-30.

Frisch, R. E., and McArthur, J. W. Menstrual cycles: fatness as a determinant of minimum weight and height necessary for their maintenance or onset. *Science,* 1974, *185,* 949-951.

Gajdusek, D. C., Leyshan, W. D., Kirk, R. L., and others. Genetic differentiation among populations in western New Guinea. *American Journal of Physical Anthropology,* 1978, *48,* 47-64.

Glob, P. V. *The Bog People: Iron-Age Man Preserved.* New York: Ballantine Books, Inc., 1969.

Harris, M. *The Rise of Anthropological Theory.* New York: Thomas Y. Crowell Co., 1968.

Heider, K. G. *The Dugum Dani: A Papuan Culture in the Highlands of West New Guinea.* Chicago: Aldine-Atherton, Inc., 1970.

Hewes, G. W. Primate communication and the gestural origin of language. *Current Anthropology,* 1973, *14* (1-2), 5-24.

Howell, F. C. Observations on the earlier phases of the European lower Paleolithic (Torralba-Ambrona). *Recent Studies in Paleoanthropology, American Anthropologist Special Publication,* 1966, 111-140.

Howell, N. Toward a uniformitarian theory of human paleodemography. In Ward, R. H., and Weiss, K. M. (eds.). *The Demographic Evolution of Human Populations.* New York: Academic Press, Inc., 1976.

Janssens, P. A. *Palaeopathology: Diseases and Injuries of Prehistoric Man.* London: John Baker, 1970.

Johanson, D. C. Lecture, Denver Museum of Natural History, Denver, 1977.

Johanson, D. C., and White, T. D. A systematic assessment of early African hominids. *Science,* 1979, *203,* 321-330.

Johnston, F. E., and Selby, H. *Anthropology: The Bio-cultural View.* Dubuque, Iowa: William C. Brown Co., 1978.

Jones, G. W. Medicine in Virginia in revolutionary times. *Journal of the History of Medicine and Allied Sciences,* 1976, *31*(3), 250-270.

Katz, S. H. Biological factors in population control. In Spooner, B. (ed.). *Population Growth: Anthropological Implications.* Cambridge, Mass.: The M.I.T. Press, 1972.

Kerley, E. R. Recent advances in palaeopathology. Clarke, M. E. (ed.). *Modern Methods in the History of Medicine,* London: Athlone, 1971.

King, J. L., and Jukes, T. H. Non-Darwinian evolution. *Science,* 1970, *164,* 788-797.

Koch, K.-F. *War and Peace in Jalémó: The Management of Conflict in Highland New Guinea.* Cambridge, Mass.: Harvard University Press, 1974.

Kolata, G. B. Human evolution: hominoids of the Miocene. *Science,* 1977, *197,* 244-245.

Kolata, G. B. !Kung hunter-gatherers: feminism, diet and birth control. *Science,* 1974, *185,* 932-934.

Kunitz, S. J., and Euler, R. C. *Aspects of Southwestern Paleoepidemiology.* Prescott, Ariz.: Prescott College Press, 1972.

Laderman, C. Malaria and progress: some historical and ecological considerations. *Social Science & Medicine,* 1975, *9,* 587-594.

Langer, W. L. The next assignment. *American Historical Review,* 1958, *63,* 283-304.

Lea, D. Stress and adaptation to change: an example from the East Sepik District, New Guinea. In Brookfield, H. (ed.). *The Pacific in Transition: Geographical Perspectives on Adaptation and Change.* New York: St. Martin's Press, Inc., 1973.

Leakey, R. E., and Lewin, R. *People of the Lake: Mankind and Its Beginnings.* Garden City, N.Y.: Anchor Books, 1978.

Lee, R. B., and DeVore, I. *Man the Hunter.* Chicago: Aldine-Atherton, Inc., 1968.

Leroi-Gourhan, A. The flowers found with Shanidar IV, a Neanderthal burial in Iraq. *Science,* 1975, *190,* 562-564.

Lewontin, R. C. An estimate of average heterozygosity in man. *American Journal of Human Genetics,* 1967, *19,* 681-685.

Lewontin, R. C. *The Genetic Basis of Evolutionary Change.* New York: Columbia University Press, 1974.

Lewontin, R. C., and Hubby, J. L. A molecular approach to the study of genic heterozygosity in natural populations. *Genetics,* 1966, *54,* 595-605.

Livingstone, F. B. Anthropological implications of sickle-cell gene distribution in West Africa. *American Anthropologist,* 1958, *60,* 533-562.

Longacre, W. A. Population dynamics at the Grasshopper Pueblo, Arizona. In Swedland, A. C. (ed.). *Population Studies in Archaeology and Biological Anthropology: A Symposium.* Memoirs of the Society for American Archaeology, No. 3, 1975.

Maddocks, I. Medicine and colonialism. *Australian and New Zealand Journal of Sociology*, 1975, *11*(3), 27-33.

May, J. M. Medical geography: its methods and objectives. *Social Science & Medicine*, 1977, *11*, 715-730.

Mayr, E. The nature of the Darwinian Revolution. *Science*, 1972, *176*, 981-989.

McNeill, W. H. *Plagues and Peoples.* Garden City, N.Y.: Anchor Books, 1976.

McNickle, D. Indian and European: Indian-white relations from discovery to 1887. In Walker, D. E. Jr. (ed.). *The Emergent Native Americans: A Reader in Culture Contact.* Boston: Little, Brown and Co., 1972.

McNicoll, G. and Mamas, S. G. M. *The Demographic Situation in Indonesia.* Papers of the East-West Population Institution, No. 28, Honolulu, 1973.

Meggitt, M. *Blood is Their Argument: Warfare Among the Mae Enga Tribesmen of the New Guinea Highlands.* Palo Alto, Calif.: Mayfield, 1977.

Monge, C. *Acclimatization in the Andes: Historical Confirmations of "Climatic Aggression" in the Development of Andean Man.* Baltimore: Johns Hopkins University Press, 1948.

Moodie, R. L. *Paleopathology: An Introduction to the Study of Ancient Evidences of Disease.* Urbana, Ill.: University of Illinois Press, 1923.

Nelson, G. S. Schistosome infections as zoonoses in Africa. *Transactions of the Society of Tropical Medicine and Hygiene*, 1960, *54*, 301-316.

Newbury, C. Trade and plantations in Eastern Polynesia: the emergence of a dependent economy. In Ward, R. G. (ed.). *Man in the Pacific Islands.* Oxford: Clarendon Press, 1972.

Paul, B. D. The Maya bonesetter as sacred specialist. *Ethnology*, 1976, *15*(1), 77-81.

Petersen, W. A demographer's view of prehistoric demography. *Current Anthropology*, 1975, *16*, 227-245.

Pfeiffer, J. E. *The Emergence of Man*, ed. 3. New York: Harper & Row, Publishers, 1978.

Pirie, P. Population growth in the Pacific Islands: the example of Western Samoa. In Ward, R. G. (ed.). *Man in the Pacific Islands.* Oxford: Clarendon Press, 1972.

Rappaport, R. A. *Pigs for the Ancestors: Ritual in the Ecology of a New Guinea People.* New Haven, Conn.: Yale University Press, 1968.

Rosen, G. Health, history and the social sciences. *Social Science & Medicine*, 1973, 7, 233-248.

Sanders, R. *Lost Tribes and Promised Lands: The Origins of American Racism.* Boston: Little, Brown and Co., 1978.

Sarma, A. *Approaches to Paleoecology.* Dubuque, Iowa: William C. Brown Co., 1977.

Schultz, A. The specialization of man and his place among the catarrhine primates. *Cold Springs Harbor Symposium on Quantitative Biology*, 1950, *15*, 37-52.

Slobodkin, L. *Growth and Regulation of Animal Populations.* New York: Holt, Rinehart and Winston, Inc., 1964.

Smith, G. E. Population growth and education planning in Papua New Guinea. *New Guinea Research Bulletin*, 1971, *42*, 58-80.

Smith, M. M. The "real expedición marítima de la vacuna" in New Spain and Guatemala. *Transactions of the American Philosophical Society*, 1974, *64* (part 1).

Solecki, R. S. *Shanidar: The First Flower People.* New York: Alfred A. Knopf, Inc., 1971.

Stanhope, J. M. Patterns of fertility and mortality in rural New Guinea. *New Guinea Research Bulletin*, 1970, *34*, 24-41.

Svejda, M. Personal communication, 1978.

Teitelbaum, M. S. Relevance of demographic transition theory for developing countries. *Science*, 1975, *188*, 420-425.

Van Amelsvoort, V. F. P. M. *Early Introduction of Integrated Rural Health into a Primitive Society.* Assen: Van Gorcum, 1964.

Van Arsdale, P. W. Activity patterns of Asmat hunter-gatherers: a time budget analysis. *Mankind*, 1978a, *11*(4), 453-460.

Van Arsdale, P. W. Population dynamics among Asmat hunter-gatherers of New Guinea: data, methods, comparisons. *Human Ecology*, 1978b, *6*(4), 435-467.

van de Kaa, D. J. Estimates of vital rates and future growth. *New Guinea Research Bulletin*, 1970, *34*, 1-23.

van de Kaa, D. J. The future growth of Papua New Guinea's indigenous population. *New Guinea Research Bulletin*, 1971, *42*, 16-30.

Vayda, A. P. *War in Ecological Perspective: Persistence, Change, and Adaptive Processes in Three Oceanic Societies.* New York: Plenum Publishing Corporation, 1976.

Weiss, K. M. *Demographic Models for Anthropology.* Memoirs of the Society for American Archaeology, No. 27, 1973.

Wells, C. *Bones, Bodies, and Disease: Evidence of Disease and Abnormality in Early Man.* New York: Praeger Publishers, Inc., 1964.

Wilson, A. C., and Sarich, V. M. A molecular time scale for human evolution. Proceedings of the National Academy of Sciences, 1969, *63*(4), 1088-1093.

CHAPTER 4

Health determinants during early phases of the human life cycle

We have already made the point that the survival of large groups depends on their adapting to a great variety of pressures in their environment; Chapter 3 supports this view of the development of the human species with evidence from the evolutionary record and from later history. The same can be said for the development of the individual, the organismic unit in the model of the human ecosystem (p. 16); interaction among body organ systems and behavioral elements defines development across an individual's life span. The stage of development at any particular age influences the individual's adaptive capacity, susceptibility to sickness, and ability to use available resources for defending health. These activities, which begin at conception and reach their end at the time of death, comprise the continuum of the human life cycle.

Our focus in the following two chapters is on the individual's health and how it is influenced by both the biological nature of the individual and the external forces that emanate from the cultural setting. Health itself is, or should be, a constant accompaniment to life, reflecting the harmonious functions of these complex interactions within ourselves and the successful adaptations to our culture that each of us tries to achieve.

Individuals may react very differently to the culture that surrounds them, even though their biological endowment is very similar. Persons who may begin life by sharing biological characteristics may then be changed in a variety of ways by the culture itself. Such easily measured factors as increased height and weight during childhood have been used to illustrate this phenomenon, often observed in first-generation ethnic groups who have migrated to the United States (Roche, 1976). Health problems formerly encountered in later adult life may be diminished in the new homeland or may be replaced by another kind of disease. Examples of this type illustrate how health is a product of both one's constitution and culture.

Finally, we offer evidence for close connections between life events and important transition periods that are sustained throughout life's course; these connections underlie our premise that health is a continuous process linked to the cumulative impact of life events. The remainder of this chapter centers on the earliest phases of human life when the foundations are laid for much of each person's future health.

A THEORETICAL MODEL OF THE HUMAN LIFE CYCLE

Infant mortality is used as one important index of health in a society. Measured as deaths under 1 year of age per 1000 live births, it seems to reflect the capability of the culture to successfully provide its succes-

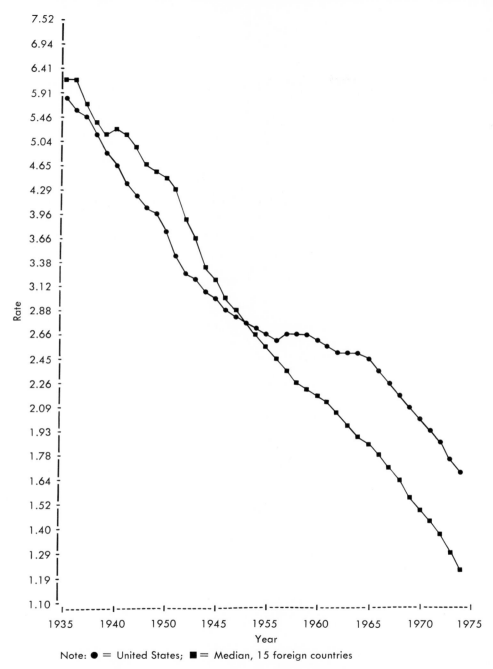

Note: ● = United States; ■ = Median, 15 foreign countries

Fig. 4-1. Infant mortality (deaths under 1 year per 100 live births) have not declined as rapidly in the United States as in fifteen other countries (3 year moving average). (From Fuchs, 1978.)

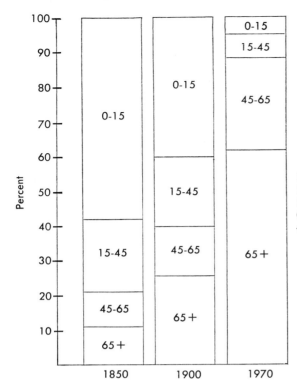

Fig. 4-2. The percentage of deaths by specified age intervals for the years 1850, 1900, and 1970. The majority of deaths have moved from the ages under 15 to over 65 years during this time span. (From Spierer, H., 1977: 40.)

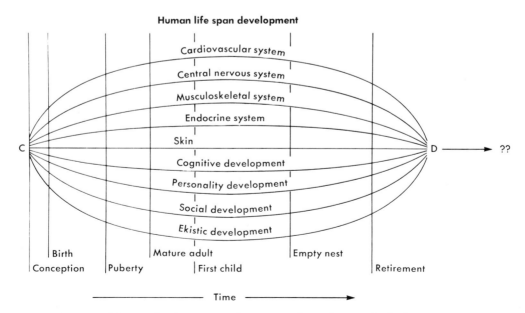

Fig. 4-3. Human life-span development can be envisioned as a "watermelon" whose stripes comprise numerous organ and behavioral systems. (Aldrich, 1976.)

sors. In a sense, it may indicate whether or not the adults are being good ancestors. Low infant mortality is a major goal of virtually all parents today, so that contemporary international meetings on health or children commit much of their time and efforts to discussing ways of improving infant survival. High infant mortality, on the other hand, is thought to be undesirable; it is considered evidence that a society in which this occurs has poor health. While a great many factors that affect infant mortality have been identified, there still are mysteries, as shown in Fig. 4-1 in which U.S. infant mortality between 1936 and 1974 is compared to the median of fifteen other countries. No verifiable explanation has been brought forth for the failure of U.S. infant mortality rates to continue to parallel those in the selected foreign countries between 1955 and 1964. After 1964 the rate fell rapidly again, evenly following that in other countries (Fuchs, 1978). What was happening in the United States in those years that was not happening elsewhere? Perhaps a cultural explanation will be discovered.

Historically, in the United States there are enormous changes in the percentages of deaths by age group (Fig. 4-2). The rapid drop in infant and childhood death rates over 120 years (1850 to 1970) are largely responsible for changing the pattern from one where most deaths occurred among the young to one where most deaths occurred among the elderly. When more infants and children survive to middle age and old age, the demographic picture in the United States changes, and the consequences of such changes affect the lives and future of all.

The integrated nature of biological and behavioral processes of development and the relationships apparent among developmental stages and different age groups have led to proposing a model of human life-span development (Fig. 4-3). This theoretical model

can serve as a unifying concept for human development that can be applied to different environments, cultures, and genders. Additional biological and behavioral systems can be added to those shown in Fig. 4-3. Ekistic development deserves further definition because it may be an unfamiliar term to most readers.* We use the term "ekistic development" to refer to the process by which one's habitat, or human settlement, impacts on other processes, critical transition periods, and life events. For example, a boy 5 years of age who lives in a rural community with a population of 5000 receives a qualitatively and quantitatively different set of experiences than would be the case if he were living in a metropolitan area like Chicago, New York, or Houston. His "grasp" of the way society works would be likely to be fragmentary when derived from a big city, but clearer and more complete if gained from a small town (Sidney, 1976). At the other end of the age spectrum, the elderly cannot function to their maximum abilities when faced with speeding cars, automatic traffic signals with short intervals, or apartments that are up

---

*Ekistics (modern Greek: ΟΙΚΙΣΤΙΚΗ) is derived from the ancient Greek adjective οἰκιστικός, more particularly from the neuter plural οἰκιστικὰ (as "physics" is derived from φυσικὰ, Aristotle). The ancient Greek adjective οἰκιστικός meant: "concerning the foundation of a house, a habitation, a city or a colony; contributing to the settling." It was derived from οκιστής, an ancient Greek noun meaning "the person who installs settlers in place." This may be regarded as deriving indirectly from another ancient Greek noun, οἴκισις, meaning "building," "housing," "habitation," and especially "establishment of a colony, a settlement or a town" (already in Plato), or "filling it with new settlers"; "settling," "being settled." All these words grew from the verb οἰκίζω, "to settle," and were ultimately derived from the noun οικος, "house," "home," or "habitat."

The English equivalent of οἰκιστική is *ekistics* (a noun). In addition, the adjectives *ekistic* and *ekistical*, the adverb *ekistically*, and the noun *ekistician* are now also in current use. The French equivalent is *ékistique*, the German *ökistik*, the Italian *echistica* (all feminine).

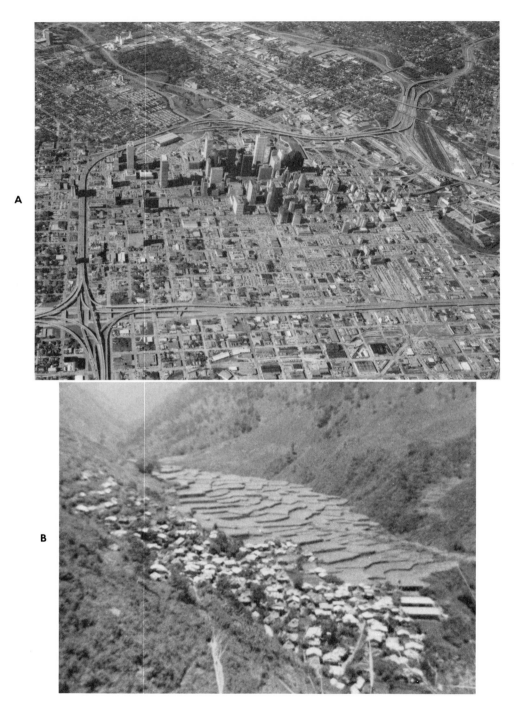

Fig. 4-4. A, A view of downtown Houston, Texas, a city for which the extraction and processing of energy on a massive scale figures importantly. **B,** Terraced fields and a village occupy adjacent sites in a Philippine setting and exhibit a different arrangement for extracting energy from the environment than that seen in Houston. (**A,** Courtesy Utility Data Corporation; **B,** courtesy M. B. Drysdale.)

several flights of stairs. These factors alone can lead to withdrawal from the neighborhood society. Thus, "habitat" does make a difference; its effect depends on both the characteristics of the human settlement itself and the stage in life of the person living there.

An examination of the earliest human settlements is useful for learning about the individuals who constructed them since the settlements reflect the culture and technology of the time (Leakey, 1978). Human beings continue to play the roles of both guinea pig and research director insofar as their settlements are concerned. Modern technology creates situations that exceed human scale and in several ways pass beyond the capacity of people to adapt. A modern metropolis in the United States may be posing a serious threat to its residents by dangerous traffic, air and water pollution, noise, and limitations on mobility because of limited transportation systems, to mention just a few problems (Fig. 4-4, *A*). Human settlements in ancient times had to be on a human scale, matching the innate physiological and psychological capabilities of those living there (Fig. 4-4, *B*).

In order to learn about human beings and their settlements, methods of qualitative and quantitative analysis are being discovered (Doxiadis, 1976) and applied to both ancient and modern sites. The basic theories underlying ekistics (Doxiadis, 1968) are being shaped and modified in ways that make it possible to apply modern technology so that the built environment preserves human scale in a manner appropriate for the times. Application of these concepts and principles to the life-span model is very helpful in gaining perspective on the effect of social trends on housing, transportation, neighborhoods, and health services distribution. Such current trends as single-parent families, unmarried couples living together, and decreasing family size are better understood in this concep-

tual framework. Likewise, the concepts of ekistics are being used to study the causes of vehicular accidents to small children in cities and the concentration of educable mentally retarded children in impoverished city neighborhoods, as shown in Fig. 4-5 (President's Committee on Mental Retardation, 1968).

In the life cycle model the critical transition periods are times when major change takes place over which individuals have little or no influence; for example, conception, birth, puberty, and death. The other vertical lines mark life events. Only a selected few that a person might encounter are shown in Fig. 4-3. Women differ from men in some of their life events or in the timing of their occurrence. "Recording" one's own life events is easy to accomplish and may provide many insights about one's own development. Numerical values can be assigned to life events in direct proportion to their impact. The loss of a spouse consistently has a high number in all samples of people tested, meaning that this has a great impact on the bereaved partner. When several events with high numbers occur within a short period of time, there appears to be increased susceptibility to illness (Holmes and Masuda, 1973).

As the foregoing suggests, culture and community have great influence over health; this influence persists throughout life, for better or for worse, and often is beyond the individual's immediate control. Although the relationships between the biological, behavioral, and social processes are sufficiently complex without the addition of environmental and community effects, such a synthesis is essential if human beings are to live in the future in harmony with their environment and are to make appropriate use of technology to serve human values on a human scale. The difficulty of achieving this synthesis was anticipated some years ago in an essay entitled "Science and Complexity"

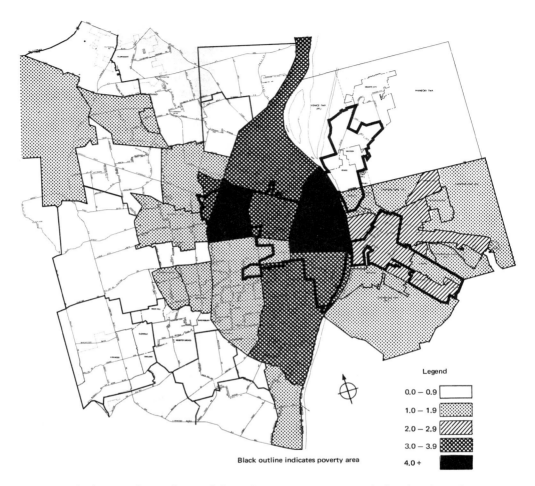

Legend

0.0 – 0.9	
1.0 – 1.9	
2.0 – 2.9	
3.0 – 3.9	
4.0 +	

Black outline indicates poverty area

Fig. 4-5. The location of mentally retarded people in St. Louis is not evenly distributed in urban areas. There are more children classified as functionally mentally retarded in urban poverty areas than in the suburban sections. This pattern in St. Louis is repeated in map data prepared on Bridgeport, Los Angeles, Harrisburg, and Seattle. (President's Committee on Mental Retardation, 1968.)

in which the concept of "organized complexity" was considered as an approach to understanding human development even though it requires a wide range of disciplines and cooperation among the professionals engaged in research (Weaver, 1948).

The remaining sections of this chapter and the next are based on our model of the human life span. We begin with the prenatal period and, in this chapter, move through

birth, infancy, and childhood. Selected aspects of each section go into greater depth where there are important new concepts about health and the role that culture plays in it.

CONCEPTION

The growth of world population ranks high among fundamental international issues. World population growth appears related to

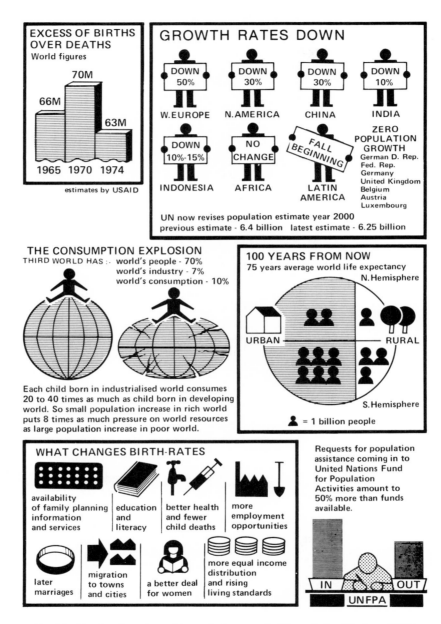

Fig. 4-6. The slowdown in world population growth. (From United Nations, 1977.)

other issues, such as food, energy, clean water, and urbanization. Therefore, discussion of conception ought to consider the factors that govern fertility in different cultural contexts. Where fertility-regulating technical methods have been introduced, their success or failure has depended on whether or not the particular technology was acceptable to the society (Polgar and Marshall, 1978).

In recent years, in India, plastic intrauterine devices have been rejected by women because of unacceptable side effects. Similarly, massive efforts to promote vasectomy led to failure. By way of contrast, in northern Thailand, fertility regulation by injections of a steroid hormone (Depo-provera) gained rapid and widespread acceptance, primarily because the injections were culturally desirable there (McDaniel and Tieng, 1978). These examples suggest that fertility regulation may be dependent on the beliefs and values held by a society. As Polgar and Marshall (1978) state,

Improved technology is an independent factor in the equation, important in its own right, but having no effect on the need to have children. Beliefs and values regarding the desirability of avoiding or postponing the next birth will be changed only by real changes in the world surrounding the decision-maker; a recognized drop in child mortality, for example, and the provision of functional equivalents for children will create a situation in which the people are able to consider adopting improved fertility regulating methods.

What has happened to world population and fertility in recent years? According to Rafael Salas (1978), "There are encouraging indications of a steep fall in infant mortality in certain areas of the Third World"; and in another section of the same report he says, "There are clear signs of a decline in fertility." Reduced fertility paralleling decreases in infant mortality suggests the operation of

internal population growth–regulating mechanisms. Other factors that contribute to a decline in world population growth include effective family planning programs, greater literacy and educational levels, improved status of women, older age at marriage, international migrations, urbanization, and rising incomes.

While it must be recognized that reliable statistics about a nation are not always available, there are suggestions of lowered birth rates to be found in three to four dozen countries, probably representing from 40% to 60% of the developing world (United Nations, 1977) (Figs. 4-6 and 4-7). Reports are accumulating that indicate China's birth rate has fallen to twenty-five per 1000 with a 20% decline occurring in the past 10 years (United Nations, 1977). Similar recent reports of declining fertility have come from India, Indonesia, and some Central and South American countries (Chile, Colombia, Costa Rica, Dominican Republic, Guyana, and Mexico). National policies with regard to fertility also are changing. The number of nations that view their fertility rates as being too high rose from forty-two to fifty-four between 1974 and 1976. Eighteen of these are in Asia, eighteen in Africa, sixteen in Latin America, and two in the Middle East; representing about 82% of the developing world.

Assuming that these trends will continue, which is by no means assured, we can expect to find increasing emphasis on quality of each newborn accompanied by expanded efforts, through applied knowledge and new research into prenatal life, aimed at preventing mortality and morbidity of the embryo, fetus, or newborn.

Development of ovum and sperm

The human female at birth is endowed with all of the ova that she will ever have. These cells have been formed in her ovaries during her own prenatal life. Like other cells

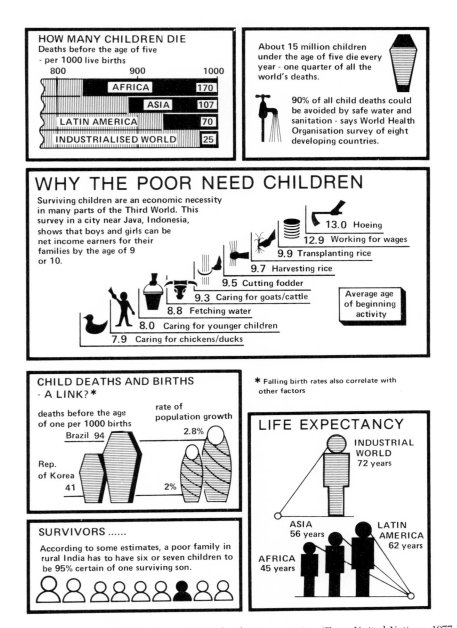

Fig. 4-7. Factors affecting childhood mortality in developing countries. (From United Nations, 1977.)

in her body, these ova are subject to many internal and external events, and for this reason the health of ova should be one of the goals for normal conception and embryogenesis. It is known that infectious agents, x-rays, some chemicals, and poor nutrition may affect the ovaries and the ova they carry during childhood and over the period of maturity and fertility. There are approximately 500,000 ova in the immature ovaries; this number undergoes attrition during a reproductive lifetime with only 400 to 500 being shed during the reproductive years (from about the ages 12 to 48). The oversupply of reproductive cells in the female is dwarfed by the much greater number of male sperm cells that are formed continuously after reaching puberty. Normally, 200 to 300 million spermatozoa are present in an ejaculation. These cells are much smaller than the ovum, which can just be seen with the naked eye (0.1 mm in diameter). A sperm is smaller (0.06 mm in length), with a long motile tail that propels it through the uterus and into the fallopian tubes, where the ovum is met and conception occurs, probably within 20 to 24 hours after the sperm enters the uterus (see Fig. 4-10).

The preconception phase of reproduction is important since factors stemming from this period influence the subsequent growth and development of the fetus. Cultural and environmental factors govern the exposure of both ova and sperm to hazardous influences. Since each reproductive cell contains the genetic material in its chromosomes that will make up the genetic characteristics of the fertilized ovum, it is important to protect it from damaging influences (Smith, 1973). Equally significant is the fact that the ovum must contain sufficient nutrients for the fertilized ovum to continue to move toward the uterus where it implants itself in the uterine wall and quickly creates a nutritional source from the forming placenta. Widespread use of chemicals and radioactive materials may have cumulative effects over long periods of time that may alter chromosomal material in either the sperm or ovum and thus induce genetic disorders in the child.

Cultural factors also play an important role in determining whether conception will occur and in influencing the selection of sexual partners, the frequency and timing of intercourse, and the availability of contraceptive measures that prevent conception. Furthermore, cultural values affect the desirability of having children as well as the number and the sex of the children that are wanted. Such values influence the attitudes of prospective parents and the kind of treatment accorded the child.

Fertilization

Sperm cells swimming through the uterus and entering the fallopian tubes each carry twenty-three chromosomes. After penetrating the outer layer of the ovum, the sperm's chromosomal material unites with the twenty-three chromosomes of the ovum, including the female (X) sex chromosome. Sperm cells carry either an X chromosome or a Y chromosome. Depending on which is carried by the fertilizing sperm, the gender of the fertilized ovum and, therefore, of the child is determined. A female will result if there are two X chromosomes; if there is one X and one Y chromosome, a male will result. At the time of union of sperm and ovum, changes, called capacitation, take place in the sperm. Capacitation permits the sperm to penetrate the clear outer layer of the ovum, called the zona pellucida. Interest in the precise details of fertilization and capacitation has moved from the laboratory to the public domain in view of the first "test tube baby" born in London in 1978. For many years the in vitro fertilization of a human ovum has been an objective of scientists studying human reproductive biology. Aside from the scientific merits of such an achievement, motivation came also from clinicians seeking to help couples who wanted a child but could not conceive because of an anatomical obstruction to the sperm's travel to the fallopian tubes. The "test tube" baby procedures start with the removal of a mature ovum from the ovary and the addition of the father's sperm in a meticulously prepared solution, so that fertilization and the first few cell divisions can occur. The conceptus is then introduced into the uterus where it implants in the uterine wall. The birth of a "test tube" baby has raised ethical issues and national debate about reproductive research of this kind and particularly about whether the termination of such a procedure constitutes an abortion.

Chromosomal disorders

With each division of the fertilized ovum, the number of chromosomes (46) should remain the same in each cell. However, mistakes can occur when the chromosome pairs are separating during the process of cell division. There are several abnormal configurations that can occur and can be identified by comparison with the set of chromosomes in the normal karyotype (Puck and Robinson, 1968). For example, one common disorder is trisomy 21. One can see by inspection of the normal karyotype (Fig. 4-8) that the twenty-first position in the abnormal karyotype (Fig. 4-9) has three instead of two chromosomes— hence the nomenclature "trisomy 21."

The features of a child born with trisomy 21, or Down's syndrome, (also called mongolism) are quite characteristic and are nearly always diagnostic at birth. Several organ systems are affected by this single chromosomal abnormality. The child is short in stature; the head is flattened at the base (occiput); the eyes have narrow palpebral fissures and prominent epicanthal folds that make the facial expression appear somewhat "oriental." The tongue is unusually large and

often protrudes; it is frequently deeply furrowed. Inside the mouth, the palate can be seen to be narrow and high. The joints in the body are very flexible; the hands are broad and flabby with the little fingers curved inward. Palmar creases are also shifted to an abnormal position. There are other manifestations, such as cardiac anomalies, speckling of the iris, underdeveloped external genitalia (especially in males), and a distinctly reduced ability to overcome infections. The primary disturbance, however, is reduced ability to learn, leading to a diagnosis of mental retardation (Forfar and Arneil, 1973).

For many years it has been customary to advise women over 35 years of age who become pregnant that there is an increased risk that their child will have a chromosomal disorder when compared to the risk in younger mothers (Hammerton, 1971). However, recent evidence provides proof that the male may also be the source of the extra twenty-first chromosome, and this introduces a broader sense of responsibility for the parents, as well as invalidates contemporary tables of relative risks for Down's syndrome based solely on the mother's age (Holmes, 1978). Furthermore, there are data showing that the average age of mothers of infants with Down's syndrome is decreasing. "Women under 35 are having over 90 percent of the infants and 65 to 80 percent of the infants with Down's syndrome" (Holmes, 1978:142).

The arrival of a retarded child with trisomy 21 in a family creates a complex set of reactions among siblings and parents. A major issue arises over whether the child should be reared at home or elsewhere in either an institution or a foster home. During the 1930s and 1940s in the United States, it was common for these children to be institutionalized as infants in either state-operated or private facilities for the retarded. Only limited efforts were made during this period to provide them with education and training.

Life expectancy during this period was shortened by infectious disorders that now can be arrested with antibiotics. In the 1950s there was a growing concern for preventing mental retardation of all types, as well as for providing education and health and social needs due mentally retarded persons as fellow citizens (President's Panel on Mental Retardation, 1962). Methods for prenatal diagnosis of some forms of mental retardation, such as trisomy 21, and other genetic disorders are available using the technique of

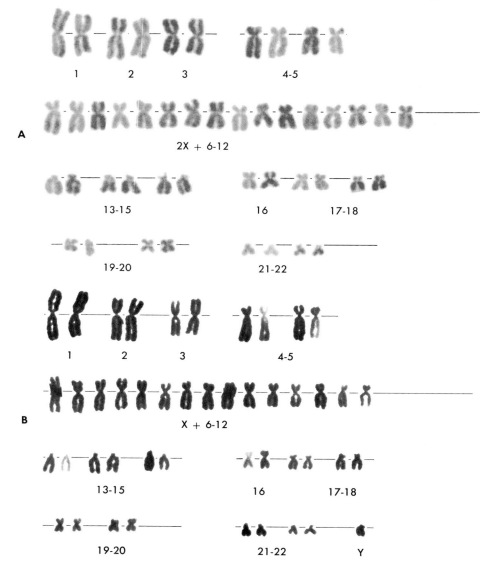

Fig. 4-8. The human karyotype, grouped and numbered according to the Denver system. **A,** Female; **B,** male. (From Reisman and Matheny, 1969.)

amniocentesis, in which fetal cells are cultured and inspected for the presence of genetic abnormalities. Prenatal diagnosis with amniocentesis permits parents to make a decision about completing the pregnancy or ending it, according to their beliefs and the values of the culture in which they live (NICHD National Registry, 1976).

Any handicapping condition, including mental retardation, has an impact on the family, its social network, and the community. Growing public awareness of the genetic origins of many handicaps should reinforce the research efforts that are required to discover how these genetic disorders happen and what can be done to prevent them.

A major determinant of health is found in the earliest division of the fertilized ovum when chromosomal patterns are formed. Defects at this stage of life are permanent, sometimes affecting several organ systems and processes. Nevertheless, there are other vulnerable times in early human development. Embryogenesis, or the generation of form, is one such period.

The generation of form (embryogenesis)

Once released from the ovaries, the ovum takes about four days to get to the uterus, during which time it can be fertilized. If fertilized, the cells begin to divide, forming a solid cluster that soon hollows out to form a blastocyst not much bigger than the ovum was at the time of fertilization. In the second week the trophoblast, the cells that are going to become part of the placenta, begin to multiply. These cells are on the outside of the blastocyst and possess the capability to penetrate the inner uterine lining. They invade and establish a connection between the mother and the embryo at the site of the placenta. It is also in the second week that the protective amniotic cavity containing clear fluid forms. Differentiation of the three principle tissues of the embryo—ectoderm, mesoderm, and endoderm—becomes visible, as shown in the sequence in Figs. 4-10 to 4-15 (Smith and Der Yuen, 1973).

Embryonic growth follows the cephalocaudal law that gives the head first priority for growth and differentiation, with the lower

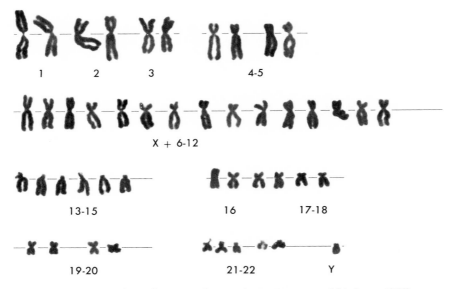

Fig. 4-9. Karyotype of Down's syndrome in a human. (From Reisman and Matheny, 1969).

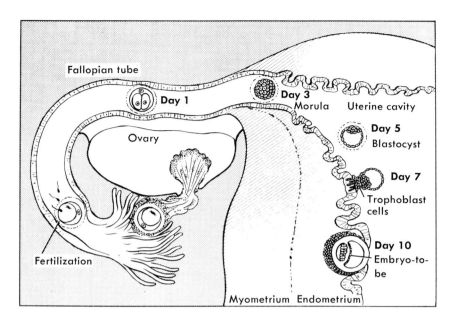

Fig. 4-10. Normal progression during the first 10 days, from fertilization in the fallopian tube to implantation in the uterus. (From Smith and Der Yuen, 1973:33.)

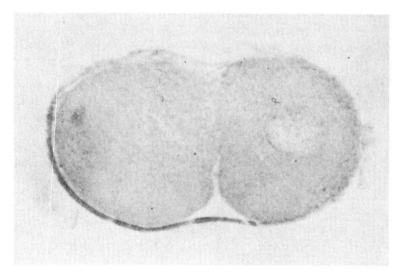

Fig. 4-11. Two-cell stage, with zona pellucida. The early divisions are reliant on the maternal cytoplasm of the ova for nutrition and occur without enlargement of the ovum. (From the Department of Embryology, Carnegie Institute of Washington, Baltimore. In Smith and Der Yuen, 1973:34.)

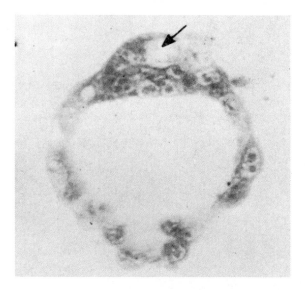

Fig. 4-12. The 4 to 5 day blastocyst stage. Differentiation has now begun. The embryonic cell mass shows the first indication toward an amniotic space (arrow). The cells above it will become trophoblasts, capable of invading the lining of the uterus. At this stage there are about 108 cells, of which eight will become endoderm and ectoderm, the initiation of the embryo-to-be. (From the Department of Embryology, Carnegie Institute of Washington, Baltimore. In Smith and Der Yuen, 1973:34.)

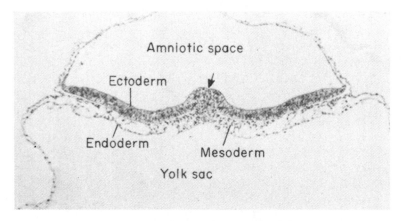

Fig. 4-13. The embryo at 17 to 18 days is now a flat disc, shown here in transverse section. Mesoblast cells migrate from the ectoderm through Hensen's node (the hillock marked by the arrow) and the primitive streak to specific locations between the ectoderm and endoderm, there constituting the high versatile mesoderm. The formation of most organ tissues results from an interaction between mesoderm and adjacent ectoderm or endoderm. Anterior to Hensen's node the notochord develops, providing axial support and influencing subsequent development such as that of the overlying neural plate. (From Smith and Der Yuen, 1973:36.)

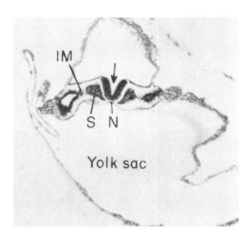

Yolk sac

Fig. 4-14. At 21 to 23 days, the midaxial ectoderm has thickened and formed the neural groove (arrow), partially influenced by the underlying notochord (N). This groove will fuse dorsally to form the neural tube. Lateral to it the mesoblast has now segmented into somites (S), intermediary mesoderm (IM), and somatopleura and splanchnopleura as intervening stages toward further differentiation. Vascular channels are developing in situ from mesoderm; blood cells are being produced in the yolk sac wall; and the early heart is beating. Henceforth, development is extremely rapid, with major changes each day. The next 3 to 4 weeks are the era of major organogenesis, during which incomplete or faulty development may leave the individual with residual malformation. (From Smith and Der Yuen, 1973:36.)

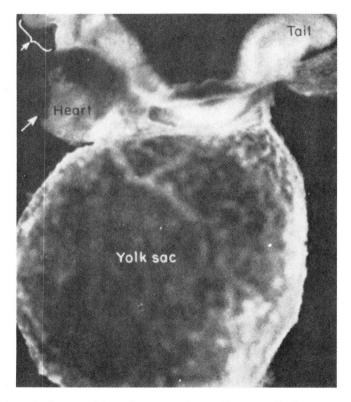

Fig. 4-15. At 24 days, the forepart of the embryo is growing rapidly, especially the anterior neural plate. The lateral portions are growing downward while the head and tail are curling downward also in their growth. Soon the body wall will be fused and the embryo will be in a C-shaped position. The cardiac tube (lower arrow) under the developing face (upper arrow) is now functional. The yolk sac will now rapidly regress. (From Smith and Der Yuen, 1973:37.)

extremities following last. It is perhaps an interesting clinical fact that wounds to children or adults heal more rapidly if on the face or head than on the lower leg or foot.

By the end of the third week, the embryo is about 2 mm long. By the fourth week, the embryo shows segmentation into what are called somites. The neural tube, including the brain, is visible all the way down to the tail by the end of the fourth week, and there is evidence of vascular circulation. The age of the embryo can be estimated by the number of somites present. On the twenty-first day there is only one pair but by the twenty-third day there are ten; by the twenty-sixth day there are twenty, and by the twenty-eighth day about twenty-five. After 1 month,

the frontal part of the brain and the forebrain are developed, and the heart is forming. The embryo is still only 4 mm long, but the head, trunk, and tail regions are all quite distinct; the heart is beating, and blood is circulating (Figs. 4-16 and 4-17).

Between the fifth and eighth weeks all of the organs become very well defined, and the embryo begins to look distinctly human. It grows during this period from about 5 mm in length to about 30 mm, and there are a number of other features that become noticeable by the fifth week. The well-differentiated central nervous system shows eyes in an early form, and there is active growth of the nerves that are going up into the limb buds for the arms and legs. The eyes continue to

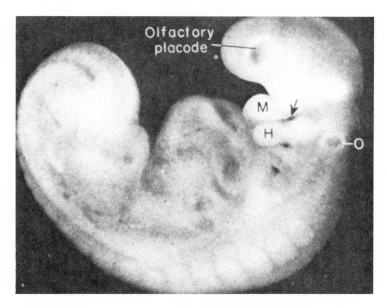

Fig. 4-16. At 26 days, the olfactory placode has begun to invaginate to form the nasal pit. Between it and the mandibular process is the area of the future mouth, where the buccopharyngeal membrane, with no intervening mesoderm, is breaking down. Within the recess of the mandibular (M) and hyoid (H) processes, the future external auditory canal will develop (arrow), and dorsal to it the otic placode (O) is invaginating to form the inner ear. The relatively huge heart must pump blood to the developing placenta as well as to the embryo proper. Foregut outpouchings and evaginations will now begin to form various glands and the lung and liver primordia. Foregut and hindgut are now clearly delineated from the yolk sac. The somites, which will differentiate into myotomes (musculature), dermatomes (subcutaneous tissue), and sclerotomes (vertebrae), are evident into the tail, which will gradually regress. (From Smith and Der Yuen, 1973:38.)

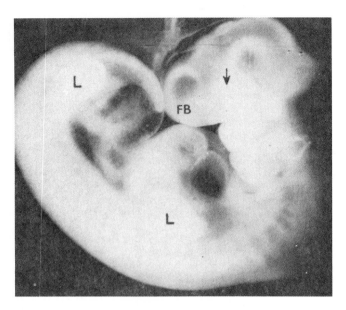

Fig. 4-17. At 30 days, the brain is rapidly growing, and its early cleavage into future bilateral cerebral hemispheres is evident in the telencephalic outpouching of the forebrain (FB). To the right of this is the developing eye, with the cleft optic cup (arrow) and the early invagination of the future lens from surface ectoderm. From the somatopleura the limb swellings (L) have developed. The loose mesenchyme of the limb bud, interacting with the thickened ectodermal cells at its tip, carries all the potential for the full development of the limb. The liver is now functional and will be a source of blood cells. The mesonephric ducts, formed in the mesonephric ridges, communicate to the cloaca, which is beginning to become septated, while the yolk sac is regressing. (From Smith and Der Yuen, 1973:39).

form all through the second month. The ears begin to form in the fourth week and are finished by the eighth week, as are the nose and other facial characteristics (Figs. 4-18 and 4-19).

The rapid linear growth and differentiation taking place in human embryos over the first 3 months are accomplished by an amazingly well-orchestrated series of physiological and biochemical changes. They are timed with such precision that even a brief period of disruption can damage the formation of an organ. An example of a chemical agent having a direct effect on the human embryo is that of thalidomide. This substance, first used in West Germany, was responsible for thousands of babies being born with missing limbs (phocomelia). The discovery of this

relationship served as an excellent example of the profound impact that chemicals can have in early life and spurred basic research into human teratology (birth defects) (Woollam, 1962). Cultures like those in the Western world, where there is widespread use of chemicals as medications, food additives, or drugs evoking behavior modification—narcotics, alcohol, tranquilizers, and sedatives—can expect to evidence influences following their use during pregnancy, especially in the early weeks before the mother is aware she is pregnant.

Infectious agents, particularly rubella (German measles), are a cause of defects in the embryo, often accompanied by blindness from cataracts, deafness, heart malformations, mental retardation, microcephaly, fa-

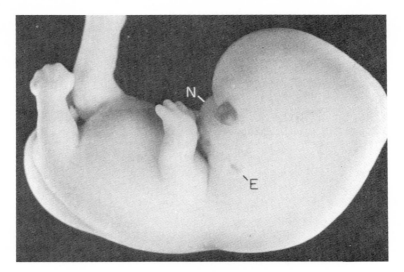

Fig. 4-18. At 41 days, the nose (N) is relatively flat, and the external ear (E) is gradually shifting in relative position as it continues to grow and develop. A neck area is now evident, the anterior body wall has formed, and the thorax and abdomen are separated by the transverse septum (diaphragm). The fingers are now partially separated, and the elbow is evident. The major period of cardiac morphogenesis and septation is complete. The urogenital membrane has now broken down, yielding a urethral opening. The phallus and lateral labioscrotal folds are the same for both sexes at this age. (From Smith and Der Yuen, 1973:41.)

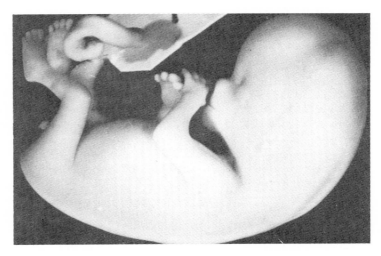

Fig. 4-19. A 10-week male. The eyelids have developed and fused, not to reopen until four or five months. Muscles are developed and functional; normal morphogenesis of joints is dependent on movement; and primary ossification is occurring in the centers of developing bones. Ossification begins at 7 weeks in the clavicle, and by birth all the primary centers are ossified with only the secondary centers at the knee being ossified by that time. In the male the testicle has produced testosterone and has masculinized the external genitalia with enlargement of the genital tubercle, fusion of the labioscrotal folds into a scrotum, and closure of the labia minora folds to form a penile urethra; these structures are unchanged in the female. (From Smith and Der Yuen, 1973:41.)

cial or dental defects, and general failure to thrive. Rubella was the first clear-cut example recognized in human beings of a nongenetic developmental deformity initiated after conception (Michaels and Mellin, 1960). Similarly, exposure to radiation or to other toxic substances and infectious agents that are part of the environment surrounding pregnant women may induce embryonic damage. The contemporary public outcry against increasing pollution of the environment is in part stimulated by the evidence that damage from pollutants is by no means limited to adults. Vigorous efforts are made to avoid medical x-rays to the abdomen of a pregnant woman and to restrict other sources of exposure to radioactive sources.

The falling birth rate in the United States is accompanied by growing numbers of people who delay having children. The changing status of women further contributes to this social shift in the timing of pregnancy as well as in the number of children planned. Expectations that each infant will be of good quality are held among potential parents. We can see convergence in U.S. culture of powerful forces aimed at assuring quality pregnancies and unblemished offspring. One very sensitive period in pregnancy, embryogenesis, has been explored primarily in terms of American culture and environment, which contain several known and, undoubtedly, other unknown hazards to the embryo. The remaining prenatal period is mainly characterized by further growth and the development of function in preparation for birth and infancy.

PREBIRTH AND BIRTH AS BIOLOGICAL AND CULTURAL EVENTS
The fetus

After embryogenesis is completed in the first 8 weeks of gestation, the developing organism is known as the fetus. No new organ systems develop during fetal life, but rapid growth and development of existing organ systems occur in preparation for birth. It is interesting that birth is the marker Western cultures apply to the beginning of one's life, while other cultures, such as the Chinese, consider the infant to be already a year old at birth and thus date the beginning of life approximately at the time of conception. The embryo is only an inch long at the end of embryogenesis, but here the pattern of growth changes. In early fetal life weight and size increase impressively under normal conditions (Fig. 4-20). Intrauterine weight for human beings as well as for other mammals increases as the cube of time since conception from the first trimester onward (Roberts, 1906). However, there are a number of factors that can influence fetal growth and development and, therefore, deserve emphasis.

A previously held view in Western obstetrics was to liken the fetus to a benign tumor or a parasite, capable of easily deriving the necessary nutrients from the mother. Such a view supported restricting maternal weight gain to approximately 15 pounds and identifying infants as premature at birth on the basis of birth weight alone. Curiously, gestational age was not thought to be obtainable, for mothers were not expected to know the date of conception or the date of their last menstrual period, approximately 2 weeks after which conception would be expected to occur. Asking women such questions and using a simple neurological examination of infants now routinely provide a means of differentiating between infants that are growth-retarded ("small-for-date") and those that are born too early ("premature").

One of the earliest studies demonstrating that fetal growth could vary was a study of infant birth weights at high altitude in Leadville, Colorado (elevation 10,200 feet) (Lichty and others, 1957). Infant birth weights were low (Fig. 2-8), and this was attributed to a

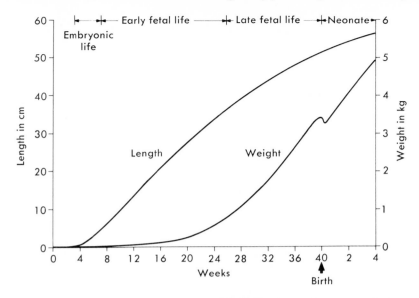

Fig. 4-20. The most rapid linear growth is during midfetal life, whereas the most rapid advancement in weight is in late fetal life. (From Smith and Der Yuen, 1973:44.)

reduction in fetal growth rate rather than to shortened gestational age. Subsequent studies at high altitude have confirmed these earlier observations on infant birth weight and have pointed to reduced oxygen availability as the likely cause (Chapter 2, first case study).

Other factors also may retard fetal growth, possibly through the same mechanism of limiting oxygen availability. Infants born to mothers who smoke during pregnancy evidence a reduction in birth weight of 150 to 180 g (Comstock and others, 1971; Hytten, 1973). Air pollution may be an additional hazard to the developing fetus. In a study controlling for the effects of maternal smoking, maternal body size, and parity, infants born to mothers residing in highly polluted areas of Los Angeles were, on the average, 200 g lighter than infants born to mothers living in less polluted areas (Williams, Spence, and Tideman, 1977).

Nutritional deprivation may also lead to fetal growth retardation as well as to other problems manifest at birth. A fetal alcohol syndrome has recently been described that is caused by excessive alcohol use by mothers during pregnancy. These infants exhibit malformations, as well as failure in postnatal physical and mental development (Jones and Smith, 1973). Children born during the widespread famine in Holland during the World War II occupation by Nazi troops were more likely to be stillborn, to be of low birth weight, or to have complicated births (Stein and others, 1975). Brain cell growth and development also may be impeded by nutritional deprivation during fetal and early postnatal life. Infants weighing 2000 g or less at birth who died of malnutrition during the first years of postnatal life showed a 60% reduction in total brain cell number, and full-term infants who died of food deprivation during the first year has a 15% to 20% reduction in total brain cell numbers (Winick, 1976:15). Winick also cites possible long-term effects of fetal malnutrition in surviving infants, such as derangement in nitrogen metabolism and increased incidence of behavioral abnormalities later in life (1976:30). Controversy continues as to whether "catch-up" brain cell growth is possible in infants surviving severe malnutrition in utero (Winick, Meyer, and Harris, 1975).

Infants that are small-for-date or are premature have higher rates of infant mortality than infants that are full-term or of normal size for gestational age. A great deal of the difference in infant mortality between affluent and poverty areas in the United States and between developed and developing countries can be accounted for by a higher proportion of premature or small-for-date infants (Rush and others, 1974). In fact, low infant birth weight is the single most important factor in accounting for infant mortality in the United States. Thus, factors that reduce fetal growth or the length of gestation are important to recognize and to remedy in order for infant mortality to be decreased. Currently, an average maternal weight gain of 25 pounds is recommended for a previously well-nourished mother (National Academy of Sciences, 1973). Pregnant women are advised not to smoke, and perhaps precautions against exposure to air pollution also should be taken. In present U.S. culture, the epidemic of teenage pregnancy, coupled with the custom in that age group of eating "junk foods" as part of a relatively nonnutritious diet, gives further grounds for concern about the nutrition of mother and fetus. In view of the potential dangers from malnutrition to the fetus in utero and to the surviving infant, food supplements and other aid programs that do not violate cultural taboos should be made available to pregnant women in areas where nutritional deprivation exists (WHO Scientific Group, 1972).

The parents

Pregnancy does not only involve the development of the fetus. Adaptations also occur on the part of the mother and the father that illustrate the extent to which pregnancy is part of a larger, cultural process.

Pregnancy elicits dramatic biological changes in the mother. Hormonal responses occur immediately after conception, but the woman may not be aware of being pregnant for several weeks or even months. Some women experience morning sickness during the first trimester; this is a collection of symptoms of nausea, loss of appetite, and dizziness. The cause of morning sickness is not precisely known, although it is thought to be linked to the increased levels of the hormone progesterone. The incidence of morning sickness varies in different environmental and cultural settings; further study is warranted to investigate the cause of such variation. Physiological adjustments to pregnancy occur in the mother in response to hormonal and other stimuli. Elevated progesterone levels prompt increased ventilation in the pregnant woman. The number of red blood cells increases, but an even greater expansion in total blood volume results in the so-called "physiological anemia" of pregnancy. The amount of blood pumped by the heart increases early in pregnancy, but controversy exists about whether levels remain elevated or return to prepregnant values during the later phases of pregnancy. The expansion of the uterus in the third trimester may restrict the mother's breathing and contribute to shortness of breath (dyspnea) in some women.

The mother is aware of fetal movements beginning the second trimester. In the third trimester interaction between mother and fetus increases as each responds to the other's movements. Fetal heart rate and fetal movements respond to noise and to maternal discomfort and pleasure. The mother feels the fetus, often quite acutely as a blow from a fist or a foot!

Maternal attitude about the pregnancy is

related to her situation at the time that she became pregnant, the extent to which the pregnancy was desired, cultural attitudes about pregnancy, and the view of the father and his willingness to accept and accommodate the pregnancy. If morning sickness is present during early pregnancy, its passage during the second trimester may result in a more positive attitude toward the pregnancy. The quality of the marital relationship may also have a bearing. Couples with fewer marital problems and who actively desire the pregnancy have a lower incidence of problems associated with pregnancy as well as with labor and delivery (Newton and Modahl, 1978).

Attitudes and behaviors during pregnancy are also influenced by the culture in which the pregnancy occurs. The traditional perceptions about fetal development and the behaviors that are appropriate for pregnant women in the Mexican community of Ajijic (population of 8000), located on the shores of Lake Chapala near Guadalajara, illustrate the importance of cultural beliefs. Their view of gestation is characterized by marked variation, depending on the personal orientation of the mother or the specialist from whom the information is obtained and also depending on the attributes of the fetus. Some believe that the male fetus develops from the essence of the mother, is positioned to the right in the uterus, and grows much more rapidly than the female who is formed, conversely, from the father's essence and is located to the left in the uterus. They believe the first child requires 9 months for development; only 8 months and 20 days are needed for subsequent children, and 11 to 12 months may be needed for twins to develop. The fetus, it is thought, breathes through the mouth and anus via the open mouth of the uterus. Should the mouth of the uterus close from any cause, the fetus will suffocate. Injections are thought to close the mouth of the

uterus, so women will refuse injections while pregnant. Other maternal behaviors also influence the fetus. Certain foods, such as an excess of "cold" foods, are avoided because they are thought to cause illness in the newborn. Sibling jealousies, excessive drinking by the father, eclipses of the sun or moon, sudden fright (*susto*) or anger (*choraje*) in the mother, certain herbs, and accumulated semen from sexual intercourse also are believed to harm the developing fetus (McClain, 1975).

Cultural beliefs operate analogously in other settings to prescribe the conduct of the mother and father during pregnancy. During the nineteenth century and continuing today in some sectors of American society, a woman was likely to be sequestered once she reached the third trimester of pregnancy. The sight of a woman in late pregnancy was considered embarrassing both for her and to others. Attitudes toward pregnancy may be linked to considerations affecting fertility, so strongly positive values are assigned to pregnancy in cultures where fertility is stressed. Where fertility attitudes are more mixed, childbirth is likely to be less highly valued, and attitudes toward the pregnant woman and the expectant father may be more ambivalent. In middle class American society, competing views on the desirability of having children, pressures fed by views about zero population growth, and competing economic and work-related demands thus may render the position of the expectant parents less certain.

Birthing

The initiation of labor begins the birthing process. The precise mechanisms responsible for the initiation of labor are not known, but hormone production by the fetus, mother, and their shared organ, the placenta, is thought critical for the timing of the event. Labor is usually defined by three stages. In the first stage faint contractions appear, the cervix dilates, and the baby enters the birth canal. This is generally the most prolonged phase of labor, especially in first births, and can last from 2 to 16 hours. The second stage of labor is when the contractions become more closely spaced and stronger; during this phase, essentially an expulsive phase, the baby emerges from the birth canal. Once the shoulders have emerged, the second stage of labor ends. The third stage of labor is the expulsion of the placenta, usually within 15 minutes after the baby is born. With the expulsion of the placenta, the birth process is complete.

The way in which the labor is conducted (for example, the extent to which the mother is medicated) has a dramatic impact on the immediate postpartum behavior of both mother and infant. Important carry-overs from this immediate maternal-infant relationship into later life are explored in the next section on parent-infant bonding. Current practices in the United States have reintroduced fathers into delivery rooms to be with their wives during labor and to greet their newborn babies. Medications have been greatly reduced during labor, primarily to favor an active, alert infant and mother rather than a listless, unresponsive mother and baby. There is increasing acceptance of the more natural childbirth approaches, including conversion of major hospital facilities to "homelike" suites that can accommodate fathers and other family members and friends of the parents.

Among modern industrialized nations with low infant mortality, there can be great differences in the approach to childbirth. In Sweden a high-technology system is used, while in Holland almost as many babies are delivered at home as in hospitals, and very little medication or instrumentation is used. Nevertheless, infant mortality in the two countries is nearly identical.

The approach to childbirth stems from the culture in which the birth occurs and thus varies in response to cultural changes. In the Mexican community of Ajijic, whose beliefs about gestation were discussed previously, traditional herbal preparations. Childbirth may take place either at home or in a hospital, with the assistance of a midwife or a physician or without any assistance (McClain, 1975). Cultural change appears to favor an increase in hospital births, since the number of midwives is declining. A comparison of infant mortality in Ajijic shows home births with or without a midwife's assistance had a lower incidence of mortality than physician-assisted hospital births. While other factors, such as a tendency for problem-ridden pregnancies to result in hospital births might be contributing to the higher infant mortality in hospitals; the culture change in birthing practices in this community may not be beneficial. Displacing traditional practices may bring with it disadvantages, such as the loss of close association of mother and child in a familiar setting and the loss of continuity in care provided by a midwife from the same cultural setting, without necessarily resulting in the advantage of lower infant mortality (McClain, 1975).

Parent-infant bonding

Currently, birthing practices in the United States are undergoing reexamination in response to the recognition that the time immediately after birth appears important for bonding processes to occur between the parents and the infant. Doubts have been raised about birth practices in which the valuable relationship between parents and infant may have been interfered with in the rush to apply new technologies and to defend the mother and infant from infection (Brazelton, 1969; Klaus and Kennell, 1976; Leboyer, 1976). As a result, many of the barriers to mother-infant interactions and participation in them by the father are being removed, and hospitals are changing traditional birthing facilities to more homelike situations. Recently home deliveries under supervision have begun to make a comeback, with the provision of good prenatal care and care of skilled nurse-practitioner midwives sensitive to the culture in which they are working (Arms, 1975).

Immediately after birth the mother and infant seem exquisitely prepared for attachment to each other. Although the available studies have tended to emphasize the interactions between mother and child, it is increasingly being recognized that the father is also a part of the bonding process. This period immediately after birth has been termed the "sensitive period" (Klaus and Kennell, 1976). Mother and infant communicate with each other by means of all their senses: vision, hearing, smell, taste, and physical contact. The infant receives an exacting physical examination in which all bodily parts are inspected to make sure everything is normal. The infant can focus on its mother immediately after birth, and time is spent in which mother and infant gaze at each other. The visual communication and recognition during bonding is a thrilling and significant event for both mother and father and, presumably, for the infant as well.

The continuous contact between mother and infant immediately after birth carries with it physiological as well as psychological benefits. Skin-to-skin contact aids the infant in maintaining body temperature in the markedly cooler extrauterine world. Transfer of maternal antibodies to the infant occurs through exposure to maternal nasal flora and through nursing. Colostrum, the initial fluid available from the breast, contains fatty substances thought to contain protective antibodies as well as other nutrients. Nursing stimulates the release of oxytocin, which aids in contraction of the uterus for expulsion of the placenta and resumption of the nonpregnant shape of the uterus, and prolactin, which acts to hasten the production of milk (Klaus and Kennell, 1976).

Birthing practices that facilitate bonding include, importantly, the presence of an alert mother and infant. Thus, as will be discussed shortly, the use of a general anesthetic that sedates both mother and infant is not recommended except in case of complications. Permitting access to the infant by the mother and father through "rooming-in" (in which the infant spends extended periods with the mother) and other policies that make the hospital a homelike setting where father and family can visit encourages bonding. Delaying the administration of silver nitrate, put in the infant's eyes to prevent infection but causing intense watering and discomfort, until after the first hour after birth also is a practice that facilitates bonding.

The experiences of birth and contact in the first hours that follow are likely to have occurred throughout human existence, since it is only recently in some industralized countries that means have become available for sedating and separating mother and infant. In considering how these very critical and meaningful events following birth are handled in other cultures, it is instructive to note a cultural practice that has been termed "couvade," a term derived from the French verb, *couver*, meaning to cover. The couvade is a period of time after birth when mother, father, and child are secluded. Sometimes a special house is built, at other times it can be a matter of ritual or symbolic seclusion. Early accounts of the couvade emphasized specific behaviors on the part of males. Such behaviors often entailed elaborate facsimiles of pregnancy in which the male would be treated as if he were pregnant, even to the point of fabricating a kind of guise to simulate pregnancy. The male would be fed the same foods, if there were certain foods that were culturally prescribed for the pregnant woman, and may even experience a ritualized birth.

Among the Wai Wai of Venezuela, when a woman is expecting a baby, the father and the mother begin to subject themselves to dietary and behavioral regulations. Such restrictions are intended to protect fetal development. For example, the pregnant woman and the man are both prevented from eating meat because, if it were tainted and caused either to vomit, the fetus would be harmed. Shortly before birth a hut is erected. Husband and wife move into the birth hut and are joined by the wife's mother, who will help with the birth. After birth, both parents stay in a hammock in the hut for about 2 weeks. Thus, there is a prolonged period of seclusion in which physical intimacy is assured. During this time the infant is named —frequently the name of a great grandfather or great grandmother or a dead relative who was beloved. If the infant is sick, medical practitioners come to the hut to help. After this period of seclusion, the couple, with their child, move back to the section of the community where they previously lived and carry on as before except for various prescribed postnatal activities. The women in Wai Wai society are the principal agriculturists and after delivering a child they continue to work in the field, calling on the husband, when necessary, to care for the infant. Postnatal regulations continue for 3 years. They are followed in order to protect the infant from spiritual forces that may be harmful. As long as mother and father and infant are joined together, the child is protected. If either parent leaves, the infant's spirit is thought to flee back and forth between the parents and to be at risk when in transition between parents (preceding account from Foch, 1967).

A modern interpretation for the couvade

is as a cultural practice that facilitates bonding by prescribing a prolonged period of intimacy between mother, father, and child. The various practices pertaining to the father could be interpreted as a means of connecting the father and child. The mother's link to the child is obvious; the father's requires cultural confirmation.

The contrast is striking between the "primitive" approach described above and the practices that surrounded birth in American culture earlier in this century. Births were nearly all in hospitals where technical precautions against infection of either the mother or infant had led to a very different but no less elaborate ritual than the couvade. However, these procedures, in contrast to the couvade, cannot be described as furthering opportunities for bonding. In fact, they were quite opposite in their effect.

The hospital birthing experience, historically, is an example of an appropriate health concern for preventing infection being met successfully by modern technology but, in doing so, eliminating the opportunity for bonding. Now that sources of infection are better understood, other means of preventing serious infection can be used, such as antibiotics, and the need for the elaborate procedures developed in the period from 1930 to 1960 has been reduced greatly.

A good modern American hospital during the 1940s and 1950s generally conformed to procedures like these: the mother was isolated in a labor room adjacent to the delivery room; access to her while in labor was forbidden to her husband and family, who were permitted only to wait in the "father's room" that frequently was not on the same floor and was out of view and hearing of the labor and delivery areas. During the delivery, everyone involved was covered with surgical costumes. and only nurses and physicians were present. The mother was usually sedated, sometimes heavily—a process begun earlier during labor and intended to reduce pain and consciousness, although it also may have been a means of allaying the mother's anxieties and fear at being alone during labor. Both mother and newborn were sleepy during the delivery because of these medications, limiting the mother's cooperation and sensitivity to what was occurring and also slowing to some extent the infant's responses, such as taking the first breath at the moment of birth. An entire medical technology developed during these years that was aimed at infant resuscitation, a need that was created in part by the sedation of the mother. The newborn infant was whisked off to a bassinet in a corner of the delivery room as soon as the umbilical cord was cut; seldom was the mother given time to see, feel, and bond with her new child. For many years, it was routine to wipe away the infant's protective skin covering (vernix caseosa) and replace this protective natural substance with oils (which later studies showed were not as protective). The baby was then moved to the newborn nursery, which usually was some distance from the mother's postpartum hospital room, thus removing the infant from the mother's sight and hearing. In this regard, it is interesting to recall that frequently a mother's first question to nurses and physicians was, "Where is my baby?" The questioner wanted to know more than the fact that her baby was in the newborn nursery; she wanted to know the precise geography of the hospital floor so that she would have a spatial orientation to her newborn. The father's visit to his baby was limited in most hospitals to a short time for viewing through a plate glass window that was kept curtained except during viewing periods two or three times daily. The baby was brought to the mother by nurses for breast or bottle feeding as the situation warranted, and since mothers rarely were encouraged to walk before the third postpartum day, there was little chance

to get to see and hold their babies except during these intervals when the infants were brought to them. Fathers were effectively excluded from intimate contact with their new children until the great day came when mother and child could go home a week or so following birth. Thus, serious obstacles prevented contact between mother, father, and infant in the first hours; and bonding was delayed beyond the optimal time (Klaus and Kennell, 1976).

The modern technology of newborn care had other unforeseen health consequences that should be mentioned briefly. Retrolental fibroplasia, a permanent disorder that affects the retina of the eyes resulting in scarring and loss of vision, became epidemic in the United States among premature infants. The cause was unknown in the early 1950s but the epidemic was growing so rapidly that it commanded national attention. A careful study by a Surgeon General's Task Force identified excessive oxygen as the cause. Oxygen in high concentrations had become at that time a routine part of premature infant care in modern hospitals. Today it is rarely used in concentrations over 40% and, with this change, the occurrence of retrolental fibroplasia became rare. We cite this as another example of a health-care practice having unforeseen consequences to a critical organ (Silverman, 1977).

Recognition of the undesirable effects of heavy sedation and other birth-related processes and the availability of alternatives for preventing infection are thus leading to changes in birthing practices designed to facilitate bonding. Such changes tend to return birthing to a human scale. Some proponents recommend even greater change, such as home births, which are common in such countries as Holland. However, substitution of home births for hospital births is not simple; an auxilliary system has developed in Holland by which vans equipped with emergency medical equipment are on hand should an emergency occur.

Bonding is unquestionably of value for the immediate adjustment of the infant to the extrauterine environment. Long-term effects of bonding are also possible. Bonded infants may be healthier than their unbonded coun-terparts (Klaus and Kennell, 1976). Failure-to-thrive syndrome and battered child syn-drome are less common where bonding and effective caretaking and attachment between parent and child have occurred (Fig. 4-21). Perhaps behavioral disturbances in which values such as trust are never established

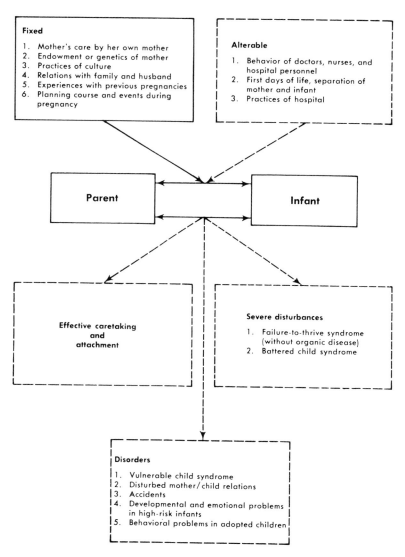

Fig. 4-21. Hypothesized diagram of the major influences on maternal behavior and the resulting disturbances. Solid lines represent unchangeable determinants; broken lines represent alterable determinants. (From Klaus and Kennell, 1976.)

may also have links to bonding and other early-in-life events. Hopefully, continued research on the long-term consequences of the failure of adaptations such as bonding and on adjustments to pregnancy and childbirth will be forthcoming and will entail productive collaboration between anthropologists, physicians, and other health scientists.

INFANCY

So far in this chapter, we have progressed through the earliest stages of the human life course, stressing the continuity of processes during embryonic and fetal life in expectation of birth. Preparation for departure from the protective uterine environment includes the maturation of vital functions that permit the infant to operate independent of maternal life support systems. Physiological functions of heart, kidneys, lungs, digestive tract, skin, brain, and special senses such as hearing are ready at birth to adapt to the greatest environmental change that an individual ever experiences—the change from life inside the mother to the external environment.

Babies are human beings

The newborn is equipped with reflexes ready to spring into action that are necessary for survival. Every normal human infant can cough and remove mucus from the throat or lungs. Respiration is regulated by mechanisms that guarantee a supply of oxygen and at the same time assure elimination of carbon dioxide. The newborn baby can sneeze and yawn by reflexes that seem to be necessary for optimal function of respiration in infants during the "lying down" period of life.

The infant's cry of hunger is compelling to most adults and particularly to the mother. Having called attention to this need, the infant is also equipped with a rooting reflex to search for the nipple. A touch on the cheek with a soft object or the smell of milk will bring forth the rooting reflex. Nature has assured that infants are born with the idea

that they must search for their meals. Application of a nipple to the lips is followed by suckling, and this leads to the complicated act by which milk is swallowed and goes to the stomach rather than into the lungs. Reflexes accurately allow a flap to cover the larynx during swallowing and to guide the milk into the stomach. The newborn can also gauge quite accurately when enough milk has been ingested to feel satisfied.

There are other automatic events that can be briefly mentioned here to further illustrate the baby's preparation for life after birth. The Moro reflex, or startle reflex, is characterized by an anguished expression, wild cries, a rigid, stiff body, and arms thrust upward and outward with clutching, outstretched fingers. Perhaps this reflex had some great significance in the evolutionary past. The reflex is elicited by a loud noise or sudden loss of the baby's equilibrium, such as when rolled over from stomach to back. The Moro reflex is present in the first 2 weeks of life and then fades over several months, but remnants can be seen in the adult "jump" when we are frightened. The Moro reflex is not present in infants who are severely damaged at birth.

The tonic neck reflex and the infant's defense cry at pain, discomfort, loud noises, or loss of balance are other examples of highly developed reflexes. Still others are "swimming" in a sinuous manner, which lasts for only a few months. The infant can withdraw from a pin prick, blink the eyes before a bright light, shiver when cold, or struggle vigorously if restrained. An infant can also lift its head off the table when lying on its stomach (but not when on its back), wave arms and legs around, stretch and grasp objects that touch the fingers and toes, and seem very pleased with hand-to-mouth movements in general.

Thus, we can see processes in the newborn that are ancient in origin but are framed in a modern setting. The disappearing reflexes probably represent capabilities that were useful long ago but whose need today has disappeared. Such characteristics of the newborn may have been adaptations to an environment that was different from that of our protective and sophisticated era. The adaptability of newborns should not be underestimated; they are rugged individuals (Aldrich, 1968).

Infant growth and development

The first 2 years after birth are a period of intense growth and development. The exponential growth rate experienced in utero is largely sustained during the first years of life. By age 2, birth weight has nearly quadrupled (from approximately 7 to 27 pounds). If growth continued at this rate, by age 10 years the individual would weigh 12 tons!

The pattern of growth changes from the intrauterine pattern, however, in that the extremities now undergo more rapid growth than does the body trunk. Body length averages approximately 19 to 21 inches at birth; by 2 years, length has increased by about 50% to an average of 33 inches. Subsequent growth is greatly influenced by genetic background, whereas size at birth and nutrition are major determinants during the first year (Wenner and VanderVeer, 1973).

Infancy is a critical period for brain growth. The extremely rapid increase in the number of brain cells seen during fetal life continues during the first 2 years, by which time the brain has reached 80% of adult size, representing a threefold increase over brain size at birth (Smith, 1973). This extremely rapid brain growth requires that nutrition be of adequate quality as well as quantity. Characteristics of mother's milk have evolved in concert with the nutritional needs of the infant, and, not surprisingly, it is nutritionally nearly ideal. The nature of the social environment is also vital for normal brain development.

Development during infancy proceeds from the head down (cephalocaudal), from the center of the body to the extremities (proximal-distal), and from attaining the general to the specific skill. This leads to an anatomical progression in which control of facial features is most developed at birth, relative to other body parts, and subsequently control encompasses the upper and then lower body areas. The Denver Developmental Screening Test (Fig. 4-22) outlines the normal sequence in the personal-social, fine motor–adaptive, language, and gross motor developmental areas. Development proceeds toward increasingly specific activities, such as grasping an object in the thumb and finger, uttering specific speech sounds, and briefly balancing one's body weight on one foot. Greater conceptualization and coordination are required for such acts. The variation in age for any particular activity or attribute is a reminder of the substantial amount of entirely normal individual variation. If an infant lags *far* behind developmental expectations based on age, a search for possible causes and sources of remediation is recommended in order to enhance infant development.

Culture and infant development

From the moment of conception, the developmental processes of the human life cycle take place in the context of culture. At no time is the cultural context a negligible feature in human development. However, with the passage of the infant to life outside the uterine environment, the effects of culture on life-cycle development become more obvious, although they are neither more nor less important than the influences of culture before birth. The relationships between the biological and cultural aspects of development and the health-sickness process also become more visible after birth, these relationships have been operating since conception.

The decision of whether or not to breast-

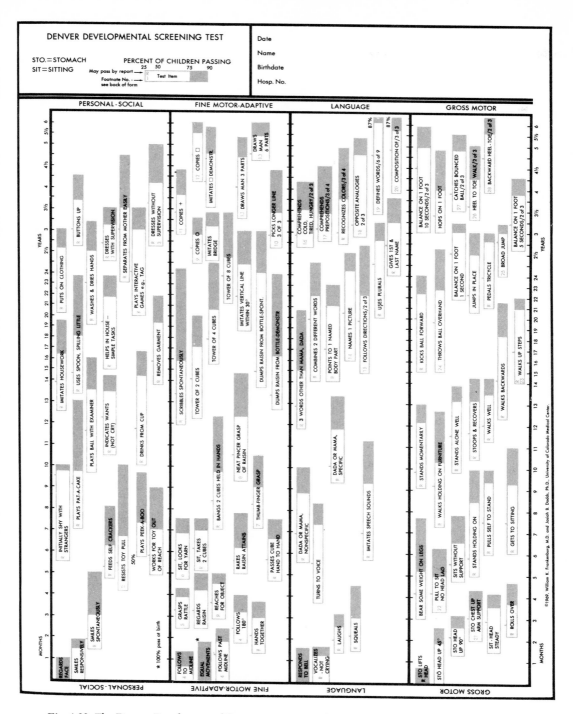

Fig. 4-22. The Denver Developmental Screening Test. Item bars are placed in relation to the age scale to indicate the age range in which 25% to 90% of the children have developed the ability to perform the item.

feed the infant is, normally, a function of cultural influence. In the United States today an increasing proportion of mothers choose to breast-feed. A trend away from breast-feeding to bottle-feeding was evident several decades ago in response to prevailing norms that favored the more "scientific" control of the infant's diet with the use of baby formulas. (It is interesting to note the use of "formula," a scientific term, in this context.) The convenience of bottle-feeding, permitting the mother a schedule that was independent of her infant's, was also an attraction. Curiously, many women today state the convenience of breast-feeding as a reason for preferring breast to bottle, since it dispenses with chores such as washing and heating bottles.

Nutritionally, breast milk meets nearly all of the infant's dietary requirements. Only the amounts of vitamin D, fluoride, and iron are inadequate in human milk. Cow's milk also lacks sufficient amounts of these substances. Human milk fulfills the infant's needs until and possibly beyond the sixth month. Besides its nutritional qualities, human milk is hygienic and inexpensive relative to other sources. Another advantage is the still unexplained contraceptive effect of breast-feeding for some women. The normal postpartum amenorrhea (lack of ovulation) is prolonged by breast-feeding; but its effect is variable, and breast-feeding is not a reliable form of contraception.

The advantages of breast-feeding are particularly pronounced in developing countries where, ironically, breast feeding is undergoing great decline. Dramatic decreases in the number of infants being breast-fed and in the length of time that breast-feeding is practiced are seen, particularly in the urban areas of Chile, Mexico, Singapore, and the Philippines (Knodel, 1977). The decline in breast-feeding is largely a product of culture change in which the bottle has become a status symbol for the "modern" way of life. Also contributing to the decline are advertising campaigns by baby food manufacturers promoting their products with slogans such as, "When mother's milk fails" or "The very best milk for baby." Manufacturers such as Nestlé have come under attack recently for promoting overseas sales with their tactics and the use of "milk nurses," women who go to villages dressed in Western-style white uniforms and dispense free samples of infant formula to nursing mothers, who are then obliged to continue using the bottle once their breast milk has dried up. A lack of opposition to such tactics from the health care community and the mechanical orientation of Western medicine have also been cited as facilitating the move from breast to bottle (Wade, 1974).

The consequences of a decline in breast-feeding in developing countries include important health and economic considerations. Whereas baby food can be purchased for a small fraction of a family's income in the United States, 20% and 50% of family income in Chile and Tanzania, respectively, are required to purchase substitutes for human milk (Wade, 1974). Often the necessary means for preparing baby food are unavailable. Unclean water may be used to dilute formula, or bottles may not be cleaned adequately. Because formula is expensive and its composition not understood, mothers have been reported to make up their own formula from a dilute flour and water mixture. The result of these efforts to "modernize" is tragic. Malnutrition, particularly marasmus, during infancy has increased, and deaths from malnutrition and such diseases as diarrhea have risen (see next section on childhood nutrition and disease). Economic problems have also been exacerbated by the high cost of baby food. The loss of the natural contraceptive effect of breast feeding has shortened the time interval between births, contributing to an overall increase in birth rates. Finally, millions of infants and mothers have been deprived of the warm, personal relationship that is fostered by breast-feeding.

The cultural environment affects infant development through a number of other kinds of influences besides those related to breast-feeding. Studies by Rene Spitz and others during the 1940s and 1950s demonstrated the importance of social stimulation for infant development. Infants raised in orphanages and given adequate nutrition and medical treatment to prevent infectious diseases were still shown to lag far behind their peers in developmental skills, such that 60% could not sit alone by age 2 years and 80% could not walk by age 4 years (Dennis and Najaran, 1957). After 2 years of residence in such a setting, 37% of the infants had died, and the survivors seemed "emotionally starved" (Spitz, 1945). The absence of stimulation from human contact seemed the overriding factor in causing these developmental abnormalities, for the conditions were reversed when contact was restored.

Preparation for parenthood is a part of male and especially female socialization in most cultures. In comparison, middle-class American society provides little in the way of formal or informal training. The experiences of an older child are more conducive for learning the values and responsibilities of adulthood than for learning about child care. Pregnancy is often a time during which couples take prenatal classes, but the emphasis is on preparation for childbirth, not parenting. Books rather than personal experience, thus, are relied on for supplying training for parenthood. Jean Liedloff, when comparing the infant-rearing practices of South American Yeguana Indians to contemporary United States practices, makes this revealing comment; "I would be ashamed to admit to the Indians that where I come from the women do not feel them-

Table 5. Expectations by high school–aged parents for child development*

Area of development	Parental expectations (wks)	
	Mother's	Father's
Social smile	3	3
Sit alone	12	6
Pull up to standing	24	20
First step alone	40	40
Toilet training (wetting)	24	24
Toilet training (bowel)	26	24
First word	32	24
Obedience training	36	26
Recognition of wrong doings	52	40

*From DeLissovoy, 1973.

selves capable of raising children until they read the instructions written in a book by a strange man" (Liedloff, 1977:18).

One effect of inadequate preparation for parenthood pertains to the expectations parents have about developmental norms. In a study of the expectations of high school–aged parents for whom preparation for parenthood had been minimal, expectations for infant development proved unrealistically high. Comparison of their expectations (shown in Table 5) with the Denver Developmental Screening Test norms (Fig. 4-22) reveals that the expectations are in advance of norms by a factor of two or three. (For example, the DDST indicates that sitting alone is possible at 20 to 32 weeks, whereas the adolescent mother's and father's expectations are set at 12 and 6 weeks.)

Health and sickness

Mortality is higher during infancy than at any other time after birth, mostly because of problems encountered in adapting to extrauterine life. At greatest risk is the premature infant, who is less prepared to make the necessary adaptations.

Hyaline membrane disease, more common

in premature than full-term infants, is among the leading causes of infant death in the United States. The precise etiology of hyaline membrane disease is not understood, but the inability of the lungs to meet the challenges of extrauterine life is the most important factor. The lungs are among the last organs to develop in utero, an environment in which the lungs do not function. With birth, the lungs begin their task of oxygenating the blood. In the infant with hyaline membrane disease, areas of gas exchange in the lungs collapse after each respiration, limiting gas exchange and making subsequent respiration more difficult. Treatment of hyaline membrane disease consists of maintaining support for respiration to minimize demands on the lungs until they have attained sufficient maturity to function normally.

Respiratory and digestive disorders are the leading causes of death from several weeks after birth to the end of the first year. Beyond the first year until middle adulthood, accidents become the leading cause of death (Wenner and VanderVeer, 1973). Tuberculosis and sudden infant death syndrome (SIDS) are forms of respiratory disease seen in infants. Tuberculosis can become more serious than in adults because the infant's defense system is immature relative to that of adults. SIDS is a particularly tragic disease because, at present, there are few known warning signs to alert parents to possible danger. A seemingly normal infant, usually in the age range of 4 to 6 months, suddenly stops breathing during sleep and, unless detected, a fatality results. Diarrhea can become a serious digestive disorder in infants because of their greater risk of becoming dehydrated. Diarrhea is particularly common in developing countries and in other situations where food and water are contaminated. In Guatemala, for example, deaths from diarrhea are twenty-five times more

common in infants than they are in the United States. (See next section on childhood nutrition and disease.

Diseases of infancy are, in many instances, distinctive because of the immaturity of the infant relative to the adult. They also tend to become potentially life-threatening more quickly as a result of decreased reserves. Thus, an active disease prevention program is particularly warranted during infancy. Well-baby clinics have become common as a means for monitoring infant development and for detecting abnormalities in developmental patterns. Immunization against childhood diseases such as mumps, chicken pox, poliomyelitis, and measles is recommended. With means for controlling such diseases available, it is alarming to note the trend toward a decreasing number of infants and children receiving immunizations (National Academy of Sciences, 1976). Accidents are another preventable cause of injury, and their rising frequency also stresses the importance of cultural and societal factors that bear on health.

A final example of the importance of the cultural environment during infancy is that of child abuse. Child abuse, or child battery, has become a more widely recognized and perhaps an increasingly frequent problem in the United States, but the phenomenon is not new. Often the parent or caregiver who batters the child was also a battered child and has limited ways of expressing feelings of anger toward the child. Most such individuals are emotionally disturbed, and the fact of child abuse is a cry for help on the part of the parent. Protection of the child is the first step in remedying child abuse. Treatment for the parent or caregiver responsible is also essential. The person responsible often has unrealistic expectations of the infant that lead to mistreatment; for instance, interpreting a persistent cry by the child as an expression of disobedience. Inappropriate expectations, as discussed earlier, are related to more widespread, inadequate preparation for parenthood, which, however, does not usually lead to child abuse. Another culturally related factor appears to be the attitudes toward the infant that were present at and before birth. In a prospective study, parents who appeared less interested in their infants at birth and who were less desirous of having the baby had a higher incidence of child abuse (Gray and others, 1976). These parents also did not bond with their infants, and a failure of bonding has been suggested as another possible factor underlying child abuse (Fig. 4-21).

CHILDHOOD

We now consider a time in the life cycle beginning about 3 age years when the child becomes increasingly independent of the parents while growing in size and acquiring complex social characteristics from the culture. Gender asserts itself very early in life, with evidences of both genetic and cultural contributions to maleness or femaleness. The nature of the environment in villages, towns, and cities influences the child's development, attitudes, values, and health. Education is prominent in the child's daily life, and it is often during childhood that special gifts or talents become evident, for example, for music, drawing, painting, athletics, poetry, or acting. Childhood is first and foremost a time for discovery of self, family, society, and environment that leads to the next transition in the human life cycle—puberty.

Child growth and development

Physical development continues during childhood in much the same pattern as was established in infancy, although the overall rate of growth is slowed appreciably. The pattern of growth continues to follow the pattern of general to specific abilities, from the center of the body toward the extremities (proximal-distal), and from the head down (cephalo-caudal). Adult head size is attained by age 5 years; the remainder of the body continues its growth through adolescence. Physiological maturation occurs in organ systems, such as the kidneys, the immune defense system, and the circulatory and respiratory systems. Maturation of the central nervous system continues through and beyond childhood, however.

The Denver Developmental Screening Test (Fig. 4-22) points to the increasing independence, complexity of capacities, and degree of coordination exhibited by the child. For example, children can dress themselves, initially with and then without supervision; copy and later draw figures; define words; and engage in tasks requiring considerable coordination, such as balancing on one foot for an extended period and walking "heel to toe."

Learning, particularly language acquisition, occupies a central place in child development. In a normal environment in which language is spoken, language development appears to be spontaneous in the child, suggesting an innate, genetically programmed capacity for language as a characteristic of the human species. Most animals possess some kind of signaling communication system, but only human beings appear to have a symbol-based system, distinguished by its flexibility, inventiveness, and abstract nature. In language, sound is separated from meaning and can be recombined in a potentially infinite number of ways to refer to objects that may or may not be present or that may be symbolic abstractions that do not exist in any concrete sense. A great many attempts to teach language to chimpanzees and other apes have revealed that apes cannot equal the speed or complexity of human beings in learning vocal or nonvocal languages (such as American Sign Language) of human invention. Washoe and other apes have shown us, however, that the capacity to learn language may not be restricted to human beings. Much more remains to be discovered about language learning, but it would appear that the genetic relationship between ourselves and the living great apes is sufficiently close to result in some degree of sharing language abilities, which used to be considered a uniquely human attribute.

During childhood, the limited vocabulary of the infant expands explosively with a command of thousands of words that can be combined in grammatically complex sentences. Marked variation in vocabulary size and word usage exists as a normal occurrence, although failure for language to develop may signal abnormal development of the brain. Girls generally acquire language at an earlier age than do boys and continue to excel in verbal abilities throughout childhood (Hamburg, 1974). Continued cognitive development during childhood leads to increasing vocabulary and familiarity with subtleties of grammar, pronunciation, and word usage along with growing memory skills and abilities to reason and perceive relationships.

The social development of the child proceeds in a variety of ways such that the child becomes instructed in the values and behaviors considered appropriate in that society. Some psychologists have concentrated on the emotional aspects of development. Erik Erikson has proposed a lifelong theory, referred to again in Chapter 5, in which attributes to be mastered during childhood are a sense of autonomy, initiative, and industry. Other child psychologists, such as Rudolf Dreikurs and B. F. Skinner, emphasize in differing ways the importance of the interaction between the child and members of the child's environment for emotional and social development. As the child grows older, the association between the child and other family members broadens so that, for example, in the United States, the school group and peers become important socializing influences.

Culture figures importantly in deciding the kinds of environmental influences to which the child is exposed. A long history of studies in anthropology directed at understanding the influences of culture on child development has evolved under the rubric of the culture and personality school of thought, or psychological anthropology as it is termed today. Leaders in the study of culture and personality, such as Ruth Benedict, sought to correlate the type of personality manifested during adulthood with the child-rearing practices of a particular culture. These are referred to as national-character studies. For example, Ruth Benedict saw the contradiction inherent in Japanese child-rearing practices in which the privilege and comfort of early childhood ended abruptly with the imposition of heavy responsibilities and severe sanctions as contributing to extreme behaviors, such as self-sacrifice and a dualistic character that combined opposites such as politeness and arrogance (1946:290-291). Criticism of the national-character studies has emphasized their tendency to oversimplify factors governing personality and to ignore consideration of individual variation and particular historical circumstance.

Subsequent efforts, such as those of John Whiting and Irvin Child, attempted more comprehensive studies that viewed child-rearing practices as an integral part of culture. A universal goal of child rearing is the transformation of the child into a responsible adult who obeys the rules of society. The techniques employed, the precise character of the rules to which the child must conform, and the age at which conformity is expected vary, however. For example, a survey of seventy-five cultures, representing a broad cross section of geographical areas, revealed marked variation regarding nursing and weaning, toilet training, sex education, independence training, aggression, and the over-all indulgence or severity with which practices were carried out. Nursing indulgence ranged from permitting the child to nurse on demand through the age of 3 or 4 years to more severe practices in some cultures, such as among the Marquesans, who believed that nursing makes a child hard to raise and not properly submissive, and so feeding was conducted at the convenience of adults. Ages for weaning ranged in this multiculture sample from less than 1 year to over 3½ years and from 1 to 5 years for toilet training. Middle-class European and American cultures are among the most severe in exerting pressure on the bodily and emotional development of the young child (Whiting and Child, 1953).

Child-rearing practices in the United States have also been the concern of Urie Bronfenbrenner, who sees patterns of age segregation and a lack of emphasis on cooperation as potential problem areas. The model of the rugged individualist, aggressive and successful by virtue of getting ahead of one's peers, is seen as a source of antisocial, violent tendencies (1970:117). The changes occurring in the state of children and their families in the United States today are discussed further in Chapter 5 (in the section on family formation, change, and variation).

Thus, the process of child growth and development is guided by cultural norms and expectations along with the operation of influences controlled by genes and the physiological maturation of organs and organ systems. Health-related consequences of these biological and cultural factors are discussed in the next two sections.

Nutrition and disease

Nutritional problems are common during childhood, but the nature and severity of the problems vary markedly. Among the poor and in developing cultures, the pressing problem is malnutrition. In middle-class America, obesity is the more common nutritional problem during childhood. Discussion here centers on malnutrition and its relationship to childhood mortality and morbidity.

Children and infants are particularly susceptible to malnutrition in areas of the world where the rapid rate of population growth limits food supply. Malnutrition stems fundamentally from an inadequate food intake, but a host of other factors influence food intake and the development of malnutrition (Fig. 4-23). The decline in breast-feeding cited earlier is of major importance in the etiology of malnutrition, particularly in the infant and young child. Natural disasters, social upheavals caused by wars or political unrest, and maldistribution of wealth and food habits influence food intake. Digestive disorders, most commonly diarrhea, resulting from unclean food or water or other disease states also may reduce food intake or the amount of substances taken up by the body (malabsorption). Other coexisting diseases or defects may also help promote malnutrition.

There are two principal forms of malnutrition: marasmus and kwashiorkor. Marasmus, a Greek word that means "wasting," results from inadequate intake of protein and calories. Marasmus typically affects younger children and infants, particularly after they have been weaned. In situations where breast-feeding has declined, the onset of marasmus occurs at an even earlier age. Marasmus may be difficult to detect because its onset is slow and obvious physical signs are usually lacking. The face may appear pinched. Both weight and stature are retarded, but unless the child's age is known, the child may simply be mistaken for being younger. Kwaskiorkor usually affects children over 2 years of age and stems from protein deficiency in the presence of normal caloric intake. The onset of kwashiorkor, com-

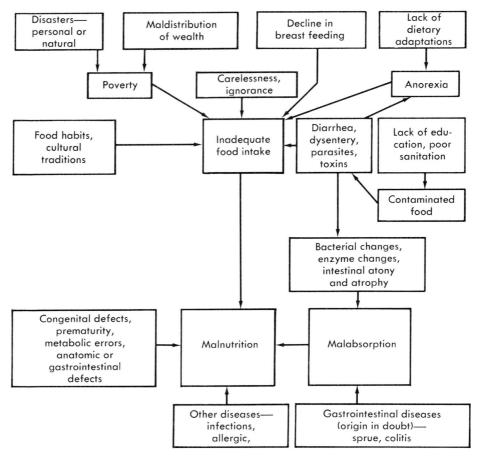

Fig. 4-23. Factors influencing the development of malnutrition in children. (Adapted from Williams, 1962.)

pared to marasmus, is rapid and obvious. Swelling (edema) is seen in the hands, legs, and face, leading to the diagnostic "moon" face. Protein deficiency prompts a loss of pigmentation, producing lightened hair color in dark-haired people and patchy, flaky discolorations of the skin. A distended belly may give the child with kwashiorkor the appearance of being well fed, or even overfed; the distention is a reflection of edema and other metabolic disturbances of malnutrition. Growth is retarded by kwashiorkor as well, but because of the edema, only stature and not body weight may be abnormal.

Either marasmus or kwashiorkor can by itself be fatal. Alternatively and more commonly, they may lead to secondary disorders of anemia, vomiting, and diarrhea. Vomiting and diarrhea aggravate the malnutrition further through loss of fluids and scarce nutrients. Diarrhea, not always associated with malnutrition, is the leading cause of child deaths and sickness in Guatemala, as well as in many other areas of the world. Childhood mortality from diarrhea is more than 500 times higher in Guatemala than in the United States (Logan, 1973). Cultural traditions may exacerbate the diarrhea in that one of the

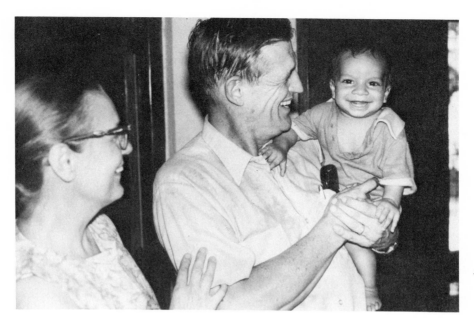

Fig. 4-24. Nutritional inadequacies can be corrected in certain instances. Soya added to the food of this child from India brought his weight up to normal within a few weeks. (Courtesy United Methodist Church, Joint Committee on Communications.)

treatments in highland Guatemala is to withhold fluids so as to solidify wastes, but the resultant dehydration increases mortality. Other treatments include the elimination of possible causes, such as unclean water, and objects that may have intruded into the body (for example, parasites) (Logan, 1973).

The rapid brain growth and development that occur during infancy and childhood render the brain a particularly vulnerable organ under conditions of malnutrition. This is reflected in the hyperirritable, apathetic, and unresponsive behaviors of the infant or child with marasmus and the apathetic, inert, and anorexic disposition of the child with kwashiorkor. If the child who has experienced sustained and severe malnutrition survives, permanent stunting of brain growth and mental retardation are likely (Winick, 1976). However, controversy continues as to whether "catch-up" growth is possible. Available evidence suggests that an adequate diet

has to be sustained for an extended period and that periodic supplements are insufficient for normal brain growth to be restored (Winick, Meyer, and Harris, 1975) (Fig. 4-24).

Child health in developed countries

Children in developed countries exhibit illness patterns in which disorders are caused mainly by accidents, infections, behavior difficulties, congenital malformations, and malignancies (Figs. 4-25 and 4-26). Importantly, as the birth rate in the United States has declined to barely replacement levels, American parents exhibit greater concern about the quality of each offspring while their expectations for their children have increased. Children's performances in learning, social adaptation, and personality formation receive daily attention in all forms of electronic and printed media and also occupy much of parents' conversation and thoughts. In other words, the purely physical aspects of health have become relatively minor worries, bringing the social-behavioral development of children into first rank among health priorities.

Child mortality in nearly all developed countries is at or below a level of one per 1000. The predominant causes tend to be accidents and congenital malformations. Accidents account for more than 40% of male and 30% of female mortality among children. By way of contrast, accidents account for usually less than 10% of childhood mortality in developing nations (Marcusson and Oemisch, 1977).

Motor vehicle accidents rank first among fatal accidents to children, followed by accidental drowning. The trend from 1955 to 1971 shows a decline in mortality for both sexes during the younger years (ages 1 to 4 years) but an increase in older age groups (5 to 9 and 10 to 14 years) because of increased numbers of deaths from motor vehicle accidents (Marcusson and Oemisch, 1977). Accident prevention is a societal con-

cern that requires participation by parents and community and civic leaders, not just by health authorities. Such efforts have been undertaken in Sweden and the German Democratic Republic and have been aimed at prevention (for example, popularizing learning how to swim, ways of ensuring road safety, fire protection) and at investigating accident-caused deaths. Keeping children off roads and impressing on them the need to pay attention to traffic are also vital for reducing traffic fatalities (Marcusson and Oemisch, 1977). Also, instruction of parents on the importance of always using car safety seats for infants and children is needed because an automobile accident that has only minor impact for an adult could be fatal for an infant or child.

Another example of the importance of environmental features in governing the health of children in developed countries is that of mental retardation. Causes of mental retardation are numerous, and knowledge about such causes is likely to increase in the future. One classification divides "organic"

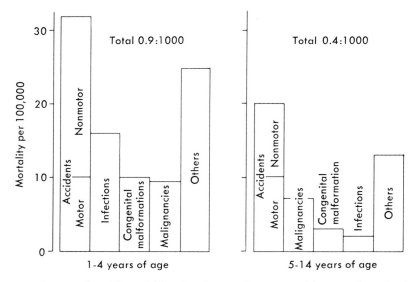

Fig. 4-25. Mortality in early and later childhood in the United States, 1965. (From Holm and Wiltz, 1973: 125.)

from "functional" causes. The former include genetic, metabolic, infectious, chemical, traumatic, and nutritional dysfunctions, as well as complications of gestation and parturition, such as oxygen deprivation or prematurity. On the other hand, functional mental retardation does not evidence any of these causes and is frequently identified for the first time when a child begins formal schooling. Parents who do not suspect impaired intelligence in their child are shocked and upset when informed by school authorities that their son or daughter is slower to learn than the others. Causes of functional mental retardation are still only vaguely understood, but epidemiology has suggested a relationship with poverty and the environmental conditions in which the child lives.

According to the President's Committee on Mental Retardation (1968:19), (1) "Three-fourths of the nation's mentally retarded are to be found in the isolated and impoverished urban and rural slums," and (2) "Conservative estimates of the incidence of mental retardation in inner city neighborhoods begin at seven percent." The 1968 committee report states also that, "The children of low income families often arrive at school age

with neither the experience nor the skills necessary for systematic learning. Many are found functionally retarded in language and in the ability to do the abstract thinking required to read, write, and count. An appalling number of these children fall further behind with the passing of each school year."

A map of poverty areas in St. Louis, Missouri (Fig. 4-5) shows a greater concentration of functionally mentally retarded children in urban poverty sectors than in suburbs. Similar data were developed by the committee for other large cities. Some of the reasons cited are lack of stimulation of infants and children by parents, such as very limited verbalization and limited contact as compared to that provided by middle-class parents. Among the recommended measures were installation of day care centers in poverty areas of urban centers where mothers working outside the home can leave their children in a stimulating environment. A number of social factors enter into the definition of retardation and the kinds of remedies that are available for functionally mentally retarded children. Deteriorating buildings, limited play areas, discriminatory practices limiting access to job and educational op-

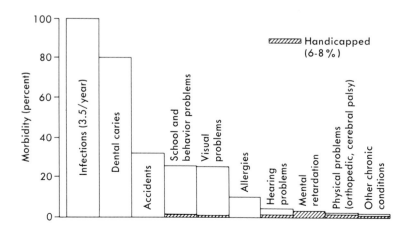

Fig. 4-26. Morbidity during childhood. (From Holm and Wiltz, 1973:125.)

portunities for parents, poor quality and inappropriately tailored schools that do not promote effective learning for ghetto children (see Kozol, 1967) all play a part.

In conclusion, child mortality results largely from preventable diseases or disorders in both developed and developing countries, although the particular causes and, therefore, remedies, vary. Child mortality over the past 2 decades is falling in both developed and developing regions, yet the differentials between the two kinds of regions continue to be more pronounced during childhood than at any other time of life (Dyson, 1977). Improvements in nutrition, sanitation, and clean water supply can be anticipated to be highly effective in reducing child mortality and morbidity in developing areas. Maternal and child health programs continue to be important, but these should be carried out while simultaneously attacking poor nutrition, insufficient sanitation, and infectious and other diseases. Parental and societal cooperation is needed to confront health problems such as accidents and to ensure the utilization of resources available for health maintenance, such as developmental screening programs and immunization.

REFERENCES

Aldrich, R. A. A life science for epoch B. In Oberttress, H. (ed.). *The Nature of a Humane Society.* Philadelphia: Fortress Press, 1976.

Aldrich, R. A. Normal growth and development of infants and children. *Ekistics,* Oct. 1968, pp. 378-381.

Arms, S. *Immaculate Deception, A New Look at Women and Childbirth in America.* New York: Bantam Books, Inc., 1975.

Benedict, R. *The Chrysanthemum and the Sword.* Boston: Houghton-Mifflin Co., 1946.

Bronfenbrenner, U. *Two Worlds of Children.* New York: Russell Sage Foundation, 1970.

Brazelton, T. B. *Infants and Mothers.* New York: The Delacorte Press, 1969.

Breslow, L., and Somers, A. R. The lifetime health-monitoring program. *New England Journal of Medicine,* 1977, 296(11), 601-608.

Comstock, S., and others. Low birth weight and neo-

natal mortality rate related to maternal smoking and socioeconomic status. *American Journal of Obstetrics and Gynecology,* 1971, 3, 53-59.

DeLissovoy, V. Child care by adolescent parents. *Children Today,* 1973, 2(4), 22-25.

Dennis, W., and Najarian, P. Infant development under environmental handicap. *Psychological Monographs,* 1957, 71, 436.

Doxiadis, C. A. *Anthropopolis—City for Human Development.* Athens, Greece: Athens Publishing Center, 1974.

Doxiadis, C. A. *Ekistics—An Introduction to the Science of Human Settlements.* London: Oxford University Press, 1968.

Doxiadis, C. A. How can we learn about man and his settlements? In Rapoport, A. (ed.). *The Mutual Interaction of People and Their Built Environment.* Paris: Mouton Publishers, 1976.

Dyson, T. Levels, trends, differentials and causes of child mortality—a survey. *World Health Statistics Report,* 1977, 30(4), 282-311.

Foch, N. South American birth customs in theory and practice. In Ford, C. S. (ed.). *Cross Cultural Approaches.* New Haven, Conn.: Human Relations Area File Press, 1967, pp. 126-144.

Forfar, J., and Arneil, G. *Textbook of Pediatrics.* London, 1973, pp. 880-881.

Fuchs, V. R. *The Great Infant Mortality, or What Caused the Slump?* Unpublished manuscript, used with permission, 1978.

Gray, J., Cutler, C., Dean, J., and Kempe, C. H. Perinatal assessment of mother-baby interaction. In Helfer, R. E., and Kempe, C. H. (eds.). *Child-Abuse and Neglect: The Family and The Community.* Cambridge, Mass.: Ballinger Publishing Co., 1976, pp. 377-392.

Hamburg, B. The psychobiology of sex differences. In Friedman, R., Richart, R., and VandeWiele, R. (eds.). *Sex Differences in Behavior.* New York: John Wiley & Sons, Inc., 1974.

Hammerton, J. L. *Human Cytogenetics, vol. 2.* New York: Academic Press, Inc., 1971.

Holm, V., and Wiltz, N. A. Childhood. In Smith, D. W., and Bierman, E. L. (eds.). *The Biologic Ages of Man.* Philadelphia: W. B. Saunders Co., 1973.

Holmes, L. B. Genetic counseling for the older woman: new data and questions. *New England Journal of Medicine,* 1978, 298(25), 1419-1421.

Holmes, T. H., and Masuda, M. Life change and illness susceptibility. In Scott, P., and Senay, E. (eds.). *Separation and Depression.* Washington, D.C.: American Association for the Advancement of Science, no. 94, 1973, pp. 161-186.

Hytten, F. E. Smoking in pregnancy. *Developmental Medicine and Child Neurology,* 1973, 15, 355.

Jones, K. L., and Smith, D. W. Recognition of the fetal alcohol syndrome in early infancy. *Lancet*, 1973, *2*, 999.

Klaus, M. H., and Kennell, J. H. *Maternal-Infant Bonding: The Impact of Early Separation or Loss on Family Development*. St. Louis: The C. V. Mosby Co., 1976.

Knodel, J. Breast-feeding and Population Growth. *Science*, 1977, *198*, 1111.

Knowles, J. H. Introduction to doing better and feeling worse: health in the United States. *Daedalus, Journal of the American Academy of Arts and Sciences*, 1977, *106*, 1-7.

Kozol, J. *Death at an Early Age*. Boston: Houghton-Mifflin Co., 1967.

Leakey, R. E., and Lewin, R. *People of the Lake: Mankind and Its Beginnings*. Garden City, N.Y.: Anchor Press, 1978.

Leboyer, F. *Birth Without Violence*. New York: Alfred A. Knopf, Inc., 1976.

Lichty, J. A., and others. Studies of babies born at high altitude. *American Journal of Diseases of Children*, 1957, *93*, 665-669.

Liedloff, J. *The Continuum Concept*. New York: Alfred A. Knopf, Inc., 1976.

Logan, M. H. Digestive disorders and plant medicinals in highland Guatemala. *Anthropos*, 1973, *68*, 538-547.

Marcusson, H., and Oemisch, W. Accident mortality in childhood in selected countries of different continents, 1950-1977. *World Health Statistics Report*, 1977, *30*(1), 57-92.

McClain, C. Ethno-obstetrics in Ajijic. *Anthropological Quarterly*, 1975, *48*, 38-56.

McDaniel, E. B., and Tieng, P. Acceptability of an injectable contraceptive in a rural population in Thailand. In Logan, M. H., and Hunt, E. E. (eds.). *Health and the Human Condition*. N. Scituate, N.Y.: Duxbury Press, 1978, pp. 328-340.

Michaels, R. H., and Mellin, G. W. Prospective experience with maternal rubella and the associated congenital malformations. *Pediatrics*, 1960, *26*, 200.

National Academy of Sciences. *Proceedings of a Workshop on Nutritional Supplementation and the Outcome of Pregnancy*. Washington, D.C.: National Academy of Sciences, 1973.

National Academy of Sciences. *Toward a National Policy for Children and Families*. Washington, D.C.: National Academy of Sciences, 1976.

Newton, N., and Modahl, C. Pregnancy: the closest relationship. *Human Nature*, March 1978, pp. 40-49.

NICHD National Registry for Amniocentesis Study Group. Midtrimester amniocentesis for prenatal diagnosis: safety and accuracy. *Journal of the American Medical Association*, 1976, *236*, 1471-1476.

Polgar, S., and Marshall, J. F. The search for culturally acceptable fertility regulating methods. In Logan, M. H., and Hunt, E. E. (eds.). *Health and the Human Condition*. N. Scituate, N.Y.: Duxbury Press, 1978, pp. 328-340.

President's Committee on Mental Retardation 68: *The Edge of Change: A Report to the President on Mental Retardation Program Trends and Innovations, With Recommendations on Residential Care, Manpower, and Deprivation*. U.S. Government Printing Office, Washington, D.C., 1968.

President's Panel on Mental Retardation. *Report to the President. National Action to Combat Mental Retardation*. U.S. Government Printing Office, Washington, D.C., 1962.

Puck, T. T., and Robinson, A. Some perspectives in human cytogenetics. In Corre, R. E., (ed.). *The Biologic Basis of Pediatric Practice*. New York: McGraw-Hill Book Co., 1968.

Reisman, L. E., and Matheny, A. P., Jr. *Genetics and Counseling in Medical Practice*. St. Louis: The C. V. Mosby Co., 1969.

Roberts, R. C. On the uniform lineal growth of the human fetus. *Lancet*, 1906, *170*, 295-296.

Roche, A. F. Physical growth of ethnic groups comprising the U.S. population. *American Journal of Diseases of Children*, 1976, *130*, 62-64.

Rush, D., Stein, Z., Christakis, G., and Suser, M. The prenatal project: the first 20 months of operation. In Winick, M. (ed.). *Current Concepts in Nutrition*, vol. 2. New York: John Wiley & Sons, Inc., 1974, p. 95.

Salas, R. M. The state of world population 1978. *United Nations Fund for Population Activities*. United Nations, New York, 1978.

Sidney, H. Why small town boys make good. *Time Magazine*, 1976, *107*(22), 17.

Silverman, W. A. The lesson of retrolental fibroplasia. *Scientific American*, 1977, *236*(6), 100-107.

Smith, D. W. Growth. In Smith, D. W., and Bierman, E. L. (eds.). *The Biologic Ages of Man*. Philadelphia: W. B. Saunders Co., 1973, pp. 1-16.

Smith, D. W., and Der Yuen, D. Prenatal life and the pregnant woman. In Smith, D. W., and Bierman, E. L. (eds.). *The Biologic Ages of Man*. Philadelphia: W. B. Saunders Co., 1973, pp. 32-61.

Spierer, H. *Major Transitions in the Human Life Cycle*. New York: Academy for Educational Development, 1977.

Spitz, R. Hospitalism: an inquiry into the genesis of psychologic conditions in early childhood. *Psychoanalytic Studies of the Child*, 1945, *1*, 53-74.

Stein, Z., and others. *Famine and Human Development*. New York: Oxford University Press, 1975.

United Nations. *Levels and Trends of Fertility Through-*

out the World. 1950-70. United Nations, New York, 1977.

Wade, N. Bottle-feeding: adverse effects of a Western technology. *Science,* 1974, *184,* 45-48.

Weaver, W. Science and complexity. *The American Scientist,* 1948, *6,* 536-544.

Wenner, W. H., and VanderVeer, B. Infancy: the first two years. In Smith, D. W., and Bierman, E. L. (eds.). *The Biologic Ages of Man.* Philadelphia: W. B. Saunders Co., 1973.

Whiting, J., and Child, I. *Child Training and Personality.* New Haven, Conn.: Yale University Press, 1953.

WHO Scientific Group. Human development and public health. *WHO Technical Report,* Series No. 485, Geneva, 1972.

Williams, C. D. Malnutrition. *Lancet,* 1962, *2,* 342-344.

Williams, L., Spence, M., and Tideman, S. Implications of the observed effect of air pollution on infant birth weight. *Social Biology,* 1977, *24*(1), 1-9.

Winick, M. *Malnutrition and Brain Development.* New York: Oxford University Press, 1976.

Winick, M., Meyer, K. K., and Harris, R. C. Malnutrition and environmental enrichment by early adoption. *Science,* 1975, *190,* 1173-1175.

Woollam, D. H. M. Thalidomide disaster considered as experiment in mammalian teratology. *British Medical Journal,* 1962, 5299, 236.

World Health Statistics Annual, 1973-1976. Geneva: World Health Organization, 1976, pp. 774-775.

CHAPTER 5

Health determinants during later phases of the human life cycle

The realization that the health of the 1-year-old infant may have important bearing on the health of the same child at 2 or 5 years of age is well appreciated. It is not so common to realize the interrelationships among phases of the life cycle as they extend into adulthood. The later phases of the life cycle, beginning at puberty and extending until death, have been less thoroughly studied than the earlier phases of the life cycle. The reasons are clear; the signs of biological change are less obvious with the completion of physical growth, at least until we approach the end of the life cycle. Until recently, American society has resisted the recognition of aging during adulthood, preferring to emphasize the notion of continuity and so contributing to a denial of the fact of aging (Butler, 1975). As proportionately more of American society reaches old age and as the average age of the American population increases, interest in the adult phases of the life cycle is growing.

Cultures vary in the extent to which they recognize continued development during the later phases of the life cycle. A form of recognition that exists in a great many cultures is the rite of passage. The notion of rite of passage was advanced by a French anthropologist, Arnold Van Gennep, as a means of understanding change in age status. Age may be determined by time; alternatively, age may be reckoned by position or standing in soci-ety, termed "age status." Van Gennep undertook an exhaustive survey of the available literature, recording the occurrence of rites of passage that he regarded as "ceremonies whose essential purpose is to enable the individual to pass from one defined position to another which is equally well defined." (Van Gennep, 1960:2-3). These ceremonies marked the appearance and the resolution of "life crises" that occur at birth, puberty, maturity, marriage, old age, and death—times analogous to many of the life events depicted in Fig. 4-3. Further, the ceremonies always shared three major phases—separation, transition and incorporation—although each phase may not be equally elaborated in each kind of life crisis. The regularity and order apparent in these ceremonies impressed Van Gennep, as did the fact that the rites of passage provided "transitional periods which sometimes acquire a certain autonomy" (Van Gennep, 1960:191-2). Rites of passage, then, serve to make explicit the individual's membership in a certain age group in society and the individual's transition to subsequent age groups.

The notion of rite of passage is used in this chapter to help delineate the later phases of the life cycle, for society plays a particularly key role in defining these periods of development. This chapter also continues the theme of the previous one; namely, that each phase of the life cycle, while different, is linked to previous and subsequent phases and that the factors affecting each phase have important ramifications for health. We continue to draw on information from human biology and cultures to develop these themes.

PUBERTY AND ADOLESCENCE

The clearest sign of the end of childhood and beginning of adolescence is puberty, the attainment of sexual development. Puberty completes the process of sexual identification that began with the chance occurrence of the fertilization of the ovum by a sperm bearing either an X or Y chromosome.

Biological and psychological changes

Puberty is initiated by the adolescent growth spurt, a speed-up in the rate of growth seen in all human populations (Tanner, 1973). The adolescent growth spurt occurs on the average 2 years earlier in girls than in boys for still unknown reasons. The growth spurt primarily results from increased levels of testosterone secreted by the developing reproductive organs of both sexes and, to a lesser extent, from increased estrogen secretion by the female ovaries. Testosterone is a potent anabolic steroid, meaning that it stimulates protein synthesis. Because greater amounts of testosterone are secreted in the male, the male experiences a relatively greater growth spurt than does the female (Tanner, 1973). Increased estrogen secretion in the female at puberty is associated with an increase in the proportion of body fat. Adolescent growth produces an obvious increase in skeletal height, but it also is accompanied by expansion of the vascular bed, increase of the muscle mass, alteration in muscle distribution, and increase in nutrition demands. The occurrence of these changes differs not only in degree but in kind between the sexes. For example, broadening of the shoulders is seen in males, whereas a widening of the hips occurs in females.

The alteration of biological systems dur-ing puberty is profound. Not only are the musculoskeletal and cardiovascular systems affected, but also affected are the other systems of human development (Fig. 4-3). The growth of pubic and axillary hair occurs along with increased oily secretions of the sebaceous glands, prompting the problem of acne in some adolescents. Changes in the endocrine system stimulate maturation of the male and female reproductive systems. Hormonally triggered, the monthly menstrual cycle is begun in which the ovaries release one of the eggs (now matured but present from embryonic life) and the inner lining of the uterus builds up and later is expelled during menstruation if fertilization has not occurred. The growth of the testes is accompanied by maturation of cells producing sperm. Even though girls begin their adolescent growth spurt on the average 2 years earlier than boys, the occurrence of sexual maturation tends to be closer together in time (Eveleth and Tanner, 1976). Within each sex, there is great individual variation in the age of attainment of sexual maturity. Consequently, some teenagers may have completed their sexual development before their peers have yet begun.

Menarche or the age at which menstruation begins is the most obvious and also the most commonly recorded sign of puberty. Menarcheal age exhibits pronounced historical as well as cultural variation. Within the United States and western Europe, median menarcheal age is currently nearly 2 years earlier than it was at the beginning of this century and some 4 years earlier than 100 years ago (Fig. 5-1). The current age of menarche in the United States, 12.8 years, is among the youngest recorded in the world (data from MacMahon, 1973, cited in Eveleth and Tanner, 1976). In populations studied throughout the world, the menarcheal age is earlier in urban segments than in rural segments, as seen in Fig. 5-2. Also girls from wealthy families attain menarche earlier than

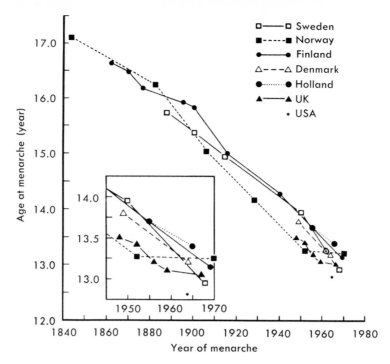

Fig. 5-1. Trend toward earlier median age of menarche in Europe from 1840 to 1970. (From Eveleth and Tanner, 1976:28.)

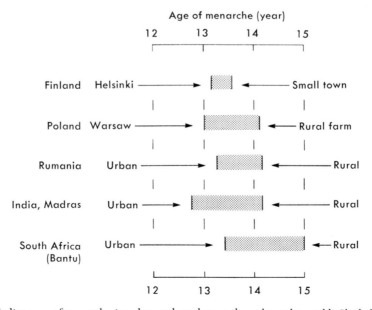

Fig. 5-2. Median ages of menarche in urban and rural areas throughout the world. Shaded areas show difference between median ages in each geographic area. (From Eveleth and Tanner, 1976:259.)

do girls from poor families within the same population (Eveleth and Tanner, 1976). The causes of variation in age of menarche are not precisely known, although nutrition and possibly the attainment of a critical amount of body fat are thought to play a role (for recent review, see Trussel, 1978, and reply by Frisch, 1978). However, differences in menarcheal age between populations in studies controlling for environmental factors would appear to support additional cultural and genetic influences (Eveleth and Tanner, 1976).

Puberty is marked by important changes in personality and social development as well. Erik Erikson (1950) proposed that adolescence was a period of conflict between developing a stable identity versus role confusion. To develop a sense of identity, the adolescent looks for congruity between sense of self and appearance to others. Adolescents may seem preoccupied with and outwardly confident about their appearance, but inwardly they are often uncertain whether something is wrong.

Becoming free of parental domination or renegotiating parental authority may occur at this stage and, in some cases, may lead to problems of juvenile delinquency, and rebellion against parental and other kinds of authority. The move away from the family is generally replaced not by reliance on self but rather by dependence on the peer group for authority. The adolescent may also seek new or heightened physical sensations by pushing oneself to the limits of one's endurance, finding out how much or how little one can eat, or experiencing the effects of drugs and alcohol. The demands placed on the self may seem contradictory, at times leading to self-denial and at other times to overindulgence in pleasures such as food, drink, or sexual relationships. The adolescent's sense of morality may also seem exaggerated, seeking the absolute and ideological solution rather than the best compromise (Werkman, 1974).

Rites of passage

In many cultures, rites of passage at the time of puberty serve to redefine the position of the individual in the society from that of a child to that of an adult. Descriptions of rites of passage at the time of puberty abound. Service describes the ceremonies seen in the late nineteenth century among the Andaman Islanders of the Indian Ocean (Service, 1978: 60-61). Once menarche is attained, a girl in this society is secluded in a hut for several days. Her behavior is closely regulated by prescriptions concerning bathing, posture, speaking, eating, and sleeping. The personal name used during childhood is replaced by one taken from a plant in bloom during the ceremony and is retained until the next rite of passage (marriage). A boy reaching puberty does not experience physical isolation but is singled out by the occasion of an all-night dance held in his honor. Scarification of his back and chest further emphasizes his coming change in status. Dietary restrictions are enforced for a period of a year or more, at the end of which time the boy is given a new name.

Puberty rites serve to eliminate ambiguity in the change from childhood to adulthood by providing transition with autonomy, a process that clearly demarcates the status of a child from that of an adult. The rite of passage also serves to cement the ties between adolescents and the society that accepts them.

In the United States, evidence of rites of passage can be seen in the confirmation and bar mitzvah ceremonies of the Christian and Jewish religions respectively, in the "coming out" parties for members of the urban upper class (or by those aspiring to membership), and in the commencement ceremonies for high school and college graduations. But by virtue of the multiplicity of ceremonies and confusion over their meaning, the transition from childhood to adulthood is rendered ambiguous. The timing of rites such as confirmation has been modified in response to social demands for earlier membership in the church. But another factor that has fostered ambiguity has been the previously discussed change in the age of puberty. The high school commencement ceremony may have effectively acted as a rite of passage to the 17 year olds of 1850, but it fails to signal a change of status to the 17 year olds of today, for most of whom puberty occurred some 4 years earlier. As a result, the adolescent is in a kind of "no man's land"—not needed in the work force, an adult sexually but treated as a child in terms of access to many jobs, to marriage, and to other markers of adulthood. The educational system has become the limbo to which the adolescent is relegated, perhaps for as long as 10 to 20 years, before being permitted the passage to adulthood.

In American society, considerable turbulence is likely to accompany biological, social, and personality development during adolescence. As might be expected, health considerations during adolescence are in part related to this turbulence. Turbulence, however, is not an inevitable accompaniment in all cultures, as Margaret Mead demonstrated in her pioneering work *Coming of Age in Samoa* (1928). In Samoa, the adolescent differed from a prepuberty sibling only by the presence of bodily changes that were absent in the younger person. This difference between American and Samoan experiences was attributed to a general casualness of life in Samoa in which there were few conflicts, few choices permitted the individual, little debate about moral standards, greater openness toward sex and education in matters of birth and death, and less differentiation between the worlds of children and adults (Mead, 1928).

Health considerations

Health problems for the adolescent in American society seem to revolve around the conflicts that are inherent in the desire to make the transition to adulthood while not being formally accorded adult status. Accidents, murder, and suicides are, in that order, the leading causes of death among adolescents (WHO statistics cited by Smith and Bierman, 1973). The majority of accidents involve automobiles; the automobile for many adolescents becomes a symbol of independence, and receiving one's driver's license may be considered a rite of passage for the American adolescent. Murder and suicide reflect, in part, difficulties in making the social and psychological transition to adulthood in keeping with one's physical maturation. Mood swings, transient neuroses, and antisocial behavior are also seen in adolescents struggling to find their identity and to establish independence. In a quest for heightened physical sensations, experimentation with drugs that range from alcohol, barbiturates, amphetamines, opiates, and hallucinogens has increased among adolescents and can result in psychic dependence as well as diseases such as hepatitis from nonsterile injections.

One of the newest health-related phenomena among adolescents in the United States is the rise in teenage pregnancies. From 1940 to 1976, the birth rate among 15- to 19-year-old unmarried girls has quadrupled (from eight to twenty-four per 1000), amounting to some 500,000 teenage pregnancies annually (Fackler and Brandstadt, 1976). While debate continues on the cause of the rise in births to teenagers, factors suggested include increased fecundity and fertility resulting from earlier menarche and increased ability of the pregnant girl to reach term (Fackler and Brandstadt, 1976), the "pull" to the realm outside the classroom that is often portrayed by the communications media as more meaningful, and increased premarital sex along with incomplete knowledge about effective contraception. Getting pregnant may also be considered an attempt to achieve recognition as an adult, since having and raising children are considered marks of adulthood.

Sexual experimentation also may lead to venereal disease. While reported rates of syphilis have not changed in recent years, the rise in gonorrhea has led authorities to describe it as an epidemic. The availability of effective antibiotic treatment has done little to lessen the incidence (Kolata, 1976). Diagnosis and treatment are hindered by societal disapproval of sexual experimentation and by incomplete knowledge about the symptoms and effects of venereal disease among teenagers.

Nutritional problems also may occur during adolescence (Freiburg, 1979). Deficiencies, most commonly in protein, calcium, and iron, may be caused by substituting foods such as soft drinks and french fries for nutritionally balanced meals. Acne problems can also be made worse by a high-carbohydrate, high-fat diet. Obesity may result, exacerbating the adolescent's often fragile self-image. Approximately 10% of adolescents are obese, a condition that is defined as more than 20% above ideal body weight. Anorexia nervosa is another kind of nutritional problem, seen increasingly among adolescents, in which severe and sustained weight loss can lead to starvation. Typically, anorexic teenagers are bright, capable persons who perceive themselves as not meeting their own or their families' goals. Failure to eat, or, for the obese person, overeating can become a kind of punishment directed at an already damaged and insecure sense of self.

With the completion of puberty and the period of adolescence, the process of sex identification that began at conception is completed. Rites of passage are intended to enable the adolescent to achieve social and personal identity as an adult; although, as we have seen, ambiguity may surround and hinder this process. Health problems arise out of the changes that occur on both biological and behavioral levels. Accidents, experi-

mentation with drugs and sex, teenage pregnancies, and an array of nutritional problems may be linked to the processes used by the adolescent to establish self-identity; these processes include separation from parents, heightened physical sensations, and a search for absolute, ideal solutions to complex problems. The ever-decreasing age of menarche has acted to initiate the period of adolescence at an earlier age and to prolong the period of turbulence, during which the adolescent attempts to reconcile the social and psychological with the biological stages of development.

FAMILY FORMATION, CHANGE, AND VARIATION

The family is the social unit charged with the responsibility of producing and caring for the next generation. In America, the ability of the family to carry out these functions has become a matter for increasing concern.

It is perhaps characteristic of our culture that discussions about the quality of the future are based almost entirely on technologic considerations. How the next generations of Americans will live, we are told, will be determined by the changes in our physical and natural environment. Whatever the predictions, they refer to the altered circumstances under which people will be living, not the changes in the people themselves. . . . As I see it, the competence and character of the next generation of Americans will depend less on deliberate genetic selection or modifications of the physical or natural environment than on changes in the human condition, specifically, the circumstances in which the next generation of Americans is being raised and developed. I refer to the changes that have been taking place in the structure of the family and its position in society.*

The changes being referred to concern the number and the kinds of adults in the home.

---

*Excerpt reproduced with permission from Bronfenbrenner, U.: Who cares for America's children. In Vaughan, V. C., and Brazelton, T. B. (eds.): The Family—Can It Be Saved? Copyright © 1976 by Year Book Medical Publishers, Inc., Chicago.

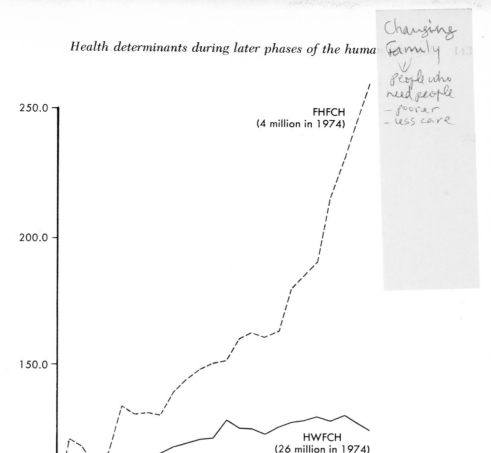

Fig. 5-3. Female-headed families with children (FHFCH) have grown much faster than husband-wife families with children (HWFCH). (From Ross and Sawhill, 1975:2.)

In the past 25 years, female-headed families with children have risen almost ten times as fast as male-and-female–headed families (Fig. 5-1). The trend, furthermore, has been accelerating. The rate of divorce has never been as high as it is at present in this country. Currently, thirty-eight out of every 100 first marriages are likely to end in divorce (National Academy of Sciences, 1976). The arrival of children, rather than preserving the marriage, as is prescribed by the commonly held myth, acts to increase the likelihood of separation. Since the 1950s, couples with chil-

dren have shown a higher divorce rate than childless couples. While large numbers of divorced people remarry, the remarriage rate remains lower for women than for men (National Academy of Sciences, 1976). This combined with the practice of awarding child custody to the mother means that the female-headed, single-parent family is a way of life, not just a stage between marriages. Also for an increasing number of women, single parenthood is not preceded by marriage. The illegitimacy ratio has risen in recent years (Fig. 5-4), reflecting the increasing propor-

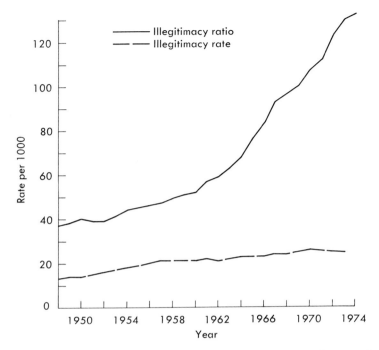

Fig. 5-4. Illegitimate births per 1000 live births (ratio) and per 1000 unmarried women (rate), 1948 to 1974. (Reproduced from *Toward a National Policy for Children and Families*, p. 20, with permission of the National Academy of Sciences, Washington, D.C., 1976.)

tion of illegitimate births relative to total births and the growing number of unmarried women of childbearing age.

Being a single parent, which nearly always means being a single mother, is part of the evolution of a new life-style for the family. Single mothers have joined together in nation-wide organizations, convinced that "nobody knows more about us than we do" (Hope and Young, 1976:vi).

We are all going through it. MILLIONS of us . . . divorced, separated, widowed, never-been-married mothers in the United States with children under eighteen. We vary in age. We are a racial mixture. Some of us are broke, some of us are rich. Together we share a unique life-style. We are solely responsible for the care and well-being of ourselves and our children. (Hope and Young, 1976:3)

Single mothers are likely to be young, nearly one-third being under 25 years of age, and poor, having a median income in 1975 of $3891 compared to a figure of $12,886 for a two-parent family, despite the fact that the overwhelming majority are in the labor force (National Academy of Sciences, 1976).

Changes in the American family are not confined to the single-parent condition. With the dramatic increase in the number of women employed outside the home, fewer adults stay at home to care for the children. The women with children under 18 years of age, and women with preschool-age children comprise the most rapidly growing sector of working women (Fig. 5-5). Even when adults are in the home, their interaction with children and with each other is limited. A study on the contact between fathers and their in-

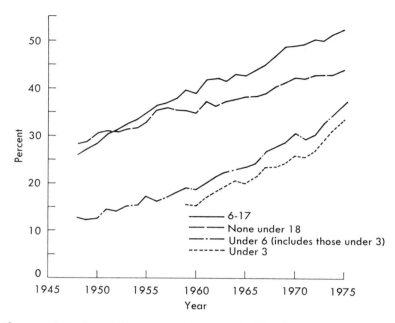

Fig. 5-5. The percentage of married women participating in the labor force has risen for each of the age groups shown from 1948 to 1975. (Reproduced from *Toward a National Policy for Children and Families,* p. 16, with permission of the National Academy of Sciences, Washington, D.C., 1976.)

fants revealed that, on the average, there were 2.7 verbal interactions per day, each lasting for 37.7 seconds (Rebelsky and Hanks, 1971). Watching television, a common family activity, has been shown to reduce personal interaction among family members. Physical and technological structures within the home, from separate rooms for each family member to television "solitaire" games, also act to isolate family members from each other. Members are also separated by societal and cultural forces, which take adults to places of work outside the home and place children in school. The result has been that the peer group, for children and adults alike, has become the principal support group. From a different perspective, segregation by age isolates family members from meaningful contact between age groups within the family and within society as a whole.

The changes described for the structure of the American family and its position in society call into question the whole notion of "the American family." The myth of the nuclear family in which husband and wife and their children live apart from other families would appear to be more of an ideal than a reality. High divorce rates, frequent but not universal remarriage, the widespread practice of couples living together without marriage, and the resulting proliferation of unwed, single, or remarried parents create a highly variable picture of American families. Marriage, rather than being a lifetime monogamous union is becoming a condition more aptly described as serial monogamy or trial marriage. Likewise, living arrangements for a child may include not only living with both parents but also, residing with a single parent, a single parent and partner, a single parent and another single parent and child, and other alternatives, as well as living with both parents.

The family need not conform to the ideal, nuclear type to be a family. Likewise, a family need not conform to definitions previously given it, such as G. P. Murdock's (1949) characterization of the family by common residence, economic cooperation, and reproduction. As a result of rethinking about the nature of the family, Lila Leibowitz (1978:11) defines the family as a recognized unit of society that links members of the opposite sex who come from different such units of society and that establishes the people with whom children from the unit can and cannot make similar arrangements. This more versatile view of the family hinges on public or societal acknowledgement and thus can accomodate unwed or serial forms of marriage, provided there is public recognition.

Family forms in other cultures

The inspection of forms of the family in other cultures reveals patterns of diversity that provide comparisons with the nature of the changes just described in American families. The two examples chosen are not intended to represent typical forms of variations of the family, nor should the descriptions be construed as complete accounts.

Medieval Europe. The history of the family in medieval Europe represents a portion of the history of American families. The period of feudalism, roughly from the twelfth to the fifteenth centuries, was a time of social unrest, characterized by a struggle between church and state over civil and moral authority.

One set of issues in this struggle concerned the basis for recognition of marriage and the role played by sexuality. In keeping with religious doctrine, the church regarded physical pleasure as evil and considered the sole purpose of sex to be procreation. Mutual consent initiated marriage, and once sexual intercourse occurred, the contract was ratified. No other formal means was required, not even parental consent (Howard, 1904:340). Civil authorities disapproved of mutual consent and sexual intercourse as the sole bases for marriage. Control of property, which included children and, for the nobility, peasants, was made difficult if marriage was simply a matter of mutual choice. The means by which the nobility were able to retain their authority was through the practice of arranging child marriages among their progeny (Howard, 1904:341) and trying to limit the choice of marriage partners among the serfs to others under their vassalage (Murstein, 1974:136).

The positions occupied by men and women in medieval society were very dissimilar. Primogeniture, inheritance by the oldest son, ensured that property, for the most part, remained undivided and in the hands of the male head of the household. A woman with property, including her dowry, was obliged to surrender it to her husband at the time of marriage. A woman's value was assessed economically, not romantically, in marriage. The Church's disapproval of sex, combined with its attributing the cause of human sinfulness to Eve's transgressions in the Garden of Eden placed the role of the wife and mother in a lowly position (Key, 1972:75). Paradoxically, the low status of women among the nobility was combined with the medieval practice of chivalry and courtly love. Chivalry decried that knights live by a code of courage, chastity, loyalty, religious faith and piety, courtesy, compassion, and obedience. Courtly love often overruled chastity, however, causing the noble knight to pursue, with burning passion, love for his lady but not for his wife (Murstein, 1974: 148). Thus, chivalry and courtly love served to exalt love and the position of women outside of marriage and the family while denigrating love and women's position within marriage and the family.

Inequality between the sexes along with an emphasis on property was more pronounced among the nobility than among the peasants or the townspeople. Women serfs worked alongside men, sharing the burdens and low status of the peasant class. As the producer of children, and thus of a labor force for the nobility, as well as a readily available source of sexual pleasure, the peasant woman's sexuality was more highly valued. Among townspeople, the household group expanded to include apprentices, journeymen, and servants, as well as unmarried or widowed kinfolk. Although the husband was master of the house, he and his wife, along with others in the household, formed a partnership in which position depended more on services rendered than on blood relationship (Queen, 1967:230).

While differences between the social institutions of medieval Europe and contemporary American society are numerous and real, two parallels may be mentioned instructively. First, both the medieval and present periods are characterized by social unrest in which the basis for marriage and the role of sexuality have come into question. Today, a church or civil ceremony is increasingly bypassed in favor of a decision to live together. Interviews with unmarried mates reveal a cautionary view of marriage as an institution that limits freedom for personal growth and impairs the quality of the relationship between partners (Whitbeck, 1976). The medieval practice of courtly love also bears resemblance to the modern-day situation in which extra-marital, including premarital, sex is viewed as capable of providing a more satisfying experience than marital sex. Second, both the medieval and present periods share an ambivalent attitude toward women. To-

day, the rising number of women in the labor force reflects more equal access to employment. However, the current failure to pass the Equal Rights Amendment to the U.S. Constitution and statistics that reveal lower pay for equivalent work and rank for women compared to men (Sawhill, 1973) indicate that equal status for women has yet to be achieved. A more egalitarian position for women continues to exist where financial rewards are the smallest, that is, in the lower classes. As in medieval times, the attitude toward women contains conflicting elements. On the one hand, their position is exalted through practices such as courtly love, beauty pageants, and the assignment of the nurturing, loving role of "mother"; while on the other hand, their position is debased by unfair employment practices and attitudes of inferiority.

The ambivalence generated creates consequences today that are potentially critical for all mothers who work outside the home, but especially for the single mother. Working mothers attempt to raise their children, in this and other ways acting in accordance with their role of motherhood, and yet unfair employment practices, the absence or inaccessibility of good day care for children, and societal disapproval stand in their way.

Central Andes of South America

The central Andean region of South America is comprised of a large number of communities at moderate to high altitudes (3000 to 4500 m) in Chile, Peru, and Bolivia. While linked by languages that belong to the Aymara language family and by a cultural past that includes Incan and Spanish influences, these communities vary in response to local conditions and traditions. However, they also share a similar process of family formation and family structure. Alternate conceptions of Aymara family formation exist, some anthropologists perceiving it as a series of "trial" marriages (Price, 1965) and others seeing it as phases of a single marriage process (Carter, 1977). In any event, family formation occurs as a result of many steps that may each take as long as several years, as described by Carter (1977). Family formation begins with courtship. Young people in their middle to late teens begin to flirt with members of the opposite sex at markets, in the fields, or wherever else they should happen to meet. Nighttime dances, the *q'achwa*, provide a more formal opportunity for courtship. Sexual experimentation varies but, overall, appears quite widespread. Girls are fearful of becoming pregnant and begin pressuring for betrothal once they become pregnant. After a period of courtship, "bride theft," actually a result of mutual consent, occurs. The girl follows the boy home, where, with great apprehension, he tells his parents of her presence. The boy's father is obliged to tell the girl's parents the following day. Each set of parents is likely to express reservation and may actively try to prevent the relationship from continuing. If it is to progress further, both sets of parents must agree on a date for a betrothal party—a time of eating, drinking, and gift-giving provided by the boy's parents. Until the necessary resources can be accumulated, the girl continues to live with the boy. If she becomes pregnant, pressure to hasten the betrothal increases, but her pregnancy is not viewed as immoral.

After the betrothal party, the "engaged" couple searches for godparents, persons of substantial means who take an active part in the coming wedding ceremony. The acceptance of presents from the boy's family signifies the willingness of the persons selected to be the godparents. The godparents and boy's parents select a wedding date. Children may be born during this interval, as again, its length is determined by the time required for gathering the necessary provisions. Before the date, public notice of the coming wedding

is given and should either partner, particularly the boy, be involved in another relationship, agreeable arrangements must be made with the other person before the wedding can proceed. A civil or a religious ceremony confers legal recognition of the marriage, but neither receives great emphasis. The party given afterward by the groom's parents is more important, the resources it requires having been important in determining the wedding date. The godparents also host celebrations for the couple. The bride continues to live with the groom's family until her parents are able to assemble a dowry and his parents have assembled a brideprice. The dowry and brideprice comprise each person's inheritance. Subsequently, the couple works to build their own house, often but not always adjacent to that of the groom's family. Both sets of parents host a roofing party to complete the structure. Then the couple establishes an independent household.

At varying times, the household may include husband and wife, their children, unmarried siblings, widows or widowers, and unrelated persons (Custred, 1977:127). Emphasis within the household accords nearly equal position to the maternal and paternal lines. Sex roles prescribe some activities for men (plowing, long-distance trading) and others to women (child care, cooking, housekeeping), but both engage in agricultural work, animal care, and spinning and weaving activities on an equal basis (Custred, 1977: 127). While male offspring sometimes receive larger inheritances, property is transmitted through both maternal and paternal lines (Isbell, 1977:92-94). The household is the functional unit for furnishing the goods and services required, not only during family formation but also as an essential part of one's lifelong existence. Reciprocal exchange is most pronounced among nuclear family members. In a wider context, it ensures the autonomy and self-sufficiency of the household unit by distributing goods among kin groups and between people in different climatic zones.

Comparisons between Andean and American familes reveal differences in the notion of marriage and in the conduct of family life. Andean marriage can be conceptualized either as multiple stages in a single process or as successive "trials" that may be terminated at any time. Reports on the rate of dissolution of marriage, once an independent household is established, are variable, but overall marital stability appears high (Lambert, 1977: 8-9). However, the notion of Andean marriage contains the recognition that marriage *develops*. Either partner can have a change of mind. Children may be born relatively early or late in the process without, seemingly, making any difference. Further, the Andean notion of marriage stresses reciprocal obligation more than does its American counterpart.

By the time the ceremonial sequence has been completed, couples have so many social obligations to kindred of bride, groom, and godparents, that they will be involved in lending and borrowing of goods and services for the rest of their lives. (Carter, 1977:210)

As a result of prior exchange, the couple's essential needs are supplied. By accepting the goods and with the expectation of future reciprocity, the bride and the group are incorporated into each other's family group while retaining ties to his or her own family. In contrast, American middle class newlyweds appear as isolates, expected to take care of themselves, surrounded by china, crystal, and other gifts. Thus, the conduct of Andean family life is influenced more by reciprocal networks of exchange and obligation than is the American counterpart. A further contrast in family life concerns the equality in sex roles cited in the Andean case as opposed to widespread (but not universal) emphasis on

the father's power seen in American families. Underlying the distinction is the more egalitarian position of Andean women, the less rigid division of labor by sex, and the tradition of bilateral inheritance.

The preceding discussion of family formation and change points to variation in the structure and process of family formation. Given this perspective, the recent changes described in American families begin to appear less remarkable. However, to underestimate their potential seriousness would be a mistake. Family structure—medieval or modern, American or Andean—is an adaptive mechanism that responds to the pressures created by social and environmental circumstances. The rise of single-parent families can thus be seen as related to conditions such as limited interaction between father and offspring, extramarital sex, and the movement to end sexual discrimination. Concern for the seriousness of changes in American families is not based on viewing the single-parent family as unnatural but as being unsupported. Societal disapproval, employment discrimination, rigid sex role differentiation, and inaccessible day care (either because it is not there or because it is too expensive) exemplify the lack of support available to single parents.

Family effect on health and vice versa

The effects of families on health and of health on families are an expression of the adaptive nature of family structure. In keeping with our ecological perspective on the determinants of health and disease, the family may be viewed as the context in which hereditary and many environmental influences are transmitted. The family is also the unit assigned major responsibility for coping with the effects of disease in its members. **Influence of heredity and family environment on health.** During reproduction, each parent transmits half of his or her genetic material to the offspring. Consequently, parents share half their genes with offspring, and siblings likewise have half of their genes in common. Decreasing proportions of genes are shared with other relatives as the degree of relationship diminishes. Specific hereditary diseases may occur in the family, depending on the particular genes transmitted from parent to offspring and the factors controlling the expression of the genes. Family pedigrees can be traced to show those persons with the disease. Fig. 5-6 shows five generations of a family with Lesch-Nyhan syndrome, a disease that results from a genetic defect that affects purine metabolism, causing mental retardation and behavioral abnormalities, such as severe biting of lips and finger tips. The gene is an X-linked recessive, and thus, the Lesch-Nyhan syndrome is more often seen in males, who have only one X chromosome, than in females, for whom it must be present on both X chromosomes before it is expressed. Fig. 5-7 shows pedigree for cystic fibrosis, which occurs in one out of 2000 births and is the most common autosomal (non–sex chromosome) recessive, inherited disease in Caucasian populations. The primary biochemical defect is unknown. Its characteristic symptoms include chronic lung disease, malnutrition, and growth failure. Death, frequently from respiratory problems, usually occurs before age 20.

Lesch-Nyhan syndrome and cystic fibrosis are two examples of diseases known as inborn errors of metabolism. Victor McKusick (1975) has identified 2336 such conditions, known or thought to be related to single genes. Genetic disorders may also occur as the result of errors in the transmission of collections of genes or chromosomes. Down's syndrome (trisomy 21), which results from an extra twenty-first chromosome, is the most common example of a chromosomal disorder (see

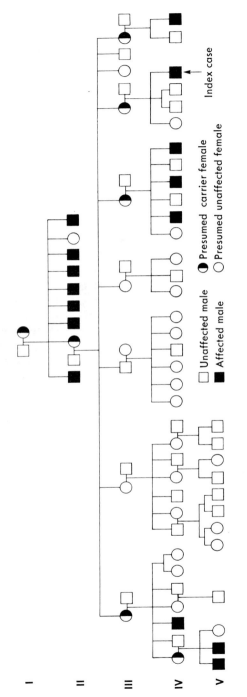

Fig. 5-6. Family pedigree of the Lesch-Nyhan syndrome. Note the pattern typical for an X-linked recessive trait in which females are carriers and only males are affected. (From Nyhan and others, 1968:1092.)

pp. 103-105 for further discussion). Other chromosomal disorders involve the sex chromosomes. Instead of the normal XX female and XY male chromosomes, people have been identified with only one X chromosome (Turner's syndrome), XXY (Klinefelter's syndrome), XXX, XYY, XXXY, XXXX, and XXYY sex chromosomes; these are associated, in most instances, with some degree of abnormality. Only a portion of a chromosome may be involved in other kinds of abnormalities, such as in the cri-du-chat syndrome. This syndrome, associated with a plaintive catlike cry and severe mental and physical disorders, results from the deletion of part of the fifth chromosome. The cause of nearly all of the chromosomal disorders just described stems from a failure of the chromosomes to divide properly during the formation of the parental sex (sperm or egg) cells; thus, they do not continue to be transmitted from generation to generation. Apart from some of the sex chromosome abnormalities, chromosomal disorders usually produce very severe disturbances in physical or mental

development. In fact, most of the possible kinds of abnormalities that could arise are probably lethal, and the individuals in whom they appear do not survive long enough for the abnormalities to be detected.

Other kinds of diseases, including cancers, cardiovascular disease and diabetes, are said to "run in families"; but the specific role of genetic factors and the mode of transmission are unclear. At least some forms of diabetes, now the fifth leading cause of death in the United States, appear to have genetic roots. It has long been recognized that people with diabetes have a larger portion of their close relatives who are diabetic than does the population at large. An array of genetic models has been proposed and, to some extent, supported for the inheritance of diabetes. Tattersall and Fajans (1975) suggested that the maturity-onset form of diabetes is transmitted by a dominant, autosomal gene. In patients with maturity-onset diabetes, 85% had a diabetic parent, and 46% showed direct transmission through three generations of their families. The other form of diabetes,

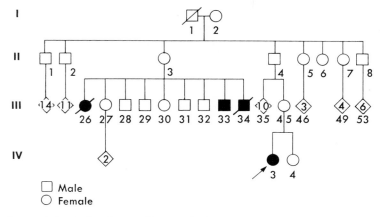

Fig. 5-7. Pedigree of a kindred with cystic fibrosis. The (patient) is IV.3. Individuals III.26 and III.34 died shortly after birth; III.33 has mild pulmonary and gastrointestinal disease at age 13. Parent I.1 died at age 65 of cancer; I.2 is living at age 80. Recessive inheritance is strongly suggested by the lack of affected individuals in generations I and II and in sibship III.35 to III.45. (From *The Metabolic Basis of Inherited Disease*, ed. 3, p. 1615, by Stanbury, J. B., Wyngaarden, J. B., and Fredickson, D. S. Copyright © 1972. Used with permission of McGraw-Hill Book Co.)

juvenile-onset (or acute-onset), has not shown strong familial tendency. However, other studies have pointed to a possible role for genes operating through genetically determined susceptibility to viral infections (Nerup and others, 1974).

Besides hereditary factors, the environment shared by family members has important effects on health. The potential range of environmental influences is very great. During prenatal life, maternally mediated influences on the uterine environment may determine later-in-life susceptibility to certain diseases. For example, diethylstilbesterol (DES), a synthetic estrogen, was administered to thousands of women in the 1940s and 1950s to prevent possible miscarriages. Female progeny from such pregnancies have been shown to have an increased risk of developing a type of cervical cancer and to have an overall increased risk of cancer later in life (Noller, 1976). Other substances that can affect the uterine environment, such as radiation, drugs, and toxins, also may have consequences for the future health of family members.

Postnatally, the range of influences of the familial environment on health expands even further. Recent studies suggest possible connections between childhood infection with mumps and Rubella (German measles) and subsequent development of juvenile-onset diabetes (Steinke and Taylor, 1974). Whether or not a child contracts these infections is likely a result of factors that are influenced or controlled by the family, such as exposure to siblings or neighbors and immunizations against diseases. Efforts to immunize each generation against preventable diseases are far from successful. A recent survey in Syracuse, New York, revealed, for example, that 55% of children aged 2 to 5 years had no discernible antibodies to type I poliomyelitis virus (National Academy of Sciences, 1976: 61). Immunization is simply one example of a health-maintaining measure that families can influence.

The kinds of resources available and allocated to maintain health and to treat illness are other important areas of the family's influence. Family life-style, goals, and behavior patterns can affect the values ascribed to health, diet, and exercise and assigned to disease prevention practices, such as hygiene and regular dental and medical checkups. The importance of these family-influenced behaviors is illustrated by studies of factors that predispose people to heart disease, the leading cause of death in the United States. Cigarette smoking, obesity, high blood pressure, elevated serum cholesterol levels, and family history are among the risk factors for heart disease. Strong correlation between parents, adopted children, and pets exists for obesity, pointing to the importance of the shared familial environment (Garn, 1976; Kolata, 1977). Dietary as well as genetic factors are implicated in the control of serum cholesterol. Some people with high cholesterol levels have a clearly genetic condition, familial hypercholesteremia; but in most instances cholesterol levels probably result from the interaction of hereditary and environmental causes. High blood pressure is another trait of complex etiology in which hereditary and environmental factors, such as diet and stress, are believed to be involved. The factors that influence cigarette smoking are, surprisingly (considering its health implications), poorly understood. Whether or not one's parents smoke is an important predictor, but additional factors are certainly also involved (Jarvik and others, 1977).

The family's importance in determining health and disease susceptibility, in sum, derives from its role in shaping both genetic and family environmental factors. In most diseases, some combination of both kinds of factors is involved. Thus the family is in a pivotal position regarding health and disease determinants.

Influence of health and disease on families. The growth and development of families express the health of its individual members and the unit as a whole. Thus, birth and the periods of infancy, childhood, adolescence, middle age, and old age reflect the individual's healthy progression through the life cycle within the context of the family. The family unit is successively reassembled, beginning with a unit in which one is a child, then a parent and a spouse, subsequently a grandparent and spouse, and then possibly a great grandparent as well as a spouse. The effects of health on families are a continuing theme throughout this and the previous chapter. To explore the effects of disease on families, we will examine an example of a chronic illness, kidney disease.

The kidneys are paired organs responsible for cleansing the plasma portion of the blood and maintaining extracellular fluid volume and osmolarity (the quantity of dissolved substances). Many diseases affect the kidneys, including bacterial infections, congenital defects, and tumors. It is currently estimated that there are 3 million undetected cases of kidney disease in the United States and from 25,000 to 75,000 deaths from kidney disease each year (Vander, Sherman, and Luciano, 1970:366). The disease can occur at any age and, if untreated, may progress to end-stage kidney disease, at which point the kidneys can no longer function. Unless help is provided, end-stage disease is fatal. Help currently exists in two forms: hemodialysis and kidney transplantation. Hemodialysis provides relief by connecting a patient's blood vessels to a machine that acts as an artificial kidney, cleansing the blood and maintaining fluid volume and osmolarity. Hemodialysis requires 6 to 10 hours, two to three times per week. It can be continued indefinitely although cost (up to $30,000 per year), incon-

venience, and discomfort (including the risk of contracting other infections) act to limit its desirability. Kidney transplantation is the only cure for end-stage kidney disease. This cure, however, depends on having a suitable donor, surviving the operation, and not rejecting the transplanted organ from the recipient's body.

The effects of end-stage kidney disease on the family vary according to the position in the family of the person with the disease and the type of treatment being received. Adults as well as children face the physical stresses of uremia (urine in the blood), especially during the period before hemodialysis; but physical discomforts persist after dialysis as well. The sick person also experiences a changed social role, described as the "sick role," which is discussed further in Chapter 6 (Parsons and Fox, 1958). Expectations are modified such that the sick person is viewed as weak and dependent but also as having a relatively privileged status that affords him or her great service. For an adult, the sick role may produce changes in life-style and self-image that conflict with one or more of the person's previous roles. The person undergoing hemodialysis may vacillate from a sick to a well role before and after treatment, producing some confusion regarding expectations among family members. Kidney transplantation offers a chance to abandon the sick role. However, the transition from sick to well is made ambiguous by the continued threat of kidney rejection and the need to continue medication to prevent it.

Simmons, Klein, and Simmons (1977) examined the social and psychological effects of end-stage kidney disease on adults and children. When a child or the husband was affected, the burden of care fell largely on the mother or wife in the families studied. If authority within the household had previously resided principally with the husband or father, this could cause a reversal of pat-

Sick
role

dependency within the household, [...]ng conflicts and potential hostility [...] depression and real fear about the [...] death. If the mother or wife was [...] member with kidney disease, the [...] for the husband to assume care-[...]ies for the children and also to care [...] often occasioned changed in fam-[...]ers' roles. Part of the treatment for kidney disease requires heavy steroids (sex hormones) that may [...]xual impotency for the husband or [...]nay create additional stress in the [...]ationship. Financial problems may arise from the inability of the patient to continue work and from costs that are related to treatment but are not covered by insurance; such complications can also cause stress as well as change in the family's socioeconomic status.

The Simmons, Klein, and Simmons study found that, overall, the effects of kidney disease were less severe in children than in adults. Partly, this was because of the tendency of children to be less sick, consistent with the likelihood that the children would have been ill for a shorter time. But, in addition, the lesser severity was thought attributable to the greater similarity between the sick role and the role of the child than between the sick role and the adult role in American society. "Both the child and the ill person are generally exempt from social responsibility and are not expected to take care of themselves" (Simmons, Klein, Simmons, 1977:113). They found that the family, especially the mother, tried to protect the child by denying to the child the seriousness of the disease. Other siblings shared in taking on concern and anxiety that might otherwise have been felt by the sick child. The shield that the family erected around the child served to protect his or her self-image but also enforced the dependency of the child on other family members. For the mother par-

ticularly, tension could develop regarding the degree to which the child should be treated as normal. The case study below (Simmons, Klein, Simmons, 1977:111-112) illustrates the inherent conflict created when a child is encouraged to pursue a normal life (going to camp) and yet is obliged to be not normal (taking medications).

Additional conflicts may be created if a decision is made to seek kidney transplantation. Family members (including relatives) are likely to be the source of the kidney, since it is possible to function normally with one kidney and since the decision regarding selection of a donor is made on genetically determined immunological similarity. If a donor is found among family members, the hesitancy the potential donor may feel about sacrificing a part of himself or herself and his or her possible refusal may occasion great

---

Case study

A 10-year-old girl received her father's kidney and was successfully transplanted. When she returned home, she did well and was able with some parental help to administer her own medications. A year later her parents decided to send her to camp, like other "normal" children. The medications at camp had to be administered through the camp nurse, and the nurse was sent these with instructions. When the child returned home, however, her blood tests indicated that she had started to reject the kidney. Upon questioning, the child indicated that when she went to the camp infirmary for her medications she could not find the nurse and did not receive her medicines for a week or more. The insidious chronic rejection of the kidney could not be halted and after a very stressful time period, the kidney had to be removed. The mother then donated her kidney to maintain the child's life.

---

conflict. Recently, a relative who was an excellent immunological match refused to donate, in this instance, bone marrow. The case was brought to court where the judge ruled that, however immoral such a decision may be viewed, the decision to donate rests with the donor (Williams and Walsh, 1978). If a kidney cannot be found among family members, waiting for a kidney to become available through the system of international registers also can be stressful. When will a kidney be found? Whose kidney will it be? Should a kidney be accepted from a dead person (which carries with it a greater risk of rejection)? Problems are not over once the transplantation is completed. The threat of rejection remains forever. Steroid treatment, which helps to avoid rejection, can have a bloating, disfiguring side effect that may interfere with improved self-image. Furthermore, resumption of a well role by the patient in the family may be hampered by having become accustomed to the sick role and by the continued possibility of kidney rejection. Finally, societal and vocational barriers exist to functioning as a well person. One's former job may no longer be available or may be inappropriate (for example, if requiring heavy, manual labor).

In spite of the possible problems, the overall impact of transplantation on both the child and adult patient is favorable (Simmons, Klein, Simmons, 1977:146). Family support is vital to successful adjustment. This example of end-stage kidney disease has emphasized the range of the disease's effects on the family. The overall, favorable effect of transplantation implies that credit for its success lies with the adjustments made within the family and the individual as well as with the technology responsible for hemodialysis, donor-matching, and the transplant operation itself.

Summary. In short, this discussion has shown that the effects of families on health

and disease and of health and disease on families are parts of the same, inseparable process. The health and disease-determining factors residing in the family's shared heredity and environment are complemented by the adaptations made within the family in response to the health and disease states of its members.

A logical question concerns the health consequences of the patterns of family formation and change in American society reviewed in the previous section. Unfortunately comparatively little is known. The importance of the immediate family as a support system is emphasized by a governmental report that notes that married people are healthier than widowed, separated, or divorced persons.* The decreasing number of adults in the home as a result of divorce, separation, births to single mothers, employment outside the home, and age segregation, which often removes the older generation from living with the family unit, can be expected to deprive family members of needed support during illness.

Urie Bronfenbrenner sees family disorganization, imposed by the external circumstances in which families find themselves, as the overriding determinant for behavior disorders and social pathology (1976:25). It would be extremely helpful to have examples drawn from other cultures on the ways in which families affect health and health affects families. The emphasis placed in Andean marriages on the ties between the nuclear family and other social units ensures the availability of support, which would be expected to aid families and family members in times of sickness. However, while concern over the state of American families appears

---

*Criteria for health in this report were presence in mental health hospitals and nursing homes, amount of restriction of activities by illness or injury, number of visits to a physician per year, and number of days in hospitals (Anonymous, 1976:9).

well founded and the lack of support networks would appear to predispose family members to problems in maintaining or restoring health and well-being at times of sickness, further study is needed to ascertain whether the variation in family structure observed is actually adaptive or maladaptive from the point of view of the health of its members.

MIDDLE AGE

The middle years have been broadly set between the chronological ages of 20 to 65 years and more narrowly between 40 to 65 years of age. Returning to the life cycle diagram (Fig. 4-3), middle age can be seen as the time of adulthood. The period of growth in biological systems characteristic of earlier phases of the life cycle has ceased, but maintenance and repair activities continue. In behavioral systems, such as personality and cognition, growth continues. Ekistic development is marked by increasing diversity of physical structures and networks that link the individual to the rest of society.

Change in body, family, and work

Development during middle age is particularly apparent in three contexts: body, family, and career.

While skeletal growth has ceased, physical changes continue. Decreasing bone density and gradual vertebral compression result in progressive shortening of the body. The functional capacities of various organ systems decline with age (Fig. 5-11), reducing physical work capacity and caloric requirements. Sedentary life-style, combined with decreased caloric needs, has led to obesity in increasing numbers of adult Americans. Declining ability of the reproductive organs to function occurs with age. Menopause, occurring between the ages of 40 and 50 years, marks the end of the ovulatory-menstrual cycle. Changes are less dramatic in men, in

whom fertility may be retained throughout life. Sexual activity may continue in both sexes, however.

Events within the middle class American family center around the departure of children, initially for school and subsequently for work and marriage. Despite the prolonged period of schooling, these events occur sooner in the lives of American couples than they did previously, as a result of having fewer children spaced more closely together. As a result, couples find themselves in their mid-forties with an "empty nest" and half of their married life span remaining. The recent trend to postpone having children until late twenties or thirties will tend to counteract "emptying the nest" so early for the next generation of middle-aged people. Increasing responsibility for the care of older generations of one's family (parents and grandparents) also accompanies middle age.

In the past, women have defined their progression through middle age with reference to events within the family cycle, whereas men have centered more on external, career-related events (Neugarten, 1968). This pattern may be expected to change with the increasing number of women pursuing careers outside the family and the redistribution of responsibilities for child care between the sexes. Work is a major focus in middle age and appears to bring both personal and financial rewards for middle class Americans. The middle years are one's most productive years. The majority of managerial and executive positions are claimed by middle-aged men. Analysis of the lives of scientists and scholars reveals that their greatest accomplishments occur in their thirties and forties (Lehman, 1968; Dennis, 1968). Despite general satisfaction and success in the work world, many middle-aged people change jobs for advancement or because of frustration or necessity. Rapid change in job-related skills has led observers to forecast that, in the future, the skills of the average worker will have only a 5-year life span (Rocky Mountain News, 1978:67).

Family and work responsibilities make the middle-aged group the "weight-bearing" generation in middle class American society. In the popular book *Passages*, Gail Sheehy (1974) describes the overlap between family- and work-related responsibilities and the potential for crises occasioned by conflict between them. Progressing through the adult years, Sheehy begins with the "trying twenties," which she visualizes as a time to work out externals, preparing for engagement in society, finding a life work, and meeting social and familial expectations. The thirties may be a time of "rooting," if priorities set in the twenties are still in effect. "Rooting" is a time of settling down, buying a house, having children, and working toward career goals. Alternatively, change may occur if the external relationships worked out in the twenties are perceived as limiting. Women may seek a career if they had not considered one earlier. The marital relationship may no longer be satisfying; the ideal of starting a family may wane. A sense of urgency may begin to develop around 35 years of age if the goals set previously have not been or are not being met. For women, age 35 has acted as a deadline for having children, although recent reports suggest that the age-associated risks for abnormalities, such as trisomy 21, may have been exaggerated (see Chapter 4, p. 103). Men, according to Sheehy, respond to this "deadline" with a "last chance" burst of energy to achieve career recognition.

Sheehy uses the term "deadline decade" for the 35 to 45 years of age time period, during which the midlife crisis frequently develops. The midlife crisis is prompted by a perception of time running out, a decrease in physical powers, the dilemma of not having absolute answers, and the necessity to reassess one's purposes and priorities. The recognition that one's remaining years are equal to or fewer than the number of years already lived is a reminder of one's perishability, one's mortality. That the recognition of one's perishability constitutes a crisis reflects the negative view of aging in American culture (an idea developed further in the old aging section of this chapter) as well as the unrealistic ideal of stability once one has "grown up." Once resolved, Sheehy contends, the midlife crises lead to a renewal of purpose and opportunity in later years. Greater satisfaction with one's self may ensue, or perhaps a more accurate assessment of one's strengths may lead to a career change. Without a reorientation in midlife, simple resignation to the rest of one's forties and early fifties may occur. For women whose preoccupation has been with children, the "empty nest" may be a release to pursue a career. A switch may take place in which men begin to emphasize a service role—through teaching, advising, and nurturing others—while women seek to meet ambitious new goals in the "outside" world.

Culture, too, plays a role in deciding the developments that occur during middle age. Comparatively little study has been directed at middle aging in other cultures. Further research is needed in order to determine the extent to which a middle-age period exists cross-culturally. One feature that has been examined cross-culturally, however, is menopause. The age of menopause has remained at 50 years of age over the past 100 years, appearing remarkably constant compared to the change in age of menarche (Diers, 1974). Cessation of reproductive functions is a universal effect of menopause, but the experience and interpretation of menopause vary widely. In a survey of 30 societies for which data were available in the Human Relations Area Files, menopause was seen as a major physical and emotional loss and an occasion for a decrease in social status in only two societies besides the United States of America,—in the Trobriand Islands and the Marquesa Islands of the South Pacific (Bart, 1969). In societies in which menopause was accompanied by a gain in social status, high value was assigned to advancing age and to reproduction; residence patterns maintained the family members in proximity to each other, and extended families were common. The emotional and physical distress (such as insomnia, nervousness, dizziness, depression, hot flashes, and sweating) commonly thought to accompany menopause in the United States are not seen in other countries, such as India, where few symptoms other than change in menstruation occur (Flint, 1975).

Middle age then is marked by changes in body, family, and career contexts. The changes act as a catalyst, entailing crisis and reorientation; but they also provide the opportunity for healthy development. Taking mortality as a measure, the middle years appear among the healthiest in the human life span. Fig. 5-8 compares survivorship in the American population from birth to age 50 with survivorship in Egypt, a less industrialized country. Low mortality throughout this period is striking in the American case. Even in Egypt, relatively low mortality during the adult (but not childhood) years is characteristic. The low mortality reflects the successful integration of the developments in biological family and career contexts during middle age. However, the low mortality may

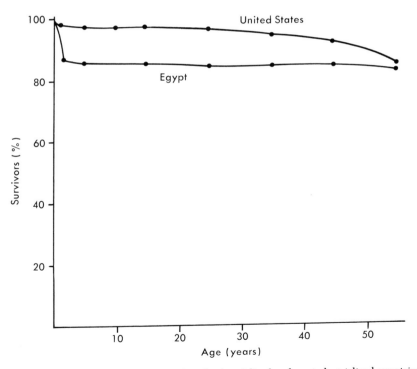

Fig. 5-8. The United States and Egypt, examples of industrialized and nonindustrialized countries, both evidence low mortality during adulthood, although childhood mortality is considerably higher in Egypt than in the United States. (Data from World Health Statistics Annual, 1973-1976:774-775.)

be deceptive insofar as chronic disease processes may be at work.

Health during middle age

Biological developments during middle age may predispose individuals to certain diseases later in life. For example, decreased energy expenditure and caloric requirements create a tendency toward weight gain. In a recent survey, 16% of ostensibly healthy middle-aged people were obese (Smith and Bierman, 1973:169). Obesity is associated with increased incidence of strokes, heart disease, diabetes, hypertension, and gall bladder disease (Kolata, 1977). Often, "middle-age spread" is seen as the price of having reached middle age and not as a link to later health problems. After obesity, hypertension is the second most common health-related problem of middle age (Smith and Bierman, 1973:169). People with high blood pressure are more likely to have strokes, heart disease, and kidney failure. However, blood pressure in the United States normally increases with age, so the definition of hypertension must take age into account. High blood pressure itself has no discernible symptoms. The cause of hypertension is unknown for 90% of the cases, but hypertension itself can be controlled through drug therapy. The leading problem in its control, however, is the unwillingness of some hypertensive people to continue taking the medication when they do not feel sick. Thus, as with obesity, hypertension is often confused with normal accompaniments of middle aging.

Part of the confusion also stems from the definition given to conditions such as obesity and hypertension. Are they diseases, risk factors, reversible conditions, or some combination of all three? Western medicine considers them risk factors and, unlike a positive family history, treatable and, therefore, akin to diseases. The absence of symptoms may lead people with these conditions not to define them as diseases and, therefore, not to follow the recommended therapy (weight loss or antihypertensive drugs).

Another reason for difficulty in detecting chronic diseases during middle age stems from the nature of the chronic disease process. Unlike acute or infectious diseases, chronic diseases do not usually have a rapid, detectable period of onset. Rather, they develop slowly often in response to multiple factors. A variety of explanations have been advanced for chronic diseases, but, fundamentally, their exact cause or causes remain unknown. Genetics, viral exposure, dietary or smoking habits, personality, stress, and the physical environment represent the range of factors proposed to account for the incidence of the two leading chronic diseases in the United States: cardiovascular disease and cancer. Work and family are the contexts in middle age in which many of these factors operate. Phrased differently, work and family developments during middle age may have an impact on the individual's future health by contributing to the processes of chronic disease.

Some effects of work on health are sufficiently clear to be termed occupational hazards. Industrial lung disease may occur as a result of exposure to dust (silica, coal dust, textile dust), asbestos, moldy hay, trace substances (such as beryllium and cadmium oxide), and various irritant and inert gases (Bouhuys and Peters, 1970). The inhaled agents may cause obstruction or constriction of airway passages and decreased capacity for gas diffusion. Lung diseases, such as coal workers' pneumoconiosis (black lung), asbestos workers' asbestosis and lung cancer, and textile workers' byssinosis, are disabling forms of illness that develop over time in ways that are still not fully understood. Many substances to which workers are exposed are only recognized as health hazards long after the period of initial exposure. For example, high doses of microwave radiation to which workers developing radar were exposed have been reported to produce headaches and cataracts. Debate continues as to whether microwave exposure may have additional central nervous system effects, including dizziness, irritability, emotional instability, depression, and reduced intellectual capacity (Brodeur, 1977). The experience of working in potentially hazardous conditions may be emotionally as well as physically stressful. The story of a plutonium worker (case study, p. 161) who accidently inhaled forty to fifty times the permissible amount reveals the emotional stress and uncertainty of becoming contaminated by industrial pollutants. Workers in industrial settings that are later identified as hazardous may face similar emotional as well as physical stresses.

The life-styles associated with different kinds of employment also have possible health effects. The amount of physical activity, smoking, and drinking, and dietary habits may vary according to income and behavior norms for occupational groups. The life-style of people with type A personalities has been reported to affect health (Friedman and Rosenman, 1974). Type A individuals are described as high achievers, constantly driving themselves, doing several things at once, eating rapidly, and wasting no time. In contrast, type B individuals are low key, less frantic but equally effective in accomplishing their tasks. High achievement has been linked to longer life expectancies (Quint and Cody, cited in Butler, 1975:365). Clearly, a multitude of factors associated with success may be responsible.

Personality is also reported to have a possible role in the development and treatment of cancer. A controversial group of studies has pointed to a possible predilection for a poorer prognosis, once cancer is present, among people less able to cope with the mental and emotional stresses of day-to-day life

(Holden, 1978). Personality thus has joined genetic, environmental, and viral hypotheses for the causes of cancer. The possibility of interaction among casual factors is emphasized by a recent study of mice exposed to a type of virus known to cause mammary tumors. Only 7% of the mice kept in a protected environment compared to 92% of the mice kept under stress developed mammary tumors (Riley, 1975). Working with cancer patients to express their emotions, to resolve stress, and thus to reverse the psychological processes underlying the disease has become a form of cancer therapy used by the Simontons and others. Additional research is needed to elucidate the role of personality in conjunction with other factors in causing cancer.

Specific effects of families on health were discussed in the previous section of this chapter. On a more general level, families act to set goals and standards that may govern the behavior of family members. Thus families may be held responsible for the difficulties as well as the successes of their members. The phenomenon of age segregation discussed before also may affect the health of family members. The physical displacement of the older generation from the family unit may deprive the family of needed help and also of the informally transmitted knowledge about the effects of career and life-style on health. Interaction with older adults may provide a valuable time perspective that otherwise is lost.

Family- and work-related developments are likely to affect the kind of environment in which the middle-aged person lives. Aspects of the environment that affect health encompass personal habits, such as cigarette smoking, as well as environmental characteristics, such as air, water, and diet. The environments occupied by individuals throughout their lives exert important influences on health. During middle age, negative environmental effects may become apparent in the incidence of cancer and other chronic diseases. It has been estimated that from 60% to 90% of all human cancers are related to environmental agents (Train, 1977; Higginson,

1969). Recently published maps of cancer mortality in the United States show large variation in cancer death rates. Fig. 5-9 presents the age-adjusted death rates from all types of cancer (liver, lungs, bladder, stom-

---

Case study*

Martin, a 21-year old with no particular skills in nuclear matters, has been employed for 2 years at the Nuclear Fuels Services reprocessing plant, performing tasks with a relatively high risk of contamination such as decontaminating equipment, loading uranium and plutonium, and taking samples for lab analysis.

On the afternoon of September 9, 1967, Martin was told to enter an area known to be heavily contaminated from leaks and spills to get samples of plutonium nitrate. Wearing the required "contamination suit"—2 pairs of coveralls, layers of plastic and rubber gloves and shoe covers, a cloth hood, and a heavy gas mask–like "respirator"—he entered the 90° F sample aisle and performed the hour-long task.

By the time he was done, he felt in such need of fresh air that instead of going through the elaborate disrobing ritual required to protect himself from the heavy concentration of plutonium dust that had accumulated on his suit, he pulled off his hood and mask and gulped fresh air.

As he approached the radiation monitors, alarms went off, and the technicians who immediately checked him found that plutonium dust covered his hair and hands and had entered his nose and throat.

Even after emergency contamination, tests indicated that Martin had inhaled forty to fifty times the maximum permissible lung burden. A week in a small local hospital followed, during which time a chelating agent was administered to aid in the excretion of the plutonium.

Returning to work in October with company assurances that he was "clean," Martin began to experience crushing headaches. His doctor (the plant physician) couldn't determine their cause, and by October 1968 Martin had left the NFS plant for a new job involving no contact with radioactivity.

Although a series of "whole-body counts" over the following years came up negative, one in July 1972 showed rib and lung deposits of about 2.5 times the maximum permissible body burden. Disturbed, Martin wrote the then Atomic Energy Commission in Washington, which quickly responded by investigating the incident and authorizing yet another whole body count. This time, Martin was told that he had retained an amount of radioactivity just equal to the maximum permissible body burden.

Although the AEC officials felt that there was very little chance of harm resulting from his exposure (and 30 years of experience with plutonium reinforces this prognosis), Martin must still live with the gnawing uncertainty, itself an emotional health hazard, shared by all such contamination victims.

---

*Adapted from Gillette, B. On inhaling plutonium: one man's long story. *Science*, 1974, *185*, 1028-1029. Copyright 1974 by the American Association for the Advancement of Science.

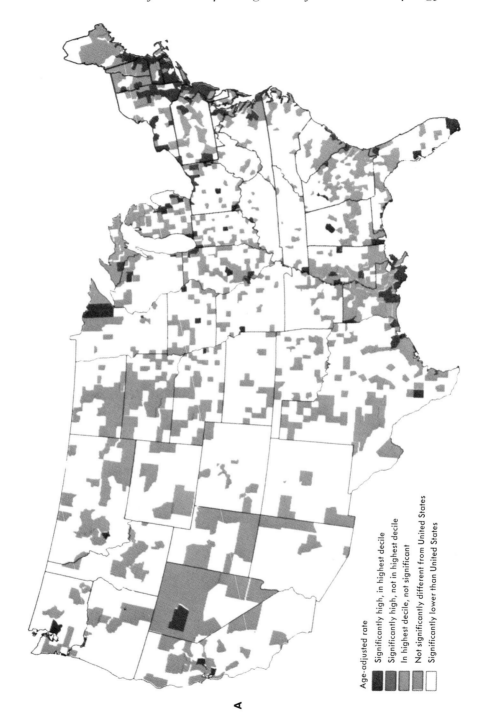

Age-adjusted rate

Significantly high, in highest decile

Significantly high, not in highest decile

In highest decile, not significant

Not significantly different from United States

Significantly lower than United States

A

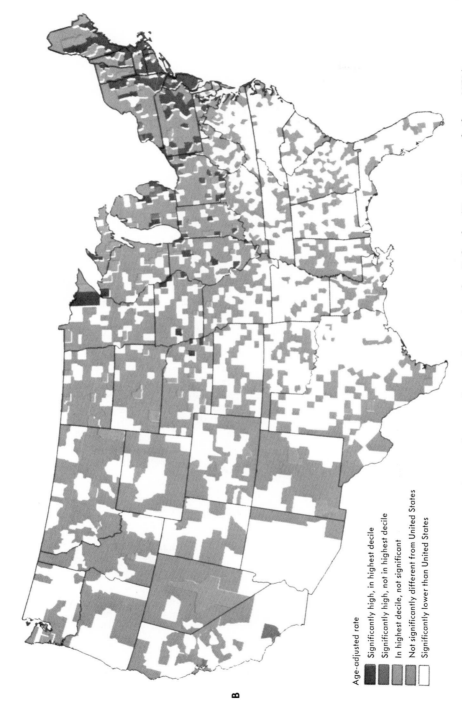

Age-adjusted rate

Significantly high, in highest decile
Significantly high, not in highest decile
In highest decile, not significant
Not significantly different from United States
Significantly lower than United States

B

Fig. 5-9. Map of cancer mortality in the United States, all types of cancer: **A**, males; **B**, females. (From Mason and others, 1976.)

ach, and others). The incidence of cancer mortality is not uniform. Mortality appears higher in urban than rural areas when adjusted for differences in population. Nonwhite males have the highest cancer mortality, followed by white males and then females (white or nonwhite) (Mason and others, 1976). The death rates for particular types of cancer suggest that local environmental influences are important. Bladder cancer, the form of cancer most closely related to occupational exposure, is clustered in industrialized areas in males working with machinery and motor vehicle manufacturing. Further examination revealed that manufacturing centers in the organic chemical industries in New Jersey had especially high death rates (Hoover and others, 1975). Environ-

mental influences on cancer include variation in natural characteristics, such as sunlight, as well as naturally and unnaturally occurring trace substances in air, water, and food supplies. The precise role of environmental influences in the incidence of cancer remains poorly understood. Possibly, the interaction of environmental with genetic, viral, or other factors holds the key. In any event, health effects of the natural and humanmade environment are a vital concern.

Effects of families combine with effects of work during middle age in the relationship between life events, stress, and illness. Life events refer to changes in personal life, such as marriage, divorce, death of a spouse, and loss or change of work. If significant and/or traumatic life events accumulate in quantity

Table 6. Social readjustment rating scale*

Rank	Life event	Mean value	Rank	Life event	Mean value
1	Death of spouse	100	23	Son or daughter leaving home	29
2	Divorce	73	24	Trouble with in-laws	29
3	Marital separation	65	25	Outstanding personal achievement	28
4	Jail term	63	26	Wife begin or stop work	26
5	Death of close family member	63	27	Begin or end school	26
6	Personal injury or illness	53	28	Change in living conditions	25
7	Marriage	50	29	Revision of personal habits	24
8	Fired at work	47	30	Trouble with boss	23
9	Marital reconciliation	45	31	Change in work hours or conditions	20
10	Retirement	45	32	Change in residence	20
11	Change in health of family member	44	33	Change in schools	20
12	Pregnancy	40	34	Change in recreation	19
13	Sex difficulties	39	35	Change in church activities	19
14	Gain of new family member	39	36	Change in social activities	18
15	Business readjustment	39	37	Mortgage or loan less than $10,000	17
16	Change in financial state	38	38	Change in sleeping habits	16
17	Death of close friend	37	39	Change in number of family get-togethers	15
18	Change to different line of work	36	40	Change in eating habits	15
19	Change in number of arguments with spouse	35	41	Vacation	13
20	Mortgage over $10,000	31	42	Christmas	12
21	Foreclosure of mortgage or loan	30	43	Minor violations of the law	11
22	Change in responsibilities at work	29			

*Reprinted with permission from *Journal of Psychosomatic Research, 11*, 213-218. Holmes, T. H., and Masuda, M., Social readjustment rating scale, 1967, Pergamon Press, Ltd.

or magnitude within a short period, the stress they generate may predispose the individual to the onset of illness. To demonstrate the relationship between life events and illness, Holmes and his colleagues (1973) developed the Social Readjustment Rating Scale shown in Table 6. Forty-three life events, ranging from marriage to beginning or ending school, were observed to cluster around the time of disease onset (Holmes and Rahe, 1967). Individuals were asked to order and assign scores to the events. The resulting ranks and mean values in Table 6 reflect the seriousness of the changes and the individual adjustment required. Comparable results from Japanese, western European, Spanish, American black, and Mexican American samples suggest an overall cross-cultural consensus as to the impact of these life events. Holmes and coworkers regard the effects of life events on disease as additive, that is, the greater the number of life events experience and the larger the total mean value score, the greater the risk of disease. They used a composite score, termed life-change units, to sum the mean values of the life events experienced in studies carried out among University of Washington physicians. Their results showed that 93% of past illnesses occurred in people having the highest life change units (more than 150 within a 2-year period), and the proportion of reported illness varied according to the life-change units accumulated previously (Holmes and Masuda, 1973). Using a similar method of scoring life events, Rahe and Romo report an elevation in life change units immediately prior to myocardial infarctions (heart attacks) in Finnish subjects. Higher life-change unit elevations had occurred for the patients who died than for those who survived the attacks (Rahe and Romo, 1974).

Recent evaluations of research on life events, stress, and illness have emphasized the strengths as well as the limitations of the findings. The relationship between a life events' score and illness has been shown to be statistically significant and indicative of the relative risk of developing subsequent illness, but the actual proportion of illnesses accounted for by life events is only around 10% (Rabkin and Struening, 1976). Relative to other risk factors for cardiovascular disease, such as high cholesterol levels, cigarette smoking, hypertension, and family history, the role of social stresses is reported to be small (Hinkle, 1974). The same kinds of life events appear to be more stressful for some individuals than for others. A variety of as yet unidentified physiological, psychological, and social factors thus may mediate the effects of stressful life events (Dohrenwend and Dohrenwend, 1974). The actual stressfulness of the event also varies according to the age and experiences of the individual. Inspecting the 43 life events (Table 6) reveals that nearly all are linked to family and career developments of middle age. This plus the fact that the life events themselves were chosen because they clustered around the time of disease onset leads to the obvious conclusion: the work- and family-related developments as well as the biological changes of middle age have potential health impact during middle age and later in life.

The effects of biological, work, and family developments of middle age differ in men compared to women. These sex differences along with the lifelong higher mortality among men make it important to examine the possible effects of sex differences on disease during middle Age. Females show an especially lower rate of cardiovascular disease. Fig. 5-10 presents data that show these sex differences. The difference is greatest during middle age, but lower mortality is retained throughout life. The overall mortality from cancer is also lower in women than in men, but sex differences in the distribution of kinds of cancer make the data difficult to in-

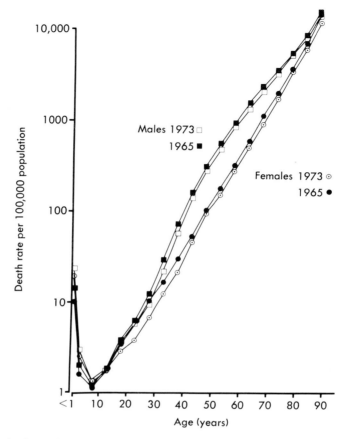

Fig. 5-10. The death rate from cardiovascular disease is higher in males than in females at every age as shown in this semilogarithmic plot of male and female mortality in the years 1965 and 1973. While cardiovascular mortality has decreased in both sexes, the difference between the sexes has remained unchanged. (Data From U.S. Vital Statistics, 1965 and 1973.)

terpret. A great many factors may be involved in the observed differences. Roles for male and female sex hormones have been advanced. The narrowing of mortality differences between men and women in cardiovascular disease after the age of menopause has supported a hormonal influence as have observations on the physiological effects of male and female sex hormones (see the first case study in Chapter 2). Male-female differences in life-style also have been implicated in differing mortality. More men smoke than

do women, although differences are narrowing. Women see their physicians more times per year than do men, perhaps reflecting a greater concern for their health and for better health care (DHEW, 1975). Different experiences in family- and work-related developments of middle age have also been examined. Greater participation in the work force among men and concomitantly greater stress also have been suggested as factors in the higher incidence of cardiovascular disease in men. However, as discussed previously, family-related developments may also be stressful, and the role of stress itself is difficult to ascertain.

Cultural variation in middle-age work and family developments is an additional, important factor that has bearing on the incidence of chronic diseases during middle age and later in life. Numerous studies have shown varying incidence of chronic diseases, such as cardiovascular disease and cancer, in different parts of the world. For example, a prospective study of heart disease in men aged 40 to 59 years in Finland, Greece, Italy, Japan, the Netherlands, the United States, and Yugoslavia points to a fourfold variation in incidence. The highest rates were seen in the United States and Finland and the lowest in Japan (Kolata and Marx, 1976). Likewise, worldwide variation in cancer incidence is pronounced (Higginson, 1969). However, variation in other factors such as diet, environmental substances, and genetic background accompanies variation in family- and work-related developments in these different cultures.

The study of diseases in populations that recently have migrated to a new culture is one technique that has been employed to study the effect of culture on disease patterns. For example, cardiovascular disease is common in Filipino immigrants to Hawaii, and mortality increased markedly from 1950 to 1970. Other chronic diseases are also common among Filipino migrants, although the type of disease appears to vary depending on the time of migration and the occupational and social circumstances into which the immigrant moved (Hackenberg, Gerber, and Hackenberg, 1978). Filipino immigrants who came prior to World War II (1906 to 1940) have higher rates of mental disorders, heart disease, hypertension, asthma, hay fever, arthritis, and rheumatism than do later immigrants. The later immigrants, Filipinos who came to Hawaii between 1966 and 1975,

have higher rates of cardiovascular disease, ulcers, and skin disease. The earlier immigrants tended to be plantation laborers in rural, low-income areas; whereas the later ones were well-educated professionals who moved into higher income, urban areas of Hawaii. Thus, the culture changes experienced may have been an important factor in predisposing both the earlier and later immigrants to this series of stress-related diseases, but the particular diseases appear to have been influenced by the socioeconomic setting into which the immigrants moved.

Summary

Despite the fact that processes of chronic diseases begin during this period, the middle years are a time of good health and relatively few recognized disease problems. In many ways, the middle years are a stable period of relatively little biological change in which family- and work-related challenges provide meaningful opportunities for accomplishment. Middle age links the period of adolescence, when physical maturity and sense of identity are being achieved, and the period of family formation with the future developments of old age. The multiple responsibilities of middle age necessitate that support be received through the social networks that link middle age with the adolescent, family formation, and old age periods. In a previous section, an example taken from the central Andes illustrated the strength of social alliance and support networks that join family groups. The contrast with the comparatively isolated and age-segregated American family emphasizes the relative absence of supportive social networks for linking age groups in American society.

The causes of the most common health problems of middle age—obesity and hypertension—are not known but are influenced by the life-style (for example, sedentary existence, smoking habits, high-cholesterol and high-salt diets) of the middle-aged person. The existence of chronic diseases such as cardiovascular disease and cancer in middle age is paradoxical insofar as their existence is generally not recognized by the individual in whom one or the other disease process has taken hold. The causes of these chronic diseases too remain poorly understood, although it is known that aspects of middle-age life play a part; among these are the physical environments in which one works and lives, life-style, personality, and life event stresses, obesity, and hypertension. The processes of chronic disease continue and, as is discussed in the next section, become apparent during old age.

AGING AND OLD AGING
Theories of aging

Aging is a continuing phenomenon throughout the human life span; it begins with conception and ends with death. As such, "aging" refers to changes in the individual that are associated with the passage of time, and so are synonymous with development. As such, old aging cannot be separated rigidly from the preceding periods of the life cycle.

To understand the process of aging, human beings have focused on the events surrounding the period of old aging in the human life cycle. In the history of Western culture, Hippocrates' writings provide the earliest theory of the aging process. Aging, he thought, was caused by an upset in the balance among the four humours—blood, phlegm, choler, and black choler. Balance among the four humours was responsible for maintaining health, and so aging was likened to illness. Hippocrates also compared the stages of human development to the four seasons of the year. In this analogy, which stays with us today, old age corresponded to the winter season of life (de Beauvior, 1973: 27). Galen, an early Roman physician, was much influenced by Hippocrates' view of aging. Aging, he believed, was caused by the loss of the inner heat that came from the four humours. Like Hippocrates, Galen considered old age closer to illness than health. When inner heat faded away, the person died. A means of retarding the aging process was to keep the body warm and well hydrated by drinking great amounts of fluid. The image of heat as life was retained, especially during the Middle Ages, when life was likened to a flame. The flame flickered if life was endangered; death occurred when the flame went out (de Beauvior, 1973:28-30). The flame as a symbol for life continues to figure importantly in Christian religious beliefs, as exemplified by the use of candles in church services and the presence of an eternal flame as a memorial at President John F. Kennedy's grave. More recently, the study of the diseases of old aging, geriatrics, and the study of the process of old aging, gerontology, have been formalized as scientific disciplines. In 1974, a National Institute on Aging was founded as a part of the National Institute of Health to plan, fund, and coordinate basic biomedical, social, and behavioral research into the process of aging and to support education and training in both research and services in the field of aging (Butler, 1975:355).

Observations that the pattern of aging is similar in all mammals and that each animal species, mammalian or nonmammalian, has a characteristic life span suggest a common basic, biological mechanism for aging. Mammalian life spans range from 3 years for mice to 110 years (± 10 years) for human beings. The life span, while difficult to determine precisely, sets the limit for the number of years that members of a specie will live. The oldest documented age for a human being is 113 years, although allegedly older ages have been reported (Acsádi and Nemeskeri, 1970). As a general rule, the smaller the animal, the shorter the life span. Life span, like other attributes of a specie and like species themselves, can evolve. Other primates have considerably shorter life spans than do human beings. The chimpanzee, perhaps our closest living relative, has a life span of about 50 years (Campbell, 1976). The present human life span has evolved to about 110 years during the course of human evolution. An individual's life expectancy is different from life span, insofar as life expectancy is the proportion of the life span that members of a specie can expect to live. Life expectancy is a function of age-specific mortality and varies among different populations; life span appears to be a genetically determined characteristic that exists for the specie as a whole.

The genetic role in aging. The existence of species-specific life spans suggests a genetic control for the length of life. Several lines of research have addressed the role of genes in the aging process more specifically. Progeria and Werner's syndrome are two rare diseases of suspected genetic origin that mimic the signs of aging (Epstein and others, 1966; Reichel, Garcia-Bunuel, and Dilallo, 1971). Children with progeria stop growing in the first decade of life; victims of Werner's syndrome begin to show signs of old aging in their twenties or thirties. In both instances, the normal aging process is telescoped. Cardiovascular problems, such as heart murmurs, arteriosclerosis, hypertension, and heart failure occur with great rapidity. The skin becomes wrinkled and takes on the parchmentlike appearance of an older person. Hair becomes gray and sparse. Other chronic diseases such as diabetes and cancer, are common. Progeria victims usually die in their twenties; individuals with Werner's syndrome die in their forties. The extremely rapid appearance of the signs of aging in these diseases suggests that some internal timing mechanism is at work that affects both

the onset and rate of deterioration in a coordinated fashion such that most organ systems appear to be aging at the same rate. The central, programmed nature of the disease is consistent with a hypothesis of genetic origin.

Another line of investigation supportive of a genetic role in the aging process comes from studies done on the cellular level by Leonard Hayflick and others (reviewed in Hayflick, 1975). This research points to a finite capacity for cell replication, whether cells were grown in controlled laboratory conditions or were transplanted to animal hosts. For embryonic human cells, the life span is about 50 doublings. Cell life span varies according to the age of the cell donor and according to the length of the species' life span; the younger the donor and the longer the length of the species' life span, the greater the number of cell doublings possible. Some cells never loose their capacity for replicating. These "immortal" cells are cancer cells. For example, cancerous cervical cells taken from Henrietta Lacks in 1951 (termed the Hela strain) have been grown in culture ever since. Cell fusion studies have pointed to a location in the nucleus for controlling the number of cell doublings. Because the nucleus contains the genetic material and because of the species-specific nature of the cell life span, the work of Hayflick and others is strongly supportive of genetic control for the aging process.

The existence of a finite cellular life span and of rare diseases of premature aging with suspected genetic origin does not explain how the functional losses associated with aging occur in biological systems. Nobody ever died of old age. Attempts to reverse the loss of function and deteriorative changes, known as senescence, that occur with old age have called forth various elixirs. Ponce de Leon searched for the fountain of youth in the 1500s. The French physiologist

Brown-Séquard believed that testicular extracts had a rejuvenating effect and attributed to them his vitality and scientific prowess. In the early twentieth century, chimpanzee testicles were grafted onto human males to prevent aging. Reproductive functions diminish with age, although great variation is seen in men, but the cause would seem to lie in hormone changes in the brain rather than in the reproductive hormones themselves (reviewed by Finch, 1975). Aslan (1974), in Roumania, reports rejuvenating effects of a special novocainelike solution that she calls Gerovital H₃." In the absence of adequate proof, such claims continue to be rejected by the scientific community.

Hormonal and immune system control. The role of hormones in the aging process continues to be an active field of research. Recent activity has centered on the pituitary-hypothalamus glands in the brain that serve as "master" glands for the regulation of the body's other hormonal systems. Caleb Finch has suggested that changes in a selected portion of the brain, such as the hypothalamus, could serve as pacemakers of hormonal aging (1975). Denckla has pointed to a possible new function for the pituitary gland. He reports that a substance is secreted from the pituitary gland that decreases the responsiveness of tissues to thyroid hormones, causing decreased tissue oxygen consumption and the hypothyroidism seen in older animals (1974).

The increase with age in the incidence of a number of diseases has led some investigators to explore the possibility that a decline in the immune system predisposes older people to illness. Some changes in the immune system, such as a decrease in thymus size, are known to occur with age. The thymus is involved with the differentiation of T cells that, in turn, play a role in conferring cellular immunity to some viruses, fungi, and other foreign substances and possibly acts

to suppress tumor growth (Adler, 1975). Changes in the immune system also may result in the increased autoimmunity (destruction of the body's own tissues by the immune system) seen in some older people. Some diseases, such as rheumatoid arthritis and maturity-onset diabetes, might be autoimmune disorders. Effects of altered nutrition on length of life also may act through the immune system. Animals fed calorie restricted but nutritionally adequate diets when young have a markedly increased length of life (DHEW, 1976).

Theories of biological aging emphasizing genetic, hormonal, or immune system control are not necessarily mutually exclusive. Hayflick has suggested that "other functional losses that occur in cells prior to the cessation of division capacity produce physiological decrements in animals much before their normal cells have reached their maximum proliferation capacity" (1975:633). The loss of function may occur in the thymus, the hypothalamus, the pituitary gland, or some other organs and, thus, may usher in the age-related changes known to occur. The debate concerns the cause of the loss of function. Hayflick accords genetic instability the major role. Genetic instability refers to the decreasing ability of genes to carry out their normal protein synthesizing function. Their loss of function may be caused by any one of a number of factors: mutations, cross-linking of molecules leading to gene repression, accumulated errors in DNA molecules, exhaustion of gene "copies," free radicals, or accumulated errors in the manufactured proteins. The opposing view held by Denckla, Finch, Adler, and others views change in the pituitary gland, hypothalamus, or thymus-immune system as primary. However, since each of these glands or systems is composed of gene-containing cells, genes may still be fundamentally responsible for initiating changes in their functioning.

Cultural and behavioral factors in aging. In addition to the biological theories of the underlying mechanisms of the aging process, additional theories of aging have attempted to explain its behavioral accompaniments.

Culture exerts important influences on aging. During past human evolution, culture acted to prolong the period of immaturity and dependence because a longer childhood was advantageous for learning tool use, tool making, social cooperation, and social organization. Culture provides a means for recognizing stages in the continuum of individual development throughout the life span. Rites of passage, as described earlier in this chapter, occur at transitions in the human life cycle to define social age, status, and role. In traditional cultures, people experiencing a rite of passage together are grouped as an "age grade." Chronological ages may vary, but the same social age is assured. Social age implicitly carries with it a set of expectations for appropriate behavior. As will be seen later in this section, means of assigning social age independent of chronological age are virtually absent in American culture.

Behavioral theories of the aging process have received relatively little attention compared to biological theories. The inherent difficulty in conducting the necessary longitudinal studies, the inappropriateness of animal models, along with the bias within American society toward ignoring aging (especially old aging) have limited the development of behavioral theories.

The disengagement theory articulated by Cumming and Henry (1961) has been the subject of a great deal of controversy, perhaps because it is one of the few behavioral theories available. According to this theory, growing old involves "an inevitable, mutual withdrawal or disengagement, resulting in decreased interaction between an aging person and others in the social system he belongs to" (Cumming and Henry, 1961:14).

According to this theory, the individual and society find the process of disengagement to be mutually satisfying. The individual accomplishes the disengagement by lowering the number, variety, and intensity of social roles and relationships. Society facilitates the process by offering freedom from constraints and proscribing and/or granting permission for withdrawal (Cumming and Henry, 1961). Some support, but mostly criticism, has been directed at this theory on the grounds that the disengagement is not inevitable, for exceptions may be found (for example, people taking on new roles), nor is it necessarily mutually satisfying. Rather than the individual wanting to disengage from the work force, for example, the individual may be forced out by social necessity based on the pace of scientific and technological accomplishment and by the need for positions to become available in the labor force.

These criticisms of the disengagement theory have resulted in the activity theory, in which older people are seen as having the same social and psychological needs as middle-aged people (Havighurst, Neugarten, and Tobin, 1968:161). According to this theory, optimal aging consists of being or remaining active. New activities are substituted for ones surrendered, new friends replace ones lost, and hobbies or new jobs take the place of jobs lost through retirement. Remaining active seems part of the appeal of retirement communities such as Sun City, Arizona, but studies reveal individual variation and great inactivity on the part of many residents (see Jacobs, 1974).

A third approach has been to emphasize personality patterns as the central dimension in the aging process. Personality is seen as a way of coping that is maintained throughout life and becomes increasingly consistent in old age. Neugarten, Havighurst, and Tobin (1968) described eight examples of personality patterns seen among a sample of 70 to 79 year olds: reorganizer, focused, disengaged, holding on, constricted, succorance-seeker, apathetic, and disorganized. These eight patterns include a range of personality types (integrated, armored-defended, passive-dependent, unintegrated), activity levels (low, medium, high); and degree of life satisfaction (low, medium, high). Included within the various categories are the kinds of people specified by the disengagement theory (that is, the disengaged pattern) and by the activity theory (that is, the integrated pattern), but additional variants are included.

A final group of theories concerned with the behavioral aspects of old aging are the stage theories of Erikson, Havighurst, and Kohlberg. Each of these theories outlines a series of developmental stages that the individual must or should reach between infancy and old age. In Erik Erikson's (1950) formulation, the development of generativity and ego integrity are associated with middle adulthood and late adulthood respectively. If these developments do not occur, stagnation (middle adulthood) or despair (late adulthood) ensues. Havighurst (1952) poses a lengthier set of tasks to be accomplished in middle age, including the achievement of civic and social responsibility, developing leisure time activities, accepting and adjusting to the physiological changes of age, and adjusting to aging parents. Kohlberg (1973) sees growth in wisdom or moral development as possibly, but not always, occurring with age. The social ages are marked by the attainment of a universal ethical principle, respect for human dignity, and cosmic perspective in which one's own life is seen as finite from an infinite perspective. In each of these three developmental theories, the continual nature of development throughout the life span receives valuable emphasis. Variation among individuals is also recognized insofar as not everyone may attain the designated stage of development. However, since each is based

on individual development, the effects of society and culture in imposing various roles and responsibilities on the individual receive comparatively little attention.

In summary, the process of aging encompasses continual biological and behavioral change throughout the life span. Aging, at the biological level, is regulated by genetic, hormonal, or immunological factors, or some combination of them. Cultural practices act to define the individual's social age. Debate continues as to whether society prescribes disengagement or continuing activity for the older person. Continuity of personality patterns in older people is recognized along with the possibility of continuing individual and moral development. Clearly, aging is a phenomenon to which a broad variety of factors contribute. Yet aging is an inevitable and, thus, ultimately predictable process. From an individual point of view, aging cannot be stopped nor should it be resented; both growth and aging are integral aspects of development. From a population point of view, aging confers the benefit of turnover, carrying with it the possibility for increasing adaptation and evolutionary change.

Biological characteristics of old age

Given the continual nature of the aging process, there is no inherent time at which old age begins. Old age can be set only arbitrarily, according to some agreed on convention. Unlike such periods in the life cycle as adolescence, old age is not signaled by any abrupt biological changes. Decreasing functional capacities characterize organs and organ systems with advanced age, as shown in Fig. 5-11, throughout the later phases of the life span. Decreasing energy expenditure is reflected in a declining metabolic rate. Lung, heart, and kidney capacities decline. Sufficient functional ability is retained in each of these organ systems for activity under normal circumstances, for each is endowed with an enormous reserve earlier in life. Normal changes in physiological parameters, such as blood pressure, glucose tolerance, and glomerular filtration rates, make it difficult to detect cardiovascular disease, diabetes, and renal disease respectively. These same changes occur to a lesser extent during middle age. Changes in the musculoskeletal system include decrease in muscle mass, relative straightening and rigidification of the spine, and reorientation of the head of the femur such that it joins the hip at more nearly a right angle. As a result, posture assumes a more stooped position and gait becomes more shuffling. Decreased senses of hearing, vision, and touch, along with poorer balance and coordination, and nervous system changes that slow reaction time, limit mobility and increase vulnerability to accidents. The older person is particularly prone to hip injury and fracture at the head of the femur. In the face of injury or stress, the comparative absence of reserve during old age limits the ability to adapt and maintain homeostasis. Thus a comparatively minor injury is more likely to trigger additional reactions and more serious problems in the older person.

While decreasing functional capacities of physiological systems is the general trend in older people, it is not the absolute rule. The presence of physiological decline accompanying age is likely to be overestimated, since the majority of studies have been done on sick and institutionalized subjects and have focused on the limiting aspects to the organism. To help correct this imbalance, an interdisciplinary study on healthy men 65 to 92 years old was begun in 1955 by investigators at the National Institute of Mental Health. A total of 47 men were studied intensively, 20 having no observable disease and 27 having observable but asymptomatic disease (chiefly, arteriosclerosis) (Birren and others, 1971). Comparison with younger age groups revealed the absence of age-associated changes in physiological parameters, such as blood pressure, serum cholesterol levels, maximum breathing capacity, and fasting blood glucose. Cerebral blood flow

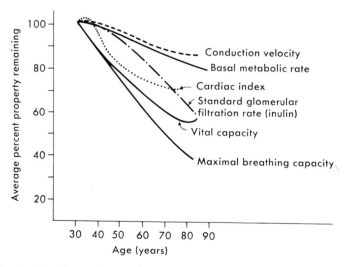

Fig. 5-11. Decline in various human functional capacities and physiological measurements with age. (From Bierman and Hazzard, 1973:20.)

and oxygen consumption were not different from those of younger men except in those older subjects with arteriosclerosis for whom decreased cerebral blood flow was observed. Vital capacity, auditory acuity in the higher frequencies, and psychomotor functioning were reduced in the older men, but, interestingly, verbal intelligence scores were higher in the older than in the younger men. A follow-up study 11 years later revealed that, among the survivors, almost one-half had diseases (most often cardiovascular) (Granick and Patterson, 1971). Blood pressure was unchanged, fasting blood sugar was increased, and cerebral blood flow and psychological test scores were decreased compared to the previous study. The people who previously had not shown any disease were more often among the survivors than those who had initially shown asymptomatic disease. This illustrates the importance of even asymptomatic illness in determining length of life. However, the length of life in the subjects, initially identified as free of disease and almost indistinguishable in health from younger people, was only slightly longer than for other men in their same age group. This points to the possible role of genetic factors for determining length of life as well as to the fact that a lengthy period of physiological decline does not necessarily precede death. Thus, while decrease in functional capacities may be present and of importance for determining length of life in some old people, physiological decline does not take place in all older persons and does not necessarily foreshadow disease and imminent death.

Another line of evidence that shows variation in the physiological trends associated with age comes from studies of aging in other cultures. Rosen and coworkers studied the hearing of the Mebaans, a group of isolated African people living in southeast Sudan (1970). These people live in a virtually silent environment, where noise levels average 35 to 40 decibals. Their culture produces little noise because guns and drums and other loud musical instruments are not present. The absence of Western technology precludes the additional noise-producing machinery of the modern age. Hearing acuity at medium and high frequencies was markedly better among the Mebaans than in people of the same age in Western cultures. Age-related declines were evident, but hearing loss in 60- to 80-year-old Mebaans approximated that in 20-year-old subjects studied in Wisconsin. The importance of their culture in protecting against age-related changes in hearing is illustrated by the observation that hearing loss develops among Mebaans living in Khartoum, the capital of Sudan.

Disease problems during old age

The picture of the health of old people in America contains what may at first appear to be contradictions. The overwhelming majority consider themselves well, live in the community, get around by themselves, and rely on family members for needed help. These findings reflect widespread, but not universal, health among elderly persons. Yet 86% of those over 65 and 72% in the 45 to 64 year old age group have one or more chronic diseases (Butler, 1975:175). Clearly, the majority of the elderly consider themselves healthy in the face of disease.

The diseases of old age are for the most part the same kinds as seen in the middle age and younger populations. These include cardiovascular disease, hypertension, arteriosclerosis, cancers, emphysema, bronchitis, arthritis, and diabetes. Some of these may result in sudden death, but in most instances the disease is present for many years before it is recognized or limits activity. As discussed with reference to middle age, cures for chronic diseases are not available because their cause or causes remain unknown. Controlling the disorders is possible, however, in many instances. Diuretics to deplete blood volume, drugs to dilate blood vessels, and drugs to decrease constriction of the blood vessels are employed for controlling hypertension. Digitalis, nitroglycerin, isoproterenol, and propanolol are among drugs used to improve heart function in people with heart disease. Insulin as therapy for diabetes and aspirin for providing relief from arthritis are well known. Variation among individuals and variation over time within the same individual limit the effectiveness of available medications, with the result that the individuals become aware, at least periodically, of their disorders.

Besides the limitations imposed by incomplete knowledge and only partial ability to control chronic diseases, the elderly face additional problems in gaining correct diagnosis and treatment. Normal physiological changes associated with aging (Fig. 5-11) complicate diagnosis. A rise in blood pressure with age hinders the diagnosis of hypertension; a decrease in glucose tolerance makes it difficult to recognize diabetes. Too, the presence of a disease over a longer period of time increases the likelihood that one or more additional disorders are present. The diagnosis of these diseases is complicated by multiple, overlapping diseases, leading to the presence of unusual symptoms. Diseases such as acute and chronic brain syndrome may be confused. Both present signs of mental confusion, memory loss, and mental disorganization. Acute brain syndrome, however, usually results from trauma, anemia, infection, alcohol, or drugs, and once the underlying problem is recognized, the condition can be reversed. If undetected, acute brain disorder can become chronic and, therefore, permanent. Chronic brain syndrome may also result from cerebral thrombosis, hemorrhage, or embolism. Correct diagnosis of and distinction between these

brain disorders is made difficult by an additional problem faced by the elderly; acting senile is sometimes viewed as an expected accompaniment of aging and, therefore, is often considered a symptom that does not require diagnosis or treatment. Chronic brain syndrome has become a "wastebasket" label applied to anyone acting senile (Butler, 1975:176). When it is applied to a person with acute brain syndrome, the results may become particularly tragic.

Medical care for the elderly became the object of major national legislation in 1965, with passage of the Health Insurance for the Aged, or Medicare, bill. Provision was made for hospital and some nursing home care (Part A) and for physician's services (Part B). Effects of Medicare are difficult to evaluate completely. The utilization of medical services by the elderly increased, principally as a result of remedying previously unmet needs. The orientation of Medicare, however, is toward providing acute care for short-term illnesses and injuries. This has created problems, given the high incidence of chronic diseases among the elderly. Payment for care of a chronic condition is excluded unless an acute exacerbation of the chronic condition occurs. Medicare also is limited in the length of time over which it pays for care of an illness. One of the most dramatic impacts of Medicare has been on health costs. Physicians are paid "usual and customary fees," and hospitals are reimbursed on a "cost plus" basis. As a result, effective limitations on health care costs have been removed, and health care costs have risen far more than has the cost of living. Before Medicare (1966) the elderly paid out-of-pocket one-half of their average annual medical bill of $468, or $234; after Medicare (1972), the elderly paid one-quarter of their average annual bill of $1100, or $276. Because of inflation and some increased use of services, out-of-pocket expenses for the elderly have actually increased under Medicare (Butler, 1975: 207).

The final set of factors, hindering effective treatment and diagnosis of disease among the elderly concerns the cultural orientation of Western medicine. As mentioned in Chapters 1 and 6, the concept of disease based on the doctrine of specific etiology was developed as an explanation for infectious diseases. The doctrine of specific etiology is still highly applicable to acute illnesses and injuries. But thus far, specific etiology has remained elusive for chronic diseases. As a result, treatment of "curable" acute disorders remains a popular part of the medical mainstream, whereas many physicians are uninterested in caring for chronic conditions (Butler, 1975:179). Stereotyping the elderly patient as a "crock," meaning an undesirable patient, is one, nonsubtle way in which preference is expressed for a patient with a curable disease. The public reinforces the traditional orientation of Western medicine by demanding instant cures for chronic diseases and by the expectation of at least "a pill" (often the treatment for an infectious disease) to remedy health problems.

The series of problems just described constitutes a vicious circle. Health care personnel share the negative view of old age present in American culture and liken aging to illness. The elderly also come to expect health problems with age and, indeed, are likely to develop one or more chronic diseases. Individually, older people are likely to view themselves as healthy. The view the elderly have of themselves as healthy makes them feel that their good health is an exception for which they should be thankful. Consequently, there is little pressure from the elderly or the general public for changes that might result in better treatment and diagnosis of disease or reorientation of the health care system more toward care of chronic conditions or toward a more positive view of old age.

Influence of culture on old age

As was mentioned in an earlier section, culture plays a central role in the old aging process. Not only does culture exert an effect on physiological changes associated with aging, but it also defines when old age begins and does much to determine the content of the old person's life. Cultures have utilized a range of means for defining old age, both formal and functional. Formal criteria are ones established without reference to any observable change in the individual, but rather according to some arbitrary convention. Functional criteria are based on a change in the ability or function of the individual in society.

In this regard, American culture operates according to a formal criteria, that is, the chronological age of 65 years. At the age of 65, the individual is obliged or expected to retire and thus becomes a senior citizen.* Defining old age by the number of years elapsed from birth is part of a uniquely elaborated concept of time in Western cultures. The formal definition of old age does not specify any tasks or roles for the old person, unlike for people in the other periods of the life cycle. It is expected that tasks will be relinquished, but no consensus exists as to what will take their place. With retirement, the role of worker ends. The role of parent is relinquished, given the pattern of family residence in which children leave home to establish their own households. Elderly persons are not expected to assume new roles, such as that of teacher, in order to pass on their knowledge, skills, and responsibilities.

Old age in America. The expected emptiness of old age is perhaps a part of the reason why many have such a negative view of old age. "Youth, I do adore thee/Old age, I do abhor thee," (William Shakespeare) still applies to a prevalent attitude. The perception

---

*With the recent change in retirement age from 65 to 70, age 70 may become the formal beginning of old age.

of old age as linked with illness is also part of the reason. As we have seen, the association of illness with old age goes as far back as Hippocrates in the cultural history of the Western world. Historical features of American culture have influenced attitudes toward old age. Until comparatively recently (especially in the West), the United States has been a frontier society. The population settling this country was young, with the parents and grandparents remaining on the other side of the Atlantic Ocean. Apart from a limited existence in agricultural regions, the extended family has never been a widespread phenomenon in the United States. The comparative absence of older people and elderly role models also may have helped foster the youth-oriented culture and the negative view of old age. Another influence has been the fact that American history almost coincides with the history of industrialization, which is marked by extremely rapid societal and technological changes. The aged in this setting can become a lost generation, possessing an outmoded culture, whose skills are rendered obsolete by "progress." Finally, the protestant tradition of the work ethic has contributed to a negative view of old age. Central to the work ethic is the idea that one achieves value as a human being through work done here and now, on this earth, and not in some future, spiritual realm. If self-worth is achieved through work, the elderly are removed from the accepted source of self-esteem. One's previous job may provide carry over, but it fades with time. A person whose health is impaired may not be able to seek new work or, even if healthy, may be perceived of as ill (by virtue of being old) and thus incapable of doing work. The factors that contribute to a negative view of aging make it not surprising that some elderly seek recourse in hair dyes, face lifts, and a continuing whirlwind of activity for holding on to the positively valued image of youth and denying the negative view of their old age.

The picture of old age in America thus contains some unpleasant aspects: the arbitrary use of chronological age to define its onset, the absence of meaningful roles for the elderly, and the negative view of old age held by older and younger Americans. However, people over 65 years of age are not uniformly bedridden, confined to institutions, and isolated from their families. Only 5% live in institutions (nursing homes, homes for the aged, hospitals); 95% live in the community, and the overwhelming majority (69%) of all the elderly live in their own homes for which the mortgage has been fully paid (Butler, 1975:108). Retirement communities are highly visible, but they house a very small proportion of the elderly. The elderly's residential location is overwhelmingly urban, as is true for the rest of Americans. Eighty-one percent of the elderly report that they are able to get around by themselves without any assistance (Butler, 1975:175). Two-thirds of the elderly consider themselves as being well. Of the services needed by the elderly, the vast majority are provided by the family. Government (local, state, federal) programs to assist the elderly have proliferated in recent years. In one urban area, for example, they include the Senior Aides Program, the Retired Senior Volunteer Program (RSVP), Older Americans Inc., the Senior Companions Program, Outreach Services for the Aging, Old Friends Visiting Program, the Senior Discount Program, Services for Seniors, and the Lost Arts Program.

Problems do exist regarding housing and governmental services available to the elderly. The force of inflation on a fixed income is such that rent, property taxes, and necessary household repairs consume a larger percentage of the elderly's income than is true for younger age groups. Age discrimination in financial lending, a shortage of low-cost housing, and deterioration in older neighborhoods create additional difficulties (see Butler, 1975.

The family continues to play an important part in the lives of older people. The majority in the United States belong to three- or four-generation families with surviving children, grandchildren, and even great-grandchildren (Shanas and others, 1968:144). Becoming a grandparent is a major marker of social life and can be an important rite of passage for elderly persons. An increase in the number of three- and, especially, four-generation families has been a twentieth century trend created by earlier age of marriage, fewer children spaced closely together, and increased life expectancy. The rise of the four-generation family has created a comparatively new situation in which 60 year olds may be caring for 80 year olds, and 40-year-old couples may potentially find themselves trying to meet the needs of two sets of parents and four sets of grandparents. With time, the elderly lose relatives among their contemporaries (siblings, brothers- and sisters-in-law, cousins) but gain family members through marriages and births among their descendants. Few American elderly (25%) live with their children; those who do tend to be widowed and living with an unmarried daughter (Shanas and others, 1968:155; Palmore, 1975:43). Thus the multigeneration family but not the multigeneration household is common in the United States. Contact with children, however, is frequent. Shanas and coworkers report that two-thirds of the elderly in the United States either lived with or had seen one of their children the previous day. Overall, daughters were seen more frequently than sons (Shanas and others, 1968:162-164).

The contradiction between the expectation based on the negative view of old age and the experience of old age as portrayed in the above statistics was made apparent in a Harris Poll (1975). Results from this survey appear in Table 7. There is an enormous gap between expectation and experience. A much larger proportion of the general public perceives problems of old age as "very serious" than the experiences of the elderly appear to justify. Likewise, when the elderly are asked to identify "very serious" problems for persons over 65, they attribute "very serious" problems more often to others of their age group than they do to themselves (Harris, 1975). The gap between experience and expectation shared by older people and the general public helps to maintain the negative view of old age and to create barriers between older people based on a false sense of personal distinctiveness.

Cross-cultural view of old age. Is a negative view of old age universal? A series of historical influences on the view of old age have been described for American culture. Have other cultures with different histories developed different views of old age? The

Table 7. Problems of old age*

Very serious problems of old age	Percent experienced by persons over 65	Percent attributed to most people over 65 by general public
Fear of crime	23	50
Poor health	21	51
Financial (problems)	15	62
Loneliness	12	60
Inadequate medical care, education, feelings of need, activity, friends, jobs, housing, clothing	3-10	16-44

*Data from The Myth and Reality of Aging in America, a study prepared by Louis Harris and Associates, Inc. for the National Council on the Aging, Inc., Washington, D.C. © 1975.

idea is often expressed that modernization leads to a decline in status for the elderly (Cowgill and Holmes, 1972). Nonindustrial societies often retain positions of power and prestige for their elderly (see Simmons, 1970, for extensive review). However, it is important to distinguish between the ideal picture of what ought to be and what actually is. Simmons reports on the ideal vision of the elderly, which may be seen in examples of old men holding central positions in Chippewa council meetings, old Kwakiutl women achieving influence as soothsayers, and Hottentot families paying deference to their elders (1970:50-81). However, heterogeneity exists in all cultures. A study by Harlan (1968) in India found considerable discrepancy between the ideal and actual circumstances of older people. As an outgrowth of Hindu principles, the cultural ideal specifies that the eldest male is the source of family authority; however, Harlan found that fewer than half of the families in three villages studied met this ideal. Instead, the authority of the eldest male was often subjugated to that of a married son, and the older family members complained of inadequate care.

Japan represents a culture in which extensive industrialization and modernization have occurred and yet where respect and high prestige for the elderly have been retained. Palmore concludes in a recent study, "In short, most Japanese think 'grey is beautiful;' most Americans do not" (1975:111). What distinguishes the process of old aging in Japan from that presented for America? Life expectancy is not different in the two settings. Cross-cultural comparisons of health are difficult because of different concepts of health and disease, but the majority of older Japanese, like the majority of older Americans, report good health (Pamore, 1975:32). In Palmore's study (1975), the primary differences appeared in work and family contexts. More than three-fourths of Japanese over 65

years of age live with their children (more frequently, a son) and typically with their grandchildren as well. Only one-fourth of elderly Americans live with their children (more frequently a daughter). The elderly provide household services, supervise meals and children, do gardening and other light tasks, and serve as advisors on family and business matters. Despite customary retirement at age 55, more than half of Japanese over 65 are employed compared to one-third of older Americans. Retirement does not necessarily mean stopping work. More often, retirement means changing jobs or staying at the same job for lower pay. Pension and social security benefits are low compared to those in the United States. But the Japanese workers more commonly report that they are motivated to work out of a sense of duty rather than financial necessity (the most common reason cited by Americans). The family provides the primary source of support for the elderly. Public recognition and respect for the elderly is fostered by Japanese language and custom, which clearly accord preference and deference to older people. Special celebration of the sixty-first birthday and a national holiday, Respect for Elder's Day, provide further recognition for the elderly. Overall, advancing age appears to bring increased satisfaction with life for the Japanese; decreasing satisfaction with life characterizes most Americans during their later years.

The Palmore study (1975) amply illustrates that modernization need not be accompanied by a loss of respect and prestige for the elderly. Instead, high status and social integration for the Japanese elderly appear to have been maintained. Palmore points to the importance of the preexisting cultural tradiions of the vertical society and filial piety. The vertical society is a system of according respect and authority by age; filial piety refers to the unconditional allegiance and support owed one's parents and is a part of Shintoism, the traditional religion of Japan. These cultural traditions accord an important place for the elderly within the family, the household, the labor force, and the society in general. The contrasts between the pattern of old aging in Japan and the United States are not caused by differences in reported levels of health, social security benefits, or governmental services. The contrasts reside in the underlying fabric of the cultures.

Summary

The process of aging and old aging is intrinsically both a biological and cultural phenomenon. Biological mechanisms control the underlying processes of aging. Current theories emphasize the possible roles of genes, the immunological system, and the hormonal systems in the brain in controlling the biological changes of aging. Society and culture play important parts in determining the way in which age is identified, the point at which old age begins, and the expected roles and status of the elderly. Personality and individual development influence the kind of adaptation to old age that occurs. In general, most people over 65 years of age in the United States appear to have made a healthy adjustment. The majority consider themselves well, get around by themselves, live in their own homes, and interact frequently with (but do not live with) members of their three- or four-generation families. The experiences of old age in America conflict with many of the expectations held by the general public. Health, financial, crime-related, and personal problems of old age appear to be exaggerated. The elderly person is expected to be disabled both physically and mentally or, at least, to be less able than younger counterparts. There is some degree of truth in this stereotypical negative view of old age, but the ste-

reotype necessarily overlooks variation. Among older people, this variation is not the exception; it is the rule.

Physiological functioning in some older people is indistinguishable from that of people in younger age groups. Where physiological decline occurs, it does not lead inexorably to disease or to a restricted lifestyle. Culture plays an important part in the existence of variation through its effects on environment, life-style, and attitudes. Japanese culture provides a contrasting example to American culture. It includes a series of cultural attributes that have preserved social prestige and integration for the elderly. The attributes of Japanese culture cannot simply be transplanted to the United States and need not be transferred in order to result in a change in our view of old age. Examining the lives and experiences of America's elderly provides the necessary stimulus to achieving a more balanced view of old age. Such an examination is needed if the social stigma attached to old age is to be removed and if the health care available to the elderly is to be improved.

DYING AND DEATH

Public discussion of dying and death has been taboo, avoided in American culture and ignored in the education of health professionals. The common view among adult Americans is that there is a fixed polarization between life and death. Being dead is the opposite of being alive; to consider death is to deny life. Perhaps the polarization between life and death is a result of a combination of cultural features: the Judaeo-Christian belief in which "body" is contrasted with "spirit"; a culturally-conditioned world view that compartmentalizes events into mutually exclusive categories (such as black-white, yes-no, past-present-future); and a technocratic society that invests heavily in educating its young, rewards the accomplishments of its adult members, and demonstrates little interest in the elderly.

Irrespective of the reasons why the American view of death has developed, avoiding the discussion of death and polarizing death and life have created a series of problems and dilemmas. Increasingly, death occurs as the result of the conscious or unconscious decision of the physician. With means available for prolonging life, such as the heart-lung machine, questions arise as to whether or not the "plug" should be pulled, who should do it, and under what circumstances it should be done.

Defining death

The well-publicized case of Karen Quinlan, in which her parents requested the discontinuation "of all extraordinary means of sustaining"* her vital processes, illustrates the complexity of the decisions that often surround death. Karen Quinlan had entered a vegetative state of "irreversible brain damage" and had no "cognitive or cerebral brain functioning." Her physician refused to comply with the parent's request since "to terminate the respirator would be a substantial deviation from medical tradition," involving a decision regarding the "quality of life" and "that he would not do so [terminate]." Judge Muir, presiding in the case, upheld the physician's decision by concluding that "the sought for authorization would result in the taking of the life of Karen Quinlan when the law of the State indicates that such authorization would be homicide."

Questions arising from the Karen Quinlan case concern the criteria for defining death, the role of the legal system in defining death, and the responsibility of the medical profes-

---

*Quotations are from Judge Muir (cited by Cantor, 1976).

sion. Does the absence of brain activity signify that death has already occurred, or is life present as long as the heart and lungs continue to function (aided or unaided)? One answer to this question has come from the practice of organ transplantation: kidney, heart, liver, lung, pancreas, and spleen transplantations have been attempted, but at present only kidney transplantation is widespread and fairly reliable. Problems arise concerning the criteria for defining death and the rights to life of both the donor and the recipient. Brain death has increasingly become the operational definition for establishing that death has occurred. Questions still remain, however, concerning justification of the costs and risks of transplants and the quality of prolonged life for the recipient.

Less publicized than the Quinlan case is the established practice within medical circles of withholding "heroic" measures to keep someone alive. The patient's right to set limits on the means to be employed for retaining his or her life has led to the formulation of the "living will" in which those limits are set. The legality of living wills is currently being questioned. Uncertainties surrounding their application include whether or not the dying person is mentally competent to create or change a living will, what happens if family members or relatives disagree with the patient's directive, and what happens if new therapy becomes available.

These dilemmas derive from uncertainties about the meaning of death as it is recognized in American culture. Death is ascribed a meaning in all cultures and, seemingly, has been throughout human existence. Solecki's research (1971), cited in Chapter 3, indicates that *Homo sapiens neanderthalensis* some 50,000 years ago was engaged in the systematic and ritualized burial of the dead. Pollen remains found with Neanderthal burials in graves at Shanidar in modern-day Iraq are from the brightest flowers in the area, such as the hyacinth. The corpses themselves indicate burial in the flexed-knee position.

The meaning of death is not the same in all cultures. Kastenbaum reports that preschool children in Western societies do not recognize death as being final. "Being dead is like being less alive" (1977:280). W. H. R. Rivers long ago presented information on death in the Solomon Islands of the central Pacific Ocean (Nagy, 1959:87-88). Inhabitants of the area had a word, *mate*, which translates as "death" yet was not conceptualized as the opposite of "life," *toa*. *Mate* was not a terminal state but a transitional period between two modes of existence. A person designated as *mate* was accorded funeral rites, but the burial itself was conceptualized as a festive symbolization of the passage from *toa* to *mate*. Life and death are part of a continuum, not polarized opposites. From an analysis of legal issues surrounding death in American society, Manning reaches a similar conclusion: "'death' is not an event but a process, is not unitary but multiple, and is not absolute but a function of the perspective of the observer" (1970:266).

Causes of death

The causes of death have also been shown to vary across human history and within different cultures. Since 1900, the major causes of death in the United States have undergone a dramatic transition. In 1900, the leading

causes of death were influenza and pneumonia, followed by tuberculosis and gastritis. Table 8 presents the proportions of all deaths accounted for by these causes in 1900 and 1973. Communicable diseases have dropped as the leading causes of death, to be replaced by the chronic degenerative diseases—heart disease and cancers. Increased life expectancy, resulting primarily from the control of childhood diseases has played a part in the shift from communicable to chronic disease insofar as the degenerative diseases predominantly affect middle aged and older people. Increased age-specific incidence and mortality for chronic diseases suggest that the still unknown factors responsible for causing the diseases may have become more prevalent.

Besides variation in the incidence of diseases, causes of death also vary according to personal and cultural interpretations of illness. Death rates drop before holidays and elections and in the month preceding an individual's birthday (Anonymous, 1977:282). The implication is that psychological factors can be brought to bear on physiological processes so that death can be postponed. In this example, cultural factors would also be important for determining the recognition accorded to birthdays and other events.

Studies of sudden death associated with voodoo and sorcery further support the importance of the culture in determining death. Townsend (1978) reports witnessing the

Table 8. Causes of death in the United States

Causes of death	1900 Percent all deaths*	1973 Percent all deaths†
Influenza and pneumonia	11.8	3.2
Tuberculosis	11.3	0.2
Gastritis	8.3	0.0
Heart disease	8.0	52.6
Cancers	4.0	17.8

*1900 data from Lerner, 1970:12-16.
†1973 data from Statistical Abstract of the United States, 1976. U.S. Bureau of the Census, Washington, D.C., 1976, p. 65 and Vital Statistics of the United States, vol. 2, part A, 1973.

death of a member of the Kru tribe in Liberia. The man died within minutes of the time that a sorcerer's curse had been directed at him at a crowded campfire, to which both local residents and Peace Corps volunteers had been invited. Greenway (1969) stresses the power of the Australian "pointing bone." In the hands of a skilled sorcerer it can be deadly. It is aimed in the general direction of the intended victim, who need not be witness to the event. However, if he learns that a curse has been cast on him, it is not uncommon for the victim to die within a week. The mechanisms responsible for causing death in these instances remain unclear. Knowledge that a curse has been delivered combined with belief in the power of the curse, inability to cope with the situation, and preexisting illness are likely to be involved.

A final example of variation in the cause of death concerns the role of volition. It is often informally reported that death has occurred as a result of people having "lost the will to live" or from having "willed" their own deaths. The ability to mobilize defenses against disease and death is poorly understood but may occur as a result of autonomic nervous system activity (see Lex, 1977) or through other still unidentified means. Observers of other cultures have long described the importance of volition in deciding the time of death. For example, Trelease tells about an Alaskan Indian woman, old Sarah, who summoned her family for a day's celebration of the Eucharist and then died at six o'clock that evening (1975).

The above examples point to the importance of individual and cultural factors in controlling dying and death. In each instance, there is acceptance of the reality and of the process of dying and death. However, the taboolike nature of the topic of death and the increasing tendency for deaths to occur in hospitals have acted to deny the reality of

death and impair the dying process for many Americans.

The process of dying

Elisabeth Kubler-Ross has written extensively about the importance of addressing the process of dying (1969, 1975). She has recognized five stages experienced by many dying people in American society: denial and isolation, anger, bargaining, depression, and acceptance. In the first stage, the person thinks that the diagnosis of terminal illness is not true. Often, the individual seeks other physicians and clinics, hoping to get a more favorable diagnosis. When denial is no longer possible, the second stage, anger, begins. Anger is often mixed with envy and resentment of others who are not afflicted with a terminal disorder. The opportunities to be missed and the friends and family to be lost create a sense of anger and frustration that is likely to be let out on those who come into contact with the dying person. The third stage is a bargaining period in which the dying person attempts to postpone the time of death. Good behavior or an agreement with God become a means of requesting an extension of life. Bringing clergymen into contact with the dying person during this stage, if not before, can be valuable. The fourth stage is depression. The dying person begins to grieve for himself as a preparation for impending separation from the world of the living. Family and friends can help by listening to the dying person's sorrow and demonstrating that the activities and interests of the dying person are continuing through the contributions made during life and through ongoing influence on others. The last stage of dying is acceptance. Anger and depression are replaced by tranquility. Meaningful contact is limited to a few people who are especially loved and trusted. The dying person is easily tired, sleeps a great deal, and is not very talkative. Throughout the previous stages, the dying person is likely to have maintained some degree of hope. The hope provides an important source of energy and courage. Hope is surrendered during the final stage of dying but with acceptance, not with despair.

Elisabeth Kubler-Ross' discussion of dying points to the failure of Western medicine to accord death the reality it deserves. Trying to ignore death hinders the process of dying. The role of family members is important throughout the dying process. Rearrangement of household activities is required. The impending loss of a family member may cause loneliness and resentment. Family members react to the announcement of impending death with the same five stages as are experienced by the dying person. Communication within the family and between family members and the dying person is essential if acceptance of death is to be achieved. Once death has occurred, family members still have to overcome feelings of bitterness, anger, and grief. Continuing counsel is needed for family members to reach final acceptance of their loved one's death.

More than two-thirds of the deaths in the United States presently occur in hospitals (Straus and Glaser, 1970:129). Yet hospitals are poorly prepared to recognize death and meet the needs of the dying patient or the patient's family and friends. The delegation of responsibility passes from the patient and the family to people who are educated in techniques of healing, not dying. Death is equated with failure in a physician's or nurse's training. Thus, "heroic" measures are employed by many health professionals to assert the purpose of prolonging life. Physicians, nurses, and other medical personnel are part of a culture that avoids death and belong to a particular society in which death is contrary to their avowed purpose. In addition, as discussed in the previous section, the fact that the dying are suffering from incur-

able, chronic diseases makes them particularly unpopular to care for by health professionals. In contrast, healers do not reject dying people in many other cultures. Other factors, such as change in the course of a disease and in the availability of effective treatment, personal attitude (optimism, pessimism), behavior of the health professionals (aggressive, conservative), and financial reward also may enter into determining the treatment received by the dying patient (Lasagna, 1970).

Adopting an impersonal attitude and avoiding the dying patient and the patient's family are therefore common practices among physicians and nurses. However, because knowledge of and much of the control over the patient's condition is vested in the physicians and nurses, the patient and family need to interact with the physicians and nurses in order to keep informed and to progress through the stages of dying. Medical personnel who do provide comfort, understanding, and help for dying patients and their families appear able to do so by virtue of their personalities rather than their education or the operation of the health care system.

The increasing attention paid to death and dying, evidenced by books such as those of Kubler-Ross, offers hope that the avoidance of and ignorance about dying and death in American culture will end. Control over the dying process needs to be shared with the dying person and the family, and in turn the dying person and the family need to be able to confront and accept death. An alternative care movement for terminally ill patients and their families, the hospice, is gaining support in the United States. The hospice is based on premises that go beyond those of the traditional medical model. The care offered extends into the community. The home is the locus of care. There, social, psychological, and spiritual considerations receive primary, not secondary, emphasis. Organizations such as the Hospice of Metro Denver, following in the footsteps of London's pioneering St. Christopher's Hospice, do use drugs for pain relief (most clients are cancer victims), but administer these as a secondary aspect of care. Emphasis is on recognition of the felt needs of clients and their families, on open communication, and on making the dying process as comfortable as possible, both medically and psychosocially. While the quotation may be heeded, "I have seldom seen anybody die with 'peace and dignity'" (Clark, 1977:288), hospice personnel—nurses, physicians, social workers, ministers, and volunteers—believe that there is such a thing as a good death. Equally as important,

they believe, is a recognition that death is not to be equated with failure (Stoddard, 1978:xvii). It is a rite of passage.

Death as a rite of passage

When conceptualized as an event that all human beings must experience, death becomes the last rite of passage in human development. Elisabeth Kubler-Ross' book, *Death: The Final Stage of Growth*, reflects the theme that death is a component of the human life cycle that is to be reckoned with along with the other phases of development.

Available information about death has become expanded by recent accounts of people who have returned to life after having been

---

Composite description of the experience of death*

A man is dying and, as he reaches the point of greatest physical distress, he hears himself pronounced dead by his doctor. He begins to hear an uncomfortable noise, a loud ringing or buzzing, and at the same time feels himself moving very rapidly through a long dark tunnel. After this, he suddenly finds himself outside of his own physical body, but still in the immediate physical environment, and he sees his own body from a distance, as though he is a spectator. He watches the resuscitation attempt from this unusual vantage point and is in a state of emotional upheaval.

After a while, he collects himself and becomes more accustomed to his odd condition. He notices that he still has a "body," but one of a very different nature and with very different powers from the physical body he has left behind. Soon other things begin to happen. Others come to meet and to help him. He glimpses the spirits of relatives and friends who have already died, and a loving, warm spirit of a kind he has never encountered before—a being of light—appears before him. This being asks him a question, nonverbally, to make him evaluate his life and helps him along by showing him a panoramic, instantaneous playback of the major events of his life. At some point he finds himself approaching some sort of barrier or border, apparently representing the limit between earthly life and the next life. Yet, he finds that he must go back to the earth, that the time for his death has not yet come. At this point he resists, for by now he is taken up with his experiences in the afterlife and does not want to return. He is overwhelmed by intense feelings of joy, love, and peace. Despite his attitude, though, he somehow reunites with his physical body and lives.

Later he tries to tell others, but he has trouble doing so. In the first place, he can find no human words adequate to describe these unearthly episodes. He also finds that others scoff, so he stops telling other people. Still, the experience affects his life profoundly, especially his views about death and its relationship to life.

---

*From Moody, 1976:21-23.

pronounced dead. A composite of many such experiences is given on p. 185. Raymond Moody in *Life After Life* (1976) analyzed several hundred reports. While each report is different, recurrent themes appear. The individuals comment that their experiences are difficult, if not impossible, to put into words. People frequently hear the pronouncement of their own death. Feelings of peace and quiet may ensue that may be punctuated by loud or unusual noises. Being pulled rapidly through a dark tunnel, passage-way, or valley is sometimes reported. A floating sensation of being out of one's body permits the calm contemplation of looking down on one's predicament. Meeting with others and with a personal being surrounded by an emanating light is described.

A rapid panoramic review of one's life may also be experienced. Some people describe a border or limit that they reach and, in turning back, regretfully rejoin the world of the living. Those who have had these experiences after death comment that their lives have been enriched and that they no longer fear death. There are seeming analogies between these personal accounts and the pictures presented by *The Bible;* Plato's *Phaedo, Gorgias,* and *The Republic; The Tibetan Book of the Dead;* and Emanuel Swedenborg's (1668 to 1772) writings. Moody offers no conclusions as to the basis of the pictures of death reported in the religious and personal accounts. Both kinds of descriptions clearly correspond to a rite of passage in which separation, transition, and, possibly,

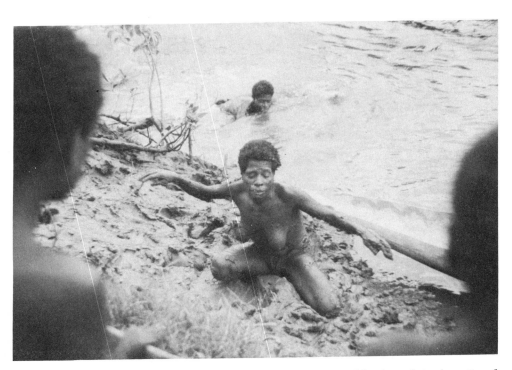

Fig. 5-12. A relative's death among New Guinea's Asmat is accompanied by the traditional practice of mourning while immersed in mud. It is thought that the mud masks the scent of the living, thus making it more difficult for the new and unsteady spirit to cause harm. (Photo by P. Van Arsdale.)

reintegration occur for the dying person.

Death is a rite of passage for the living as well as for the dying. Cultural rituals of bereavement are an adaptation to death that permit survivors to continue their individual growth and development. Bereavement rituals vary among different cultures (Fig. 5-12). The common experience of death—denial and isolation of grieving family members from other segments of the community seen in middle-class American society—contrasts with other ways of recognizing death. An example of mourning as practiced in Jewish culture in the United States shows how grief is expressed and continuity is maintained (Gordon, 1975). The dying person is always kept company, either by family or other members of the community. Once death has occurred, the mourners are responsible for making the funeral arrangements. The funeral is kept simple and realistic. Grief is openly and forcefully expressed through the practice of rending garments *(kriyah)*. A period of grieving *(shivah)* follows in which mourners express their grief and share their recollections of the deceased with community members. Grieving continues for a period of a year, divided into 3 days of deep grief, 7 days of mourning, 30 days of gradual readjustment, and 11 months of remembrance and healing. The necessity to confront, to deal realistically with, and to grieve openly for the death of a loved one permits the reintegration of the mourners into the community.

Summary

In short, the final stage of the life cycle is marked by the continuing effects of the biological and cultural factors seen in previous stages. Dying and death are not single events but the culmination of all phases of development. The diseases present result from the action of genetic as well as environmental influences on biological systems, from cultural influences on life-style, and from disease-promoting behaviors. Death entails completing a series of behavioral developments as well as terminating biological functions. Finally, acceptance and resolved grief for the dead permit continuity and development for the survivors.

REFERENCES

Acśadi, G., and Nemeskéri, J. *History of the Human Lifespan and Mortality.* Budapest, Hungary: Akademiai Kiado, 1970.

Adler, W. Aging and immune function. *Bioscience,* 1975, 25, 652-656.

Anonymous. The death-dip hypothesis. In Zarit, S. H. (ed.). *Readings in Aging and Death: Contemporary Perspectives,* New York: Harper & Row, Publishers, 1977.

Anonymous. Study reveals unwed folks healthier. *The Denver Post,* 1976, 84(325), 9.

Aslan, A. Theoretical and practical aspects of chemotherapeutic techniques in the retardation of the aging process. In Rockstein, M. (ed.). *Theoretical Aspects of Aging.* New York: Academic Press, Inc., 1974.

Bart, P. *Why women's status changes with middle age.* Sociological Symposium no. 3, Blacksburg, Va: VPI and State University, Department of Sociology, Fall 1969.

Bierman, E. L., and Hazzard, W. R. Biology of aging. In Smith, D. W., and Bierman, E. L. (eds.). *Biological Ages of Man,* Philadelphia: W. B. Saunders, 1973.

Birren, J. E., Butler, R. N., Greenhouse, S. W., Sokoloff, L., and Yarrow, M. R. (eds.). *Human Aging I: A Biological and Behavioral Study.* DHEW Publication no. ADM 77-122, 1971.

Bouhuys, A., and Peters, J. M. Control of environmental lung disease. *New England Journal of Medicine,* 1970, 283, 573-581.

Brodeur, P. *Zapping of America: microwaves, their deadly risk and cover-up.* New York: W. W. Norton & Co., Inc., 1977.

Bronfenbrenner, U. Who cares for America's children. In Vaughn, V. C., and Brazelton, T. B. (eds.). *The Family—Can It Be Saved.* Chicago: Year Book Medical Publishers, Inc., 1976, pp. 3-32.

Butler, R. A. *Why Survive: Being Old in America.* New York: Harper & Row, Publishers, 1975.

Campbell, B. *Humankind Emerging.* Boston: Little, Brown and Co., 1976.

Cantor, N. "In the Matter of Karen Quinlan"—A Comment. *Bioscience,* 1976, 26, 257-259.

Carter, W. E. Trial marriage in the Andes? In Bolton,

R., and Mayer, E. (eds.). *Kinship and Marriage.* Washington: American Anthropological Association no. 7, 1977, pp. 117-216.

Clark, M. A right to die? In Zarit, S. H. (ed.). *Readings in Aging and Death: Contemporary Perspectives,* New York: Harper & Row, Publishers, 1977.

Cowgill, D., and Holmes, L. (eds.). *Aging and Modernization.* New York: Appleton-Century-Crofts, 1972.

Cumming, E., and Henry, W. E. *Growing Old: The Process of Disengagement.* New York: Basic Books, Inc., Publishers, 1961.

Custred, G. Peasant kinship, subsistence and economics in a high altitude Andean environment. In Bolton, R., and Mayer, E. (eds.). *Andean Kinship and Marriage.* Washington: American Anthropological Association, no. 7, 1977, pp. 117-135.

De Beauvior, S. *The Coming of Age.* New York: G. P. Putnam's Sons, 1973.

Denckla, W. D. Role of the pituitary and thyroid glands in the decline of minimal O_2 consumption with age. *Journal of Clinical Investigation,* 1974, *53,* 572-581.

Dennis, W. Creative productivity between the ages of 20 and 80 years. In Neugarten, B. (ed.). *Middle Age and Aging.* Chicago: University of Chicago Press, 1968, pp. 106-114.

DHEW. *Current Estimates from the Health Interview Survey,* Vital and Health Statistics Series, no. 10, Department of Health, Education and Welfare, 1975.

DHEW. *Nutrition and Aging,* DHEW Publication no. NIH 78-1409, 1976.

Diers, C. J. Historical trends in the age of menarche and menopause. *Psychological Reports,* 1974, *34,* 931-937.

Dohrenwend, B. S., and Dohrenwend, B. P. Overview and prospects for research on stressful life events. In Dohrenwend, B. S., and Dohrenwend, B. P., (eds.). *Stressful Life Events: Their Nature and Effects.* New York: John Wiley & Sons, Inc., 1974, pp. 313-331.

Epstein, C. J., Martin, G. M., Schultz, A. L., and Motulsky, A. G. Werner's syndrome: review of its symptomatology, natural history, pathologic features, genetics and relationship to the aging process. *Medicine,* 1966, *45,* 177-221.

Erikson, E. *Childhood and Society.* New York: W. W. Norton & Co., Inc., 1950.

Eveleth, P. B., and Tanner, J. M. *Worldwide Variation in Human Growth.* London: Cambridge University Press, 1976.

Fackler, J., and Brandstadt, W. *The Teenage Pregnant Girl.* Springfield, Ill.: Charles C Thomas, Publisher, 1976.

Finch, C. Neuroendocrinology of aging: a view of an emerging area. *Bioscience,* 1975, *25,* 645-650.

Flint, M. The menopause: reward or punishment? *Psychosomatics,* 1975, *16,* 161-163.

Freiburg, K. *Human Development: A Lifespan Approach.* North Scituate, Mass.: Duxbury Press, 1979.

Friedman, M., and Rosenman, R. H. *Type A Behavior and Your Heart.* New York: Alfred A Knopf, Inc., 1974.

Frisch, R. Reply to Trussell. *Science,* 1978, *200,* 1509-1513.

Garn, S., and Clark, D. Trends in fatness and the origins of obesity. *Pediatrics,* 1976, *57,* 443-456.

Gillette, B. On inhaling plutonium: one man's long story. *Science,* 1974, *185,* 1028-1029.

Gordon, A. The Jewish view of death: guidelines for mourning. In Kubler-Ross, E. (ed.). *Death: The Final Stage of Growth.* Englewood Cliffs, N.J.: Prentice-Hall, Inc., 1975, pp. 44-51.

Granick, S., and Patterson, R. D. (eds.). *Human Aging II: An Eleven Year Follow-up Biomedical and Behavioral Study,* DHEW Publication no. ADM-77-123, 1971.

Greenway, J. Personal communication, 1969.

Hackenberg, R. A., Gerber, L. M., and Hackenberg, B. H. Cardiovascular disease mortality among Filipinos in Hawaii: rates, trends, and associated factors. R & S Report, Research and Statistics Office, Hawaii State Department of Health, 24, 1978.

Harlan, W. Social status of the aged in three Indian villages. In Neugarten, B. (ed.). *Middle Age and Aging.* Chicago: University of Chicago Press, 1968, pp. 469-475.

Harris, L., and Associates, Inc. *The Myth and Reality of Aging in America.* Washington, D.C.: The National Council on Aging Inc., 1975.

Hayflick, L. Cell biology of aging. *Bioscience,* 1975, *25,* 629-637.

Havighurst, R. J., *Developmental tasks and education.* New York: David McKay Co., Inc., 1952.

Havighurst, R. J., Neugarten, B. L., and Tobin, S. S. Disengagement and patterns of aging. In Neugarten, B. (ed.). *Middle Age and Aging.* Chicago: The University of Chicago Press, 1968, pp. 161-172.

Higginson, J. Present trends in cancer epidemiology. *Canadian Cancer Conference,* 1969, *8,* 40-75.

Hinkel, L. The effect of exposure to cultural change, social change, and changes in interpersonal relationships on health. In Dohrenwend, B. S., and Dohrenwend, B. P. (eds.). *Stressful Life Events: Their Nature and Effects.* New York: John Wiley & Sons, Inc., 1974, pp. 9-44.

Holden, C. Cancer and the mind: how are they connected? *Science,* 1978, *200,* 1363-1369.

Holmes, T. H., and Masuda, M. Life change and illness susceptibility. In Scott, P., and Senay, E. (eds.). *Separation and Depression.* Washington, D.C.: American Association for the Advancement of Science, no. 94, 1973, pp. 161-186.

Holmes, T. H., and Rahe, R. H. The social readjustment rating scale. *Journal of Psychosomatic Research*, 1967, *11*, 213-218.

Hoover, R., Mason, T. J., McKay, F. W., and Fraumeni, J. F. Cancer by county: new resource for etiologic clues. *Science*, 1975, *189*, 1005-1007.

Hope, K., and Young, N. *Momma: the sourcebook for single mothers*. New York: The New American Library Inc., 1976.

Howard, G. E. *A History of Matrimonial Institutions*. New York: Humanities Press, Inc., 1904.

Isbell, B. J. Those who love me: an analysis of Andean kinship and reciprocity within a ritual context. In Bolton, R., and Mayer, E. (eds.). *Andean Kinship and Marriage*. Washington: American Anthropological Association, no. 7, 1977, pp. 81-105.

Jacobs, J. *Fun City: An Ethnographic Study of a Retirement Community*. New York: Holt, Rinehart, and Winston, Inc., 1974.

Jarvik, M. E., Cullen, J. W., Gritz, E. R., and others. (eds.). *Research on Smoking Behavior*. Washington, D.C.: U.S. Government Printing Office, no. 017-024-00694-7, 1977.

Kastenbaum, R. The kingdom where nobody dies. In Zarit, S. H. (ed.). *Readings in Aging and Death: Contemporary Perspectives*, New York: Harper & Row, Publishers, 1977.

Key F. G. *The Family in Transition*. New York: John Wiley & Sons, Inc., 1972.

Kohlberg, L. Continuities in childhood and adult moral development revisited. In Baltes, P. and Schaie, K. W. (eds.). *Life-span Developmental Psychology: Personality and Socialization*. New York: Academic Press, Inc., 1973.

Kolata, G. B. Obesity: A growing problem. *Science*, 1977, *198*, 905-906.

Kolata, G. B. Strategies for the Control of Gonorrhea. *Science*, 1976, *192*, 245.

Kolata, G. B., and Marx, J. L. Epidemiology of heart disease: searches for causes. *Science*, 1976, *194*, 509-612.

Kubler-Ross, E. *Death: The Final Stage of Growth*. Englewood Cliffs, N.J.: Prentice-Hall, Inc., 1975.

Kubler-Ross, E. *On Death and Dying*. New York: The Macmillan Co., 1969.

Lambert, B. Bilaterality in the Andes. In Bolton, R., and Mayer, E. (eds.). *Andean Kinship and Marriage*. Washington, D.C.: American Anthropological Association, no. 7, 1977, pp. 1-27.

Lasagna, L. Physicians behavior toward the dying patient. In Brim, O. G., Freeman, H., Levine, S., and Scotch, N. (eds.). *The Dying Patient*. New York: Russell Sage Foundation, 1970, pp. 83-101.

Lasagna, L. The prognosis of death. In Brim, O. G.,

Freeman, H., Levine, S., and Scotch, N. (eds.). *The Dying Patient*. New York: Russell Sage Foundation, 1970, pp. 67-101.

Lehman, H. L. The creative productivity rates of present and past generations of scientists. In Neugarten, B. (ed.). *Middle Age and Aging*. Chicago: University of Chicago Press, 1968, pp. 99-105.

Leibowitz, L. *Females, Males, Families: A Biosocial Approach*. North Scituate, Mass.: Duxbury Press, 1978.

Lerner, M. When, why, and where people die. In Brim, O. G., Freeman, H., Levine, S., and Scotch, N. (eds.). *The Dying Patient*. New York: Russell Sage Foundation, 1970, pp. 5-29.

Lex, B. W. Voodoo death: new thoughts on an old explanation. In Landy, D. (ed.). *Culture, Disease, and Healing: Studies in Medical Anthropology*. New York: The Macmillan Co., 1977, pp. 327-331.

MacDonald, E. J., Wellington, D. J., and Wolf, P. F. Regional patterns in mortality from cancer in the United States. *Cancer*, 1967, *20*, 617-622.

Manning, B. Legal and policy issues in the allocation of death. In Brim, O. G., Freeman, H., Levine, S., and Scotch, N. (eds.). *The Dying Patient*. New York: Russell Sage Foundation, 1970, pp. 253-274.

Mason, J. J., and others. *Atlas of Cancer Mortality for U.S. Counties: 1950-1969*. Washington, D.C.: U.S. Government Printing Office, 1976.

McKusick, V. *Mendelian Inheritance in Man*. Baltimore: Johns Hopkins University Press, 1975.

Mead, M. *Coming of Age in Samoa*. New York: William Morrow and Co., Inc., 1928.

Moody, R. A. *Life After Life*. Harrisburg, Pa.: Stackpole Books, 1976.

Murdock, G. P. *Social Structure*. New York: The Macmillan Co., 1949.

Murstein, B. *Love, Sex and Marriage through the Ages*. New York: Springer-Verlag, 1974.

Nagy, M. H. The child's view of death. In Feifel, H. (ed.). *The Meaning of Death*. New York: McGraw-Hill Book Co., 1959.

National Academy of Sciences *Toward a National Policy for Children and Families*. Washington, D.C.: National Academy of Sciences, 1976.

Nerup, J., Platz, P., Anderson, O., and others. HL-A antigens and diabetes mellitus. *Lancet*, 1974, 2(2), 864-866.

Neugarten, B. The awareness of middle age. In Neugarten, B. (ed.). *Middle Age and Aging*. Chicago: University of Chicago Press, 1968, pp. 93-98.

Neugarten, B. L., Havighurst, R. J., and Tobin, S. S. Personality and patterns in aging. In Neugarten, B. (ed.). *Middle Age and Aging*. Chicago: University of Chicago Press, 1968, pp. 173-177.

Noller, K. L. DES and pregnancy: lower reproductive

tract changes in offspring. *Bioscience*, 1976, *26*, 541-547.

Nyhan, W. L., and others. Discussion of epidemiology and genetic implications. *Federation Proceedings*, 1968, *27*, 1091-1096.

Palmore, E. *The Honourable Elders*. Durham, N.C.: Duke University Press, 1975.

Parsons, T. C., and Fox, R. Illness, therapy, and the American family. In Jaco, E. G. (ed.). *Patients, Physicians, and Illness*. New York: The Free Press, 1958.

Price, R. Trial marriage in the Andes. *Ethnology*, 1965, *4*, 310-322.

Queen, F. *The Family in Various Cultures*. Philadelphia: J. B. Lippincott Co., 1967.

Rabkin, J. G., and Struening, E. L. Life events, stress, and illness. *Science*, 1976, *194*, 1013-1020.

Rahe, R. H., and Romo, M. Recent life changes and the onset of myocardial infarction and coronary death in Helsinki. In Gunderson, E. K., and Rahe, R. H. (eds.). *Life Stress and Illness*. Springfield, Ill.: Charles C Thomas, Publisher, 1974, pp. 105-120.

Rebelsky, F., and Hanks, C. Father's verbal interactions with infants in the first three months of life. *Child Development*, 1971, *42*, 63.

Reichel, W., Garcia-Bunuel, R., and Dilallo, J. Progeria and Werner's syndrome as models for the study of normal human aging. *Journal of the American Geriatric Society*, 1971, *19*, 369-375.

Riley, V. Mouse mammary tumors: alteration of incidence as apparent function of stress. *Science*, 1975, *189*, 465-467.

Rocky Mountain News. Short lifespan seen for skilled workers. *Rocky Mountain News*, October 22, 1978, p. 67.

Rosen, S. Noise, hearing, and cardiovascular function. In Welch, B. L., and Welch, A. S. (eds.). *Physiological Effects of Noise*. New York: Plenum Publishing Corp., 1970, pp. 57-66.

Ross, H. L., and Sawhill, J. V. *Time of Transition: The Growth of Families Headed by Women*. Washington, D.C.: The Urban Institute, 1975.

Sawhill, I. The economics of discrimination against women: some new findings. *Journal of Human Resources*, 1973, *8*, 383-396.

Service, E. *Profiles in Ethnology*, ed. 3, New York: Harper and Row, Publishers. 1978.

Shanas, E., Townsend, P., Wedderburn, D., and others. *Old People in Three Industrial Societies*. Chicago: Aldine-Atherton, Inc., 1968.

Sheehy, G. *Passages: Predictable Crises of Adult Life*. New York: E.P. Dutton & Co. Inc., 1974.

Simmons, L. *The Role of the Aged in Primitive Society*, Hamden, Conn.: Archon Books, 1970. (First published, 1945.)

Simmons, R. G., Klein, S. D., and Simmons, R. L. *Gift of Life: the Social and Psychological Impact of Organ Transplantation*. New York: John Wiley & Sons, Inc., 1977, pp. 111-112.

Smith, D. W., and Bierman, E. L. *The Biologic Ages of Man*. Philadelphia: W. B. Saunders Co., 1973.

Solecki, R. S. *Shanidar, The First Flower People*. New York: Alfred A. Knopf, Inc., 1971.

Stanbury, J. B., Wyngaarden, J. B., and Fredrickson, D. S. *The Metabolic Basis of Inherited Disease*, ed. 3. New York: McGraw-Hill Book Co. 1972.

Steinke, J., and Taylor, K. W. Viruses and the etiology of diabetes. *Diabetes*, 1974, *23*, 631-633.

Stoddard, S. *The Hospice Movement: A Better Way of Caring for the Dying*. Briarcliff Manor, N.Y.: Stein & Day Publishers, 1978.

Strauss, A. L., and Glaser, B. G. Patterns of dying. In Brim, O. G., Freeman, H., Levine, S., and Scotch, N. (eds.). *The Dying Patient*. New York: Russell Sage Foundation, 1970, pp. 129-155.

Tanner, J. M. Growing up. *Scientific American*, 1973, *229*(3), 34-43.

Tattersall, R. B., and Fajans, S. S. A difference between the inheritance of classical juvenile-onset diabetes and maturity-onset diabetes of young people. *Diabetes*, 1975, *24*, 44-53.

Townsend, H. Personal communication, 1978.

Train, R. Environmental cancer. *Science*, 1977, *195*, 443.

Trelease, M. Dying among Alaskan Indians: a matter of choice. In Kubler-Ross, E. (ed.). *Death: The Final Stage of Growth*. Englewood Cliffs, N.J.: Prentice-Hall, Inc., 1975, pp. 33-37.

Trussell, J. Menarche and fatness: reexamination of the cultural fat hypothesis. *Science*, 1978, *200*, 1506-1509.

Vander, A. J., Sherman, J. H., and Luciano, D. S. *Human Physiology: the Mechanisms of Body Function*. New York: McGraw-Hill Book Co., 1970.

Van Gennep, A. *The Rites of Passage*. Chicago: University of Chicago Press, 1960. (First published, 1908).

Werkman, S. Psychiatric disorders of adolescence. In Arieti, S. (ed.). *American Handbook of Psychiatry*. New York: Harper & Row, Publishers, 1974.

Whitbeck, C. Unwed stretch laws, social etiquette. *The Denver Post*, 1976, *84*(325), 25.

Williams, D. A., and Walsh, L. Bad Samaritan: cousin's refusal to donate bone marrow. *Newsweek*, 1978, *92*, 35.

World Health Statistics Annual, 1973-1976. Geneva: WHO, 1976.

CHAPTER 6

Cultural belief systems and their impact on health care

In the preceding five chapters biocultural variables have been used as the basis on which to build a central argument: that health must be viewed in total systems contexts that span gradual changes in form over generations (evolution) and changes in patterns of adjustment within generations (life cycle). We have demonstrated that ecological parameters circumscribe the biocultural processes that affect health and suggest that, while resisting biological determinism, medical anthropologists need to take careful account of human biological factors in their attempts to assess short-term adjustments and long-term adaptations. This can best be accomplished through holistic, rather than reductionistic, analyses.

Chapters 6 and 7 continue the biocultural theme. However, emphasis is shifted away from biology toward belief systems, themes, and paradigms in the study of medical systems and policy issues. The comparative and historical methods of study are stressed. Examples are used to illustrate the ultimate point that a fuller understanding of Western health care can be obtained by systematically examining non-Western practices. No one system is inherently "right" or "wrong," but rather each can be shown to exemplify certain historical themes within a particular paradigm (see McQueen, 1978). The juxtaposition of descriptions of primitive belief/ curing systems early in this chapter as well as descriptions of both minor and dominant systems currently practiced in the United States demonstrates how less-dominant medical/ curing systems can shed light on those that have become more dominant owing to sociopolitical and historical circumstances.

RELIGION, MAGIC, AND HEALING: AN OVERVIEW

Just prior to Thanksgiving Day, 1978, the world was jolted by the news that unknown hundreds of people had died in a mass suicide-murder in Guyana, South America. The dead had been members of the People's Temple, a small religious cult under the leadership of the Reverend Jim Jones. Eventually, it was learned that 912 men, women, and children had died; most had succumbed within 5 minutes after drinking a mixture of cyanide and Flavoraid that had been administered by cult medical personnel. Few members of the group's Jonestown community survived. Jones himself was found among the dead. Those who survived reported that most of Jones' followers had voluntarily swallowed the poison. Many had been observed tearfully bidding their friends and relatives goodbye before doing so.

A mass suicide-murder of this magnitude is unprecedented in the modern era, yet this is perhaps the only unusual aspect of the activities engaged in by the cult's leaders and followers. Numerous other small but active religious sects in the United States (the People's Temple was based in San Francisco) and elsewhere utilize systems of recruitment, indoctrination, and program implementation like those of Jones. Others such as the New Druids and the Divine Light Mission ask their members to display total obedience to doctrine; they might ask their members to make tremendous personal sacrifices on behalf of the group. What is important in introducing the subject of religion, magic, and healing is that one need not automatically turn to the analysis of small-scale, "exotic" societies in order to find examples in which these processes are tightly interwoven. One should not presume that only "primitives" believe in the interactive effects of religion, magic, and healing. Reverend Jones proclaimed that he could effect cures for his followers through faith healing. Although certain witnesses claimed that the "tumors" passed by some of those seeking Jones' cure were actually chicken organs, and that he once staged a fake assassination attempt against himself to demonstrate his "invulnerability," the central issue is that religion, magic, and healing all deal with manipulation and control of presumed natural-supernatural-psychological factors. The sleight of hand used by Jones in his faith healing parallels that used by a traditional Asmat curer in New Guinea. Taken out of context, both might appear to be charlatans. Yet when viewed within the context of their particular belief systems, each offers a unification of doctrine and practice that is deemed valuable by those adhering to the same belief. As a result of the interaction of psychological and physiological processes (as exemplified in the section on death and dying in Chapter 5), cures of certain illnesses can indeed be effected.

Anthropological views of religion and magic

The study of religion and magic in cross-cultural perspective has been of interest to anthropologists since the formal dawn of the discipline in the nineteenth century. Sociocultural evolutionists such as Edward Tylor and Sir James George Frazer sought to analyze religious phenomena in terms of stages of cultural evolution. These theories have since been criticized extensively. According to Frazer, humanity must pass through three stages: from magic and superstition to religion and then on to science and rationality. Frazer, following Tylor, conceptualized magic as "bastard science," with key similarities: "Both were attempts to control events, both had a strong faith in the order and uniformity of nature, both believed in invariable natural laws. Religion in contrast postulated a world in which events depend on the whim of spirits" (Wilk, 1976:254). Frazer's magnum opus, *The Golden Bough*, was first published in 1890 and was later expanded to twelve full volumes. His detailed compilations of phenomena in cultural, historical, and comparative perspective have rarely been equaled. His influence continues to be felt theoretically as well, although much of this is heuristic—his ideas have provoked scientifically fruitful disagreement.

The idea that humankind has evolved toward greater rationality, coupled with Western scientific advancement, is of importance in the present context. As the late Jacob Bronowski noted, between 1500 and 1700 A.D., it became possible to propound a unitary theory of the world. Emergent Western scientific achievements permitted the world to be seen from the perspective of a single type of explanation—one grounded in physical science and a singular logic. The contrast developed between magic and science is striking:

[Magic] is the view that there is a logic of everyday life, but there is also a logic of another world. Science is distinguished from magical views by the fact that it refuses to acknowledge a division between two kinds of logic . . . There is only one logic; it works the same way in all forms of conduct . . . (Bronowski, quoted in Medawar, 1978:124).

Along similar lines, the interest of many people in magic today has been termed "contemporary irrationalism" (Medawar, 1978:125).

Magic may indeed be a different kind of logic, but it *is* logical, especially when viewed functionally and from the perspective of the belief system of which it is a part. Bronowski is correct when he suggests that two kinds of logic can exist side by side. What must be recognized is that, although magic and science cannot easily coexist within the Western conceptual framework, they can do so within other frameworks.

Parallels also exist between science and religion. Both are concerned with the interpretation of beliefs from the vantage of a unified (although not necessarily singular) perspective. Both are concerned with attempts to elucidate cause-effect relationships. In terms of medical anthropology, both at times focus on the nature of health and the human condition (see Logan and Hunt, 1978). As Kenny (1976:332) notes, no single definition of religion is universally accepted. Most anthropologists would agree that religion is manifested in different ways. Depending on particular environmental, historical, and cultural variables, however, it can safely be regarded as an institution concerned with human interactions with superhuman beings or extraordinary powers capable of harm or aid. In all societies, religious beliefs are in some way structured, and in all societies certain individuals are present who serve as religious specialists or repositories of religious knowledge. Following the pioneering work of Malinowski (1948), who noted that religion functions in situations of emotional stress, anthropologists have continued to focus on functional analyses.

Although most anthropologists have recognized the importance of religion in a society's structuring of its relationship to superhuman or extrasensory powers, not all have accorded religion a role in a society's relationship with its environment. During the 1960s and 1970s a good deal of debate arose as to what place religion occupied in the emergent ecological schemes of anthropology. Julian Steward (1955) in particular implied that religious activities might best be regarded as somewhat peripheral epiphenomena. Others, however, have stressed the significance of ritual for regulating economic-resource activities. Citing four separate studies, Vayda assigns a "major role to religious or ceremonial features as adaptive factors in the interactions of human populations with their environments" (1968:487). Indeed, ritual can serve a regulatory function in the process of resource exploitation and long-term management of resources (for example, Rappaport, 1968). A similar argument can be made for ritual's impact on health care.

Anthropological views of medical systems

In the study of societies, many anthropologists have included as part of typical ethnographies discussions of medical systems. Some researchers have focused attention exclusively on this area of study. Here we present brief synopses of the contributions of some of the most notable socioculturally oriented scholars. These include early investigators, such as Rivers and Clements and, somewhat later, Ackerknecht and the late Steven Polgar; and present-day scholars such as Paul, Alland, Foster, Leininger, and Fabrega. Each has contributed something unique theoretically or methodologically to the field of medical anthropology.

One of the first to systematically study systems of medicine cross-culturally was W. H. R. Rivers. Much of his field work had been conducted in the southwest Pacific. As a physician and an anthropologist he attempted to classify medicine as an aspect of culture within the parameters of social organization. He stated that ". . . medical practices are not a medley of disconnected and meaningless customs" (1924:51), but rather constitute a cohesive social institution when considered in conjunction with beliefs. As a result, Rivers believed that methods appropriate to the study of social institutions in general were, therefore, appropriate to the study of medical systems (Wellin, 1977:49). Thus Rivers concluded that although primitive medical practices were unlike Western practices, the medical system of a preliterate people was based on a definite, patterned, underlying belief system. The system itself was, more importantly, an integral part of the total cultural complex.

In attempting to develop a conceptual model, Rivers proposed that the dependent variable was the observable, reported health behavior of the social group being studied. The independent variable was the group's world view. The independent variable could be delineated into three classifications: magical, religious, and naturalistic. Magical world views regarding disease causation relate to beliefs that these result from human (magical) manipulation of the forces in the universe, such as through sorcery and witchcraft. The religious views suggest that the events of life, including disease, are controlled by supernatural powers. In the naturalistic view, the phenomena are viewed as being subject to natural law; this view is characteristic of modern, Western medicine (Wellin, 1977:50).

Another early contributor to the field of medical anthropology was Forrest Clements (1932). At his time of study, the "culture area" approach was prevalent. This in turn was an outgrowth of an earlier anthropological concern with detailed trait analysis characteristic of the school of thought known as historical particularism. Clements used this type of approach to classify disease causation processes on a world-wide basis. He thus focused on tracing similar traits—beliefs, practices, rituals, and artifacts—cross-culturally both spatially and temporally. Although Clements' concepts were at times vaguely defined and atomistic, he was a pioneer in attempting to define disease in cognitive terms, and his work continues to be of heuristic value (Wellin, 1977:50).

Disease causation concepts among preliterate groups were classified by Clements for comparative purposes into five categories: sorcery, breach of taboo, intrusion by a disease object, intrusion by a spirit, and soul loss. Examples of how this classification relates to the treatment of disease have been provided by Rogers (1976):

1. Sorcery. Treatment of disease thought to be caused by sorcery also involves sorcery or some form of related magic as a nullifying force. Rogers refers to an Australian Arunta man who was hit by a boomerang during a fight. Only a minor wound resulted, but the victim believed himself to have been "sung" and became very concerned about his overall health. A sucking cure was effected only after a curer who knew the magic of the offending band was enlisted.

2. Breach of taboo. This is considered to be a common cause of disease among Eskimo peoples (see also Foulks, 1972); their shamanic therapy requires that the curer ask his own possessing spirit what taboo may

have been broken. <u>Elucidation of the problem requires confession by the patient and confirmation by those in attendance</u>.

3. Disease-object intrusion. Sleight-of-hand is frequently employed by the shaman in his attempts to convince patient and onlookers alike that the offending object has been successfully removed. For example, a Pima shaman "sucked furiously over the body of a woman suffering from poisoning in order to remove the horn of a horned toad which he said was in her heart. Finally the offending object flew into his mouth and gagged him for a moment until he could remove it" (Rogers 1976:31).

4. Spirit intrusion. Spirit intrusion was thought to have been the cause in the case of the Asmat exorcism described on pp. 218 to 219. Rogers provides an account of Chinese spirits that are thought to be equally powerful.

5. Soul loss. The treatment for disease caused by soul loss can be very complex. Rogers refers to a procedure among native Americans of Puget Sound who employ the "spirit canoe" ritual to recover the wandering soul and thus restore health. Part of the ritual pantomimes the journey of the curers to the underworld in search of the lost soul. In the village of the dead, they prowl among various houses hoping to find it. On retrieving the soul, they wrap it in a cloth and return to the patient, where the soul is at last "reinstalled," although not without difficulty.

Among these five categories, Rogers notes that the first two can be more generally classified as remote causes (those that have occurred in the patient's past experience, although the event may have been quite recent). The last three are proximate causes (those logically involved more immediately and mechanistically). Causation is not mutually exclusive; interactions can occur among causal factors (see Fig. 6-1).

Erwin Ackerknecht, trained as a physician, also concentrated on the belief systems underlying primitive medicine. Ackerknecht believed there was not just one primitive medical system but many, and these systems could best be understood in terms of cultural beliefs and definitions (Wellin, 1977: 51). The variations found among societies were associated with their respective magical and religious attributes. Thus a major contribution in the 1940s was to focus on the functional attributes of these medical beliefs within the total cultural belief system (following Benedict [1934], Ackerknecht used the term "configuration"). Many contemporary writers in the field of medical anthropology focus their efforts along lines

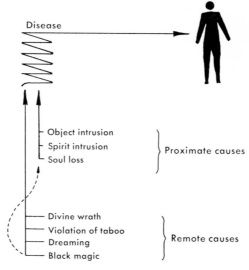

Causes of disease

Fig. 6-1. Black magic solely can be a remote cause where the suffering of the patient is attributed to magic in a general way. In other instances magic is thought of as the means of soul stealing or the instrumentality for injecting evil spirits into the body. This is a remote cause that induces a proximate cause. (From Rogers, 1976:39.)

suggested by Rivers, Clements, and Ackerknecht.

Benjamin Paul was unique in his early applied approach to medical anthropology. In his interpretation, the intricacies of cognitive terms and primitive magical beliefs became tools for practical application. This is exemplified in his 1955 "applied classic," *Health, Culture and Community*. No longer were the elements viewed merely as functional entitites, in the mode of Rivers, Clements, and Ackerknecht. Paul's introductory chapter indicates that an incipient systems approach was being employed. It was largely through his efforts to conceptualize the dynamics of medicine within a culture that researchers and those interested in applications began to deal with the process and effects of social change. Planned interventions in the medical system could be anticipated within a larger socioeconomic framework (see Wellin, 1977:53). What Paul's model lacks is the larger view of influences and effects of both biological and environmental factors on the cultural system.

It was to these issues that Steven Polgar and Alexander Alland, Jr., contributed. Polgar, influenced by his associations with the medical profession, added cross-cultural evolutionary and demographic approaches to the study of medical anthropology (1964, 1972). Alland made the most significant contribution in his synthesis of evolution, biology, and cultural aspects of human adaptation (1970). Largely through his efforts the subfield of medical anthropology moved out of the fragmented collection of interesting case studies into an integrated field with an overarching conceptual framework.

George Foster (1969, 1976), through his long involvement with studies of cultural change, acculturation, and applied anthropology, has more recently combined these interests with a disciplined approach to developing more "cognitive" taxonomies of health belief systems. Foster deals with the complexities of human cognitive systems by identifying two major frameworks that he believes are the key to cross-cultural comparisons of disease etiologies among medical systems. These frameworks are identified as personalistic and naturalistic. In the personalistic all misfortunes are explained in essentially the same way. Illness, religion, and magic are viewed as elements of a closely interwoven system. Misfortunes are caused "by the active, purposeful intervention of a *sensate* agent" (Foster and Anderson, 1978: 53). The most powerful cures have supernatural and magical powers, but the primary role of healers is diagnostic. In contrast, naturalistic etiologies explain illness in impersonal, functional, systemic ways. Disease causality has little or nothing to do with other misfortunes, thus religion and magic are in some ways unrelated to illness. Cures are primarily therapeutic. Foster's approach is comparative in the broadest sense.

A brief historical-cultural example of the so-called hot-cold syndrome as it is manifested in Mexico and Central America is interjected here because, as representative of an equilibrium model, it conforms ideally to a naturalistic system; ". . . health prevails when the insensate elements in the body, the heat, the cold, the humors . . . are in balance appropriate to the age and condition of the individual in his natural and social environment" (Foster and Anderson, 1978:53). Among all the health-illness systems, the hot-cold syndrome has been one of the most widely researched (Logan, 1977, 1978: Currier, 1966; Harwood, 1971; Kay, 1977). Analysis of the system also has been important to the understanding of acculturation processes, as illustrated here. As the Spanish *conquistadores* secured their empire in the sixteenth century, so their beliefs in humoural causes of disease (see Chapter 7) were diffused throughout much of aboriginal Amer-

treatment
ethnonursing

ica. The diff[...] easy in parts of what is now [Mexico because i]t was intimately compatible w[ith the ancient A]ztec concept of a universe o[rdered by a syste]m of balancing opposites. T[he world was vie]wed as being in an eternal w[ar between hot] and cold substances (Ne[swander and] Souder, 1977: 97). Thus, b[oth tradition an]d diffusion have shaped thei[r views. The ru]les these indigenous peopl[e use for classify]ing their diseases are in accor[dance with the r]esponses of each disease to tr[eatment. In gen]eral a hot disease responds fa[vorably to contac]t with cold, and a cold dise[ase responds pos]itively to contact with hot. Using these criteria, each disease is precisely classified according to its response to the administration of foods, herbs, baths, and medications that have properties opposite to those of the disease. If the patient responds favorably to the administration of a hot substance, the conclusion is that "the disease wants hot," meaning the disease itself is classified as a cold one. Hot diseases are caused by bodily contact with heat-producing elements, and cold diseases are caused by cold-producing elements. Malaria is an example of a hot disease, while measles is considered to be a cold disease.

Some of the more recent contributions to medical anthropology have emphasized the applied aspects of the field. Madeline Leininger, an anthropologist and a nurse, has made a major contribution to medical anthropology (or transcultural health, as she prefers to call the field) by identifying a set of concepts related to care and cure. She is the pioneer of a subfield now known as transcultural nursing. Rather than focusing on the broad issues of curing, Leininger narrows her approach to ethnonursing, which she defines as ". . . a systematic study and classification of nursing care beliefs, values, and practices as cognitively perceived by a designated culture through their local language, experiences, beliefs, and value systems. The central goal is to obtain the local, or indigenous, peoples' viewpoints, beliefs, and practices about nursing care or modes of caring behavior and processes of the designated cultural group" (Leininger, 1978:15). The process by which Leininger approaches her study is one used in much of medical anthropology, that of ethnoscience. The approach is an emic one, that is, the researcher attempts to accurately describe an illness or state of well-being from the native's (or in this situation, the patient's) point of view. The emic approach is in contrast to an etic approach, in which illnesses are described from an outside point of view, such as a physician's diagnosis of a native's ailment. Because health care providers of various types deal with individuals rather than large populations in their caring procedures, the emic approach is particularly appropriate. Thus, while the data so gathered may not easily be generalizable beyond the group nor the specific time, the principles by which they are collected have potential applicability on a universal level (see, for example Aamodt, 1978). Her contribution bridges scientific concerns with actual caregiving procedures.

The contributions of other anthropologists who have made significant impacts in the sociocultural area of medical anthropology have not been included in this overview. To mention but a few, these include Arthur Rubel, Margaret Clark, and Arthur Kleinman. We conclude by citing the ongoing contributions of Horacio Fabrega, Jr. As much as any other individual, he has succeeded in bringing the perspective of medical anthropology to the attention of both interdisciplinary and international audiences. Fabrega's *Disease and Social Behavior* (1974) stands as a synthesis of a large body of information about diseases within a behavioral model. Recently he has called attention to the need for an ethnomedical science. He defines ethnomedicine as the study of how members of different cultures think about disease and illness and organize themselves toward medical treatment and the social organization of that treatment (1975:969). Fabrega stresses the insights that a systematized ethnomedicine can offer to the health sciences through assessment of social and behavioral dynamics. Further information on changes in the way people function, behave, define themselves, and report their feelings will enable us to better understand the sequence of changes that occur in illness. A "social grammar" of illness may be discoverable, he believes, perhaps one that is relatively culture-free. More generally, he concludes that a theory of disease is needed, one that would incorporate the contributions of both biomedical and social science. This could lead to the more rational control of illness (see Fig. 6-2). Others, including phys-

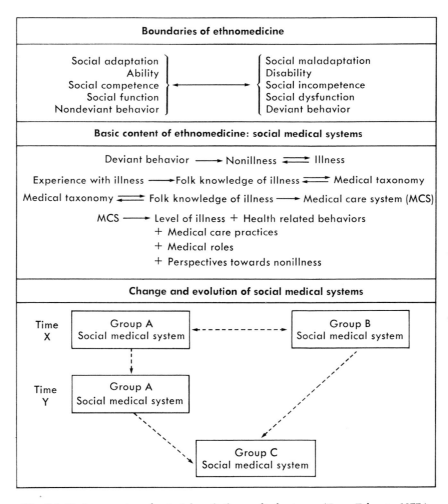

Fig. 6-2. Basic concepts and principles of ethnomedical science. (From Fabrega, 1977.)

[handwritten: Universal Treatment.]

icians, are now following the direction Fabrega has set forth (see, for example, Engel, 1977).

BELIEF SYSTEMS
The difficulties of comparative study

The belief system associated with the members of a particular society can, in the most general sense, be thought of as a reflection of their world view and of their normative patterns of behavior. Beliefs reflect perceived relationships between culture and environment, which are in turn related to ideas about the basic nature of their constituent elements. Beliefs thus pertain directly to cause-effect relationships. While attempts have been made to reduce explanations of "cause" and "effect" to some set of universal, physical denominators (see Rapoport, 1968), in the present context such an approach would be misleading. The medical anthropologist needs to assess the nature of belief in a relativistic sense, using the parameters of the particular culture under study as a guide. Causes and effects related to health and sickness need to be understood in a philosophical and sociobehavioral context as opposed to one that is purely mechanistic (see, for example, Foster, 1976).

The relativistic approach is, on the one hand, the key to the accurate within-system analysis of belief, but on the other hand presents problems when cross-cultural comparisons are then attempted. Are some set of universal, cultural denominators to be employed? What is being compared to what? What are the theoretical criteria? A consensus among medical anthropologists has not been reached, although symposia and publications have at least addressed these problems directly. A special issue of the journal *Social Science & Medicine* (April 1978) was devoted entirely to analyses of the theoretical foundations for the comparative study of medical systems. A statement by Rosenberg

sums up one view of the situation: "A of categories broad enough to really adequately things that must be cove every culture are so broad as to not alytically useful. It also has the da wrenching a particular part or compo a certain institution out of a particular per se" (Unschuld, 1978:75) and may a dilemma, as stated by Mendelsohn, believe for an instant that a concept o or disease, of healing or illness is tran across all cultural or societal bound across time" (quoted in Unschuld, 1

It becomes apparent that an asses the nature of belief is a two-edged sword. The anthropologist must analyze his or her own beliefs about the fundamentals of comparative analysis as well as the actual health-sickness beliefs of particular cultures. While recognizing the unresolved nature of these problems, the anthropologist must attempt to make comparisons, for generalizations are of importance and cannot be derived in any other way. The ecological approach offers a useful way of generalizing about the nature of belief. By recognizing the importance of a culture's own views, Arthur Rubel's suggestion is heeded: "It is a poor start to begin with the disease categories of modern medicine. One should look . . . at misfortune and see how people cope [in that culture]" (Unschuld, 1978:75). Too, the ecological approach emphasizes illness and patterns of illness behavior rather than merely disease. The concept of coping behavior is a useful bridge for comparing the beliefs, behaviors, and ecological relationships among societies. The result, as Kleinman (1978a) suggests, will be a comparison of medical systems as cultural systems, as the following examples illustrate.

Varieties of belief

Each type of society throughout history has had distinctive forms of sickness. The great plagues of the Dark Ages and the scourges of the Renaissance are replaced with influenzas and cancers of the Atomic Age. But each society in its time and place defines its own response to sickness. Priests, shamans, "witchdoctors," sorcerers, physicians, spiritualists, *curanderos*, and gurus all have served to care for societies' responses to disease and illness. Each culture in turn gives shape to its own unique view of wellness and health (Illich, 1976:128).

Cultural belief systems about health and sickness serve as the foundations of all medical care. To understand why one population treats an open wound with a wad of cow dung while another uses merthiolate requires a deep understanding of the belief systems of each society. Incantations and rituals have different meanings for different groups. The diversity of cultural beliefs clearly illustrates the tremendous capabilities and adaptations of human beings, both evolutionarily and ecologically.

A typology of religious belief systems according to culture area has been devised (Gilbert, 1976:332-334). It is based on an "ethnographic present" of 1600 A.D. The four primary categories are monotheistic (such as Judaeo-Christian), Olympian (as in central Africa), communal (such as Oceanic), and shamanic (for example, circumpolar). The interactions of religious and health beliefs are readily exemplified in the last category. The religion of the Eskimos is characterized by the activities of shamans. These specialists are believed to be able to communicate with the spirit world and by so doing to be able to assist in the curing process. Among certain Eskimo groups, the shaman is thought to possess—and be possessed by—a *tunraq* (demonic spirit). It is through such possession that one's calling as a shaman is first recognized. For this reason the shaman is a person to seek out and yet to be wary of. Illness itself results from the commission

of socially unacceptable acts. In a sense it is viewed as a form of punishment. When illness or other misfortune occurs, the shaman summons the community. Restoration of social balance is needed. Beginning with a seance, which puts him in touch with key spirits, the shaman proceeds to drum and chant. At a point where the rhythm is intense and the involvement frenzied, he may lapse into a trancelike silence. Voices of spirits can be heard by the onlookers and are likely to be manifested in the tones of the *tunraq* (for example, a wolf growl). During the period of the trance, which may last for hours, the shaman is thought to be "out of mind"— possessed, but not crazy. The possession state is a mark of curing abilities. If a cure takes place, it is thought to have been effected through restoration of religious-cosmological equilibrium (Foulks, 1972:49-53).

In less technologically developed, preliterate societies, such as the one just described, the variation in belief systems is less, and the choices are limited, in comparison with a multicultural society such as the United States. As mentioned earlier, these belief systems are generally viewed as having strong religious and magical components. Richard Ward (1977) found that among nonindustrial groups, disease was commonly explained by attributing it to supernatural forces, such as demons and spirits. Among thirteen different cultural groups from widely scattered parts of the world,* as related in the Human Relations Area Files, it is commonly believed that disease results from contact with supernatural forces. Too, in spite of "nonscientific" theories of disease causation, all the societies surveyed maintained healthy, reproducing populations; the

*Andamanese, Comanche, Kapauku, Kikuyu, !Kung, Maori, Maria Gonds, Ona, Pomo, Semai, Yanomamo, eighteenth-century England, and modern Georgians of the Soviet Union.

belief systems were adapted to the ecological needs of the groups.

By means of comparison, commonalities can be noted in the belief systems of numerous peasant peoples, and in turn of those of various industrialized populations. Differences are more pronounced among preliterate, peasant, and industrial types of belief systems than among the specific societies represented by any one of the three types; that is, intertype differences are for the most part more significant than within-type differences. Observations of this sort lead Frazer to develop the three-stage sequence mentioned earlier. However, such sequences were overly simplistic, were often based on a belief in psychic unity, and were not sufficiently critical in the use of ethnographical analogy; that is, generalizations derived from observations or records of historical or proto-historical societies at differing levels of socioeconomic and political organization were loosely applied to the unknown prehistoric eras of other societies in the hopes of illustrating their overall sequence of cultural evolution (see Chapter 3). Proper account was not yet being taken of economic resource criteria—the effect of ritual on economic regulation processes—and intrasocietal variation in human behavior. The belief system was placed in a "package" containing historical and social information without thoroughly addressing economic and ecological factors. Belief at the macrolevel was conceptualized as the independent variable, whereas (if causality be assigned) it can better be understood as a dependent variable.

How do societies arrive at their health-sickness belief systems? How are causes identified? Most often some pathological process or symptom, such as swelling, discoloration, or lack of a properly functioning sense (such as sight), needs to be explained within the cultural context. Societies that do not use scientific methods may use religious or magical concepts to help delimit the causes and parameters of the situation, thus arriving at some explanation for a problem that is likely to recur. In scientific medicine, causes are established for disease and death out of a body of knowledge that has developed by testing hypotheses with the scientific method; for example, the cause of a sore throat can be reasoned as being caused by infection of the tonsils and upper throat lining by streptococcus or some other bacterium. The proximate cause is seen as an internal physiological one; whereas, in a preliterate system, the cause might likely be seen as being remote—competition between neighbors, greed, or curses cast by witches. Because of the relative lack of knowledge about physiology and anatomy (with notable exceptions such as among the Aleuts [Laughlin, 1977]) the cause is generally viewed as originating outside the body. The treatment, however, is aimed at the *presumed cause* of the condition in both the Western and preliterate situations. In the case of scientific medicine, the healer attempts to eliminate the infection through drugs, nutrition, or surgical intervention. The native healers attempt to alleviate and attenuate the effects of the ghost, witch, or strained social relationships.

Belief systems exemplified

Witchcraft, sorcery, vodun ("voodoo"), and divination are subjects enjoying widespread popularity in scientific and popular writings. In many cases they are juxtaposed with discussions of health care, illness, curing, and belief systems. Such juxtaposition correctly indicates that the conceptual and activity systems each term connotes are intimately bound with other elements of society; separation even for purposes of analysis can be difficult and misleading. However, in both scientific and popular circles there is disagreement regarding the precise definitions of these terms, especially those of witchcraft and sorcery.

For example, within the Spanish-American belief system, folk medicine is highly integrated along traditional lines (especially as evidenced in Colorado and New Mexico). Foster and Anderson (1978:74-76) point out that in theory and therapy it conforms to an equilibrium model of health, which in turn can be traced to modifications in the humoural pathology tradition. *Brujería*, or *hechicería* (witchcraft), is grounded in the belief that a witch works sympathetic magic against a victim, as exemplified by *mal ojo* (evil eye). Such witchcraft can be countered, however, and equilibrium thus can be reestablished. However, Spanish-Americans disagree even among themselves whether a *curandero* (traditional curer) can also be a *brujo* (witch) (Kay, 1977:150), and whether self-identified witches should be recognized as "socially legitimate" in a cultural context that recognizes the existence of witchcraft primarily by virtue of accusation.

By way of contrast, among the pre-Columbian Aztecs, witches were thought to be much like vampires. They sucked the blood of children, frightened people at night, transformed themselves into animals, and had the ability to fly (Madsen, in Olien, 1978:402-403). These *nahualli*, as they were called, were thought to possess attributes that now can be seen as similar to those of witches in the Euro-American tradition. Other examples could be given where the terms witch and sorcerer are used interchangeably (Olien, 1978:400-401); it has also been suggested that sorcery is a subcategory within the category of witchcraft (Kenny, 1976:254).

For the purposes of this text, however, witchcraft is defined as a conceptual and activity system within a particular cultural complex wherein a practitioner (the witch) is thought to secretively attempt by magically manipulative means to effect a maladjustive change in the psychophysical condition of another adherent of the same culture complex. Such changes are thought to be effected through some mystical power inherent in the witch's personality. Indeed, as was pointed out by Evans-Pritchard in his classic work among the Zande of Africa, witches are not thought to be entirely human (Olien, 1978: 401). In most societies witches are known through the accusations of others; they are not self-identified. (An exception would be the self-proclaimed but secretive New Druid witches of Colorado, who it is speculated may have been responsible for some of the cattle mutilations in the midwest during the 1970s. Another exception would be the self-proclaimed *brujos* mentioned before.)

Sorcery is defined as a conceptual and activity system within a particular cultural complex wherein a practitioner (the sorcerer) attempts by magically manipulative means to effect a change—usually maladjustive—in the psychophysical condition of another adherent of the same cultural complex, specifically through the use of leavings or objects associated with the person toward whom the sorcery is being directed. Unlike witches, sorcerers are thought to be ordinary humans. It should be noted that, as among the Zulu, a sorcerer also may devote a certain degree of energy to the curing of patients.

Vodun ("voodoo"), although not a focal point of this chapter, is defined as a religious system characteristic of certain of the people of Haiti. It developed secretively among transplanted African slaves, who incorporated elements from traditional African belief systems, Islam, and Catholicism. Cult membership is extensive, hierarchical, and oriented in part toward interpretation of the desires of deities who make themselves known through possession of selected adherents. Divination practices likewise are not a main topic of the present chapter. Suffice it to say they are extremely widespread and, like witchcraft and sorcery, are not restricted to any one type of belief system. Divination focuses on mystical-magical-psychical attempts by trained practitioners to diagnose the conditions of patients and foresee events bearing on human welfare. Specific attention is paid by most diviners to the use of objects (such as tea leaves, animal bones, and divining rods) that serve as communication media, for transmitting the diagnostic and/or psychic message to interested individuals.

Witchcraft. Witchcraft is important in the present context to the extent that its practice and conceptual underpinnings can be used to illustrate behavioral responses to change in particular socioeconomic systems and their impact on health and sickness. It relates to social learning formulations in this regard (Spanos, 1978:419-420). Its role as a functionally adaptive mechanism is examined also. In the case that follows, it is shown that coping with illness per se is secondary to the process of reestablishing equilibrium within a system.

Witch beliefs have flourished in the Hindu belief system for centuries and continue to be important even with the onset of modernization. Scarlett Epstein (1967) spent 2 years studying witchcraft and its impact on women in a modernizing Mysore village. Her research clearly illustrates witchcraft's role as an adaptive mechanism and its role in mediating social relationships, especially those in which tensions exist.

To set the stage, mention must first be made of the changing role of the woman within the Mysore economy. Traditionally, a married woman was supposed to work diligently on her husband's land, bear many children, display obedience to her husband, and demonstrate, among other social traits, generosity to kin and beggars alike. However, with the introduction of systematic irrigation in the Mysore region, much of the land that had previously supported only subsistence farming became fertile enough for cash-crop farming, a development that was accompanied by a new struggle for status among peasant farmers. One way a man could gain prestige was to have his wife work less and exhibit greater independence than previously. A farmer was considered relatively wealthy if his wife did not need to work. Husbands also began to give gifts of money and other material wealth to their wives in order that the women could retain family prestige after their husbands' deaths.

Through this transitional economic process and role shift, women became important moneylenders within the market economy, and new social relationships and accompanying tensions emerged. In turn, the three traditional aspects of peasant witch beliefs were strengthened; witchcraft accusations (1) tend to be directed against women, (2) are intracaste, and (3) arise out of tension in interpersonal relationships.

Epstein's report of the strained relations between a young peasant woman and an elderly widow who was her relative and neighbor illustrates the point. The young woman accused the widow of having poisoned her through witchcraft. Preceding the accusation, the young woman had visited a traditional curer in another village, seeking relief for a lingering illness. Having induced her to vomit, the curer reported finding two poisonous pills, which the young woman concluded she had been fed at the widow's house shortly before becoming ill. Thus arose the accusation of witchcraft. In an attempt to relieve the tensions surrounding the incident, the case was brought before the village *panchayat* ("judge"), although a direct accusation was never made during the proceedings themselves because it is believed that "witches are women who administer poison to their victims, but cannot help doing so. Women who give poison cannot control the evil spirit within themselves which makes them poison other people" (Epstein, 1967: 138). The case was resolved—and tensions eventually relieved—through the *panchayat's* decision that the young woman pay back part of the money that the widow had lent her prior to the accusation. It seems that no payment had yet been made on the debt because the young woman believed it unnecessary because the widow was her relative. On the other hand, the widow, in her emergent role as moneylender, had been constantly badgering her about the debt, as she would any other debtor. The accusation of witchcraft had indeed resulted from strained social relationships and from a misunderstanding on the part of the young woman. Tradition-

ally, she would not have had to repay a debt to a relative. By accusing the widow of witchcraft, an activity over which women are thought to have no direct control, she was able (perhaps subconsciously) to initiate a process that eventually clarified the parameters of the socioeconomic tensions, led to resolution of the case, and left no permanent indictment against the widow. Such incidents have served to reinforce the place of witchcraft in a changing Mysore society, in part because it can serve as a socially adaptive mechanism.

Accusations of witchcraft and the importance of understanding these processes in the context of ecology and coping behavior are exemplified in a different way in the contro-

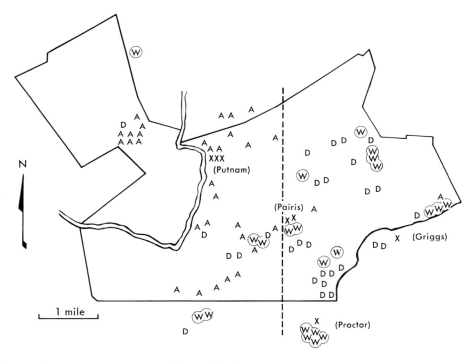

Fig. 6-3. Residence patterns, Salem Village, 1692. The names in parentheses indicate the households in which the afflicted girls were living, excluding Sarah Churchill, whose affliction is believed to have been fraudulent. The nonvillagers shown on this map are those whose places of residence lay on the fringes of the village boundaries. Residences are labeled X, afflicted girl; W, accused witch; D, defender of the accused; and A, accuser. (From Caporael, 1976:24.)

versial study done by Caporael (1976). Salem Village, Massachusetts, in the late seventeenth century was the scene of a relatively short-lived but intense siege of witchcraft accusations, as a result of which twenty persons were executed during a 2-year period. Subsequent debate has focused on several issues, one of which is of particular ecological interest here. Was socially defined deviant behavior in fact being demonstrated by certain of the accusers or were they merely seeking "societal scapegoats"? Were the accusations the product of psychophysiological factors traceable to environmental sources?

Caporael's inferential reconstructions indicate that certain members of the Salem community may have unknowingly been ingesting ergot. This parasitic fungus, which grows on damp grains, such as rye, can be responsible for a moderately severe form of poisoning known as convulsive ergotism, which is characterized by hallucinations, vertigo, disturbances in sensation, and epileptiform convulsions. Rye was a well-established New England crop in the seventeenth century. Reconstruction of farming and residence patterns (Fig. 6-3) in Salem Village indicates that a number of those who made accusations of witchcraft may have been eating ergotized rye from swampy farmlands in the western sector. Most of those accused of being witches lived in the eastern sector of the village. Caporael suggests that many of the accusers were indeed suffering from convulsive ergotism; because of preexistent, well-documented factionalism between the two sectors, the accusers seized on witchcraft supposedly perpetrated by women of the eastern sector as a cause.

No direct medical evidence exists to support Caporael's argument. And, while it is interesting for its ecological implications, Spanos and Gottlieb (1976) have compiled an impressive body of ecological and sociological

data that successfully refute it. Convulsive ergotism tends to be found in groups where severe vitamin A deficiency can be correlated with the consumption of ergotized grain. The Salem area was not likely to have suffered this vitamin-deficiency problem because of the abundance of seafood, nor do records of the period indicate that this population suffered other symptoms usually associated with vitamin A deficiency. Although Caporael does not suggest that all witchcraft accusations in the Salem area are traceable to convulsive ergotism, Spanos and Gottlieb do point out that such accusations were not confined only to areas where ergotized grain may have been consumed or marketed. The pattern is sociologically, not ecologically, delineated. They stress that all of the witchcraft phenomena in Salem Village can be accounted for via sociopsychological theory.

Just as socioeconomic change played a role in the Hindu case described earlier, Boyer and Nissenbaum (1974) suggest that it played a part in witchcraft in the Salem area. They extend their analysis beyond Salem Village, a subsistence-based outlying community, to Salem Town. By the 1690s, the latter was becoming a center of mercantile concerns, and wealth and political power were coming increasingly under the control of its merchants.

The witchcraft accusations were a continuation, on a psychological level, of the power struggle in the political, economic, and ecclesiastic arenas. According to this interpretation, the accusers were generally persons with a stake in maintaining the traditional social order of a farming community, while the accused were primarily identified with the newer values of pre-industrial capitalism. (Karlsen, 1978:703.)

That many of those accused of witchcraft lived outside Salem Village and could have been expected to have access to nonergotized grain further suggests that causes other than ergotism must be examined.

Karlsen also adheres to a theory of social learning and socioeconomic tension, but expands on the work of Boyer and Nissenbaum in an attempt to better account for the fact that most of the main protagonists (the accusers and the accused) were female. She notes that women were more than merely passive agents in the interpersonal and intercommunity struggle. Documents of the era indicate their active concerns with their roles in the society. The stresses and uncertainties associated with the socioeconomic changes mentioned may well have had an even greater impact on the women than the men; women's security was tied to a stable subsistence-based life-style in which the family was the basic socioeconomic unit. Few institutions other than the mystical were available for women to express their grievances. This situation strongly reflects the relatively marginal power position that women hold in comparison to men in many societies (Garrett, 1977). We suggest that the pattern of coping behavior chosen—witchcraft accusations—fits a preexistent Puritan belief system, one whose adherents in all likelihood did not actively recognize the magnitude and causal interactions of underlying socioeconomic variables but did actively recognize the need to deal with interpersonal tensions (see, for example, Garrett, 1977:463).

George Devereux defined the central problem for "psychiatric anthropologists," or more generally those interested in the interface of health and belief, as determination of the exact locus of culturally defined boundaries between normal and abnormal behavior (Scheper-Hughes, 1978:72). The two preceding examples from India and America indicate that such loci are indeed difficult to pinpoint, in part because socioeconomic and ecological factors that are not immediately apparent may serve as key independent variables. Those who exhibit the coping behavior themselves need not recognize all the important variables that may be operating in order for their behavior to be effective; however, the behavior must reflect aspects of the dominant belief system. Both normal and abnormal behaviors are culture- and belief-specific, and it is to these variables (rather than socioeconomic and ecological variables) that people themselves most often turn first in attempting to justify or explain their own actions. Medical anthropologists identifying socioeconomic variables do not provide better explanations, merely ones that may be less culture-bound and more oriented toward social learning and systems theories.

One problem in the identification of boundaries between normal and abnormal behavior has rested in the methodologies employed by investigating anthropologists. Too often "normalcy," while recognized as being culturally relative, has been narrowly and homogeneously defined. In fact, as DuBois clearly illustrated in her quantitative, psychologically oriented research conducted among the Alorese of Indonesia in 1938 and 1939, a great range of "normal" variation in personality exists even within very small populations (Barnouw, 1973:153-162). Assuming that behavior is at least a partial reflection of personality, it is this recognition of heterogeneity in a culturally relativistic context that allows appreciation of witchcraft as an example of "deviant behavior" in one society but "normal behavior" (yet not practiced by many) in another. In turn, it must be recognized that the overarching belief system includes some internal recognition of individual variation and differential adherence to belief.

Too often beliefs have been presented in anthropological literature without adequate recognition of deviation between the "presumed," as reported by a society's members and the "real," as practiced—but not always understood—by them. The differential between "presumed" and "real" behaviors is reflected in European witchcraft beliefs. Accusations of witchcraft in Massachusetts to some extent paralleled accusations on a broad scale in Europe during the same era. It has been estimated that as many as 500,000 people were tortured or killed as accused witches during the fifteenth through seventeenth centuries (Harris, 1974:207). Contrary to popular opinion, although the Christian Church believed in witchcraft and magic prior to the eleventh century, it primarily devoted its energies to limiting, rather than encouraging, witch superstitions; "witches were considered individual nuisances whose power was often overrated by a superstitious population" (Spanos, 1978:420). The shift in the Church's pattern of belief and practice regarding witchcraft only took place between the eleventh and fifteenth centuries, when it paralleled key social, political, and technoeconomic changes.

By the 1600s many of the best-educated people in Western Europe did indeed believe in the existence of witches. Some went so far as to suggest that the accused belonged to an international satanic conspiracy dedicated to the eventual overthrow of Christianity. The presumption was that numerous people—usually women—were in fact witches and that they flew to sabbats where "they had sexual intercourse with demons and animals as well as with one another, killed and ate children, and performed a parody of Christian rituals" (Spanos, 1978: 420). Some authorities went so far as to pass laws to thwart such activities indirectly. For example, the Irish Parliament in the twelfth century passed an act forbidding the purchase of red swine because Irish witches were believed to be turning wisps of hay into red-colored pigs and selling them in the market places (Byrne, 1967:11).

Since it is probable that exceedingly few individuals in Europe were ever self-identified, practicing witches, the discrepancy between "presumed" and "real" behaviors seems remarkable anthropologically. Yet both types exist, and it must be remembered that the discrepancy was not perceived, or at least not perceived to be great, by Europeans of that era. As in the Salem case, an analysis of both types of behavior from a historical and socioeconomic perspective indicates that Euro-American witchcraft accusations can best be understood as coping behavior. It is behavior to be understood primarily in a sociological, community-interaction framework rather than in one grounded in the psychiatric or psychophysiological analysis of supposed aberrant individuals.

For comparative purposes, it is worth noting a similar analysis, derived from the study of contemporary, self-identified practicing witches. Leininger (1973) examined witchcraft in the United States and found six significant reasons for increased interest in it; they include (1) distrust and unrest among the many different ethnic groups in the United States who have not interacted with one another until recently, (2) heightened interest in extrasensory perceptual phenomena, (3) increased use of secretive and highly symbolical forms of communication in order to relate differently and intimately with humans and nature, (4) increased belief in astrology, (5) increased use of magical explanations by people who are "nonscientifically inclined," and (6) attempts among contemporary youth to test what is reality and what is not. She notes that some witchcraft is practiced in families as a means of coping with in-group problems initiated by external societal factors (Leininger, 1973:82). It is interesting that in the United States, with witchcraft no longer primarily a phenomenon dependent on accusation for its existence, some individuals are attempting to extract, internalize, and adopt portions of this belief system in order to cope with situations of a different sort.

Sorcery. Whereas witchcraft has been defined as a belief complex based on accusation (witches rarely identifying themselves as

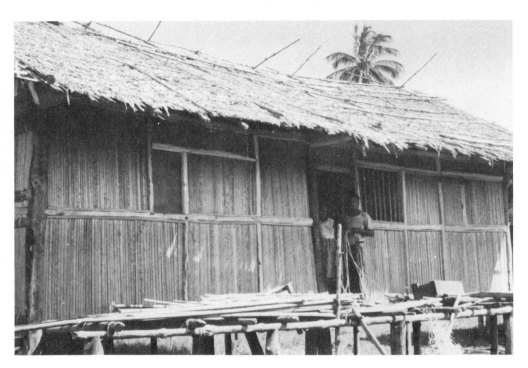

Fig. 6-4. The most powerful sorcerer in one of the coastal New Guinea Asmat villages, this man has enlisted the support of other villagers to build a house considered to be more grandiose than that of anyone in the vicinity. He also serves as leader of an active cargo cult. (Photo by P. Van Arsdale.)

such), sorcery is defined as a related phenomenon in which self-proclaimed practitioners actually exist (Fig. 6-4). Accusations are also important in sorcery and can be correlated with social control. In this regard Whiting (1950) was able statistically to support her hypothesis of a functional association between sorcery and "coordinate control" (social control in band or tribal societies where delegated authorities for settling disputes do not exist, so offenses are dealt with by kin or local groups). It should be noted that some of the societies she lists as having sorcery should be considered as having witchcraft instead, by the definitions employed here. In both types, however, the importance of social control pertains, and patterns of coping behavior associated with misfortune are apparent.

One of the best-documented cases of sorcery as defined here has been provided by Harner (1978), based on his extensive research among the Jívaro Indians of the Ecuadorian Amazon. Although he in fact uses the terms "witchcraft" and "sorcery" somewhat interchangeably (see, for example, Harner, 1978:191), he presents a strong case for the relationship of sorcery to shamanism, and in turn for the relationship that both have to inflicting misfortune and reciprocal coping behavior. His study places illness in a totally social-supernatural context.

The Jívaro believe that sorcery is the cause of most illnesses and nonviolent deaths. "The normal waking life, for the Jívaro, is simply a 'lie,' or illusion, while the true forces that determine daily events are supernatural and can only be seen and manipulated with the aid of hallucinogenic drugs" (1978:188). Thus the society places a high premium on specialists who can deal directly with both natural and supernatural beings.

Jívaro specialists are of two related types, those who act primarily as sorcerers and those who act primarily as shamanic curers. Both receive their initial training in the same manner, and both rely on the ingestion of a hallucinogenic brew referred to as *natema* that allows them to attain the trance state necessary for communication with the multitude of beings (many in animal form) that inhabit the supernatural world. Under the influence of *natema* a sorcerer is able to call upon *tsentsak* ("spirit helpers") who can be employed as "darts" to inflict illness or death from afar. It is believed that a powerful *tsentsak*, if regurgitated properly through the sorcerer's mouth, can be magically thrust entirely through a victim's body. The victim who learns in time that such an act has been perpetrated against him will attempt to enlist the help of a shaman. The cure frequently involves the sucking out of the intruding "darts."

With such powers at their command, neighboring sorcerers in Jívaro society are virtually in constant "warfare." Shamans intercede, attempting to alleviate the misfortune that has been inflicted. If properly manipulated and enticed, spirits become powerful allies; if not, their behavior can be extremely difficult to predict. Yet in all cases they are very real to the Jívaro. Victims of their activity indeed become ill and occasionally die, which would not be the case if an intended victim did not adhere to the same set of beliefs.

Sorcery and microsystem effects

It has been suggested (as in Lindenbaum, 1975) that whether sorcery or witchcraft activity are in fact practiced or are merely based on accusation, both can be related to demographic, economic, and ecological considerations. Sorcery, or its threat, occasionally can serve to even out demographic irregularities. As exemplified among the Fore of New Guinea:

A charge of sorcery allocates responsibility for the severe illness or death of members in one's own group. It is a charge of willful depletion, an affront to groups dedicated to equality. Sorcery debates consequently have a strong moral element . . . After a number of deaths in one's own group, intergroup affairs arrive at an impasse, since loss of life has reached an intolerable limit. Small New Guinea populations are vulnerable to marked stochastic events . . . Neighbours now have a potential for domination (Lindenbaum, 1975:69-70).

As with the Jívaro, a delicate balance must be struck among a complex of natural and supernatural forces. Demographic and ritual processes act as mutually reinforcing variables within the system. The group's members aid the sorcerer in focusing power by abstaining from sexual intercourse during the period when aggressive sorcery is being performed. (Abstention is also practiced while a Fore woman is in therapeutic consultation with a curer.) "That is, there is a group prohibition on intercourse during active interference in life-saving and life-taking situations, as if to deal with only one demographic variable at a time" (Lindenbaum, 1975:70-71).

Sorcery's impact on the economic structure of the highland New Guinea region is intriguing. It can be viewed in an open-systems context in that its influence is not merely restricted to symmetrical intracultural relationships. In the east-central area of the highlands, there is a tendency for traders to travel uphill. Since there also exists a tendency to fear the threat of sorcery from people downhill, asymmetrical intercultural relationships are suggested. A "downhill group" may use the fear that an "uphill group" has for its sorcery to assure safe passage on uphill trading expeditions. Fear of sorcery can be said to flow downhill, while the trade of luxury items (such as shells and feathers) flows uphill (Lindenbaum, 1975). Luxury goods are exchanged for products of intensive labor, such as axes and pigs. Thus, a holistic approach that includes consideration of religico-magical beliefs is necessary to gain an adequate understanding of economic activities.

As a final example of a demographic variable being related to accusations of sorcery, we consider the case of *kuru*, a chronic, degenerative neurological disease that severely affected certain of the Fore of New Guinea until recently. In one of the most remarkable series of medical anthropology studies ever conducted, Nobel prize–winning virologist-anthropologist D. Carleton Gajdusek of the National Institutes of Health was able to identify the causal agent as an unconventional "slow virus" and to relate its transmission to the practice of endocannibalism (the ritual consumption of the corpses of one's own group out of respect for the deceased). He found that the virus resides in human brain tissue, has a long incubation period, and—being highly infectious—can be transmitted via conjunctival, nasal, and skin contact during dissemination of a corpse's flesh and the opening of its skull. Lindenbaum (1978) and other ethnologists stress the direct consumption of brain tissue—not thoroughly cooked—by those later exhibiting the disease's symptoms. Particularly as seen among male and female Fore children and female adults, kuru is characterized by cerebellar ataxia (inability to coordinate voluntary muscular movements) and shiveringlike tremors. Specifically, there is usually clawing and gripping toe movement, breast tremor, a "tripod" sitting posture, laughter and euphoria, progressively greater difficulty in standing and walking, and eventual death

within 1 year (Gajdusek, 1977; Sorenson and Gajdusek, p. 4).

By examining the cultural context of Fore beliefs, the differential impact kuru had on adult females as opposed to males can be explained, as can its relationship to accusations of sorcery. Prior to the cessation of Fore cannibalism, women, with the assistance of their children, had been primarily responsible for the ritual dissection and preparation of the kuru victim's flesh—as they would the flesh of any other deceased relative. These same individuals were the primary consumers as well. Thus males who had escaped the disease in childhood would likely avoid becoming infected at all (Gajdusek, 1977:956; Hunt, 1978:93-94; Foster and Anderson, 1978:23-24). Having no knowledge of the biological processes involved in the origin and continued spread of the disease, the Fore frequently blamed its occurrence on sorcery. For example, in the southern Fore region in 1963 a peak of sorcery accusations was seen to coincide with especially large numbers of kuru deaths among the women. The reproductive potential of the population was being seriously curtailed. Relating this to comments made earlier, it becomes clear how demographic fluctuations can become especially pronounced within a small population and how ritual becomes a ready—if not always effective—means of coping with a little-understood situation (Lindenbaum, 1975, 1978).

In concluding this section, brief mention must be made of a classic in the anthropological study of sorcery. Approximately half a century ago, Reo Fortune conducted a detailed study of the social organization of the Dobu Islanders of Melanesia that was published in 1932 under the title *Sorcerers of Dobu*. Some of his data later were utilized by Ruth Benedict in *Patterns of Culture* (1934). In Chapter 3 of his book (reprinted in Landy, 1977), Fortune weaves together a meticulously detailed account of the interactions of sorcery, disease, and yam production, an account that can be cast in the ecological light of the present text.

Fortune's underlying premise, analogous to Foster's conceptualization of "limited good" (1967), is that social success is necessarily gained at the expense of others.

The healthy person is he who has defended himself from the black art [sorcery] of others in his pursuit of social success at the expense of others. The sick, deformed, and dying are those whose magic has not been as strong as that of those others who have felt themselves injured by their social climbing (Fortune, 1977:199).

Similarly, it is thought that an overly successful garden with an abundance of yams has been gained at the expense of another whose yams may have been stolen by magic. If suspicions of this sort arise, and Fortune suggests they are indeed common, sorcery is attempted in the hopes of causing illness or death. The yam supply can, in turn, be expected to "even out" over the long run.

Despite the contributions of Fortune's early research to subsequent study of medical anthropology in an ecological perspective, important questions remain unanswered. Was the actual practice of Dobuan sorcery as widespread as he suggests? Was account taken of the possibly large differential between "presumed" and "real" behavior patterns regarding sorcery? If it were possible to go back in time with the research methods now available (that is, a methodology such as that employed by Rappaport [1968] in his study of ritual and ecology), could changes in yam production actually be correlated with accusations of sorcery? Nonetheless, the central finding remains: sorcery, like witchcraft, helps shape social relationships. Its ongoing practice—and the threat thereof—relates to the actualization of a societal concept of illness behavior.

Culture-bound syndromes

Historical evidence suggests that "hysterical" or "atypically psychotic" people have long been known. In certain societies their position (and consequent management) is well defined, and in others established methods of coping are essentially nonexistent. In the early Christian tradition, Satanism was thought to manifest its evil in the behavior of people of this sort (Bromberg, 1975:64). The notion that such individuals were possessed by a malevolent, supernatural agent was common. In colonial America, prominent physicians, such as Benjamin Rush, stated that beatings and bloodlettings served to calm such people—the beatings through the pain inflicted and the bloodlettings, which Rush practiced, through reduction in the amount of blood in the brain. Despite this "scientific" interpretation and treatment, the underlying belief was by no means dispelled that a beating would actually drive out a possessing spirit.

Within the past century, the systematic Western study of mental illness began to gain a foothold, a development that has been correlated with the rise of psychology and psychiatry, although it is not entirely delimited by these disciplines. The study of hysteria followed this rise, with early work focusing on Euro-American case studies (White, 1964:22-25); only more recently have ethnopsychiatrists and medical anthropologists turned their systematic, comparative attention to the hysterias and "atypical psychoses" characteristic of other societies. Foulks' (1972) study of Arctic hysterias among the Eskimos is a case in point.

Given this brief background, attention can be turned to what have come to be called "culture-bound syndromes" (Kleinman, 1978b), or "ethnic psychoses" (Landy, 1977:340). At the broadest level these include the hysterias and atypical psychoses. The definition of these syndromes is a loose one, meant to include severe psychosocial or psychogenic reactions to stress that are significantly molded by the particular cultural milieu. What makes a workable definition hard to derive is that numerous different yet related terms exist in the literature. There are cross-cultural differences in the manifestation of symptoms, thus making it difficult to sort out possible physiological or genetic etiological components; and even within a given society, a particular syndrome is frequently thought to be "atypical" (Yap, 1977). In all cases an adequate understanding can only be obtained through analysis of behavioral patterns associated with the onset, climax, and (usually) disappearance of the illness. This includes the behavior of relevant others no less than that of the patient.

Latah. An issue of the journal *Culture, Medicine and Psychiatry* (Sept. 1978) presents a set of articles on the subject of culture-bound syndromes. *Latah* is a reactive syndrome that has been noted in Malaya and Indonesia since the nineteenth century (Kenny, 1978). It is primarily manifested by women who have reached or passed menopause. Local inhabitants and European observers alike agree that "shock" or "startle" is an important causal factor both in the first occurrence and in subsequent manifestations of *latah*. In some areas of what is now Malaysia, it is even thought that a woman and a tiger may have the powers to render one another *latah* through fright.

"Through obscenity the *latah* transcends the constraints of normal morality" (Kenny, 1978:219). It is through the use of obscenities that *latah* behavior is often most clearly manifested. Although there is some disagreement, prominent observers believe that spirit possession is thought to account for the obscenities. In fact since the *latah* herself is not thought to be in control, some people amuse themselves by startling the victim in the company of others in order to provoke an outburst. Apart from obscenities, speech is usually disorganized. Another behavior often seen is a compulsion to mimic the speech or actions of onlookers. When the mutual interaction (or provocation) between *latah* and onlookers subsides, so too does the episodic behavior.

Kenny's summary of numerous reports and historical records helps to place *latah* in the appropriate cultural context. The syndrome has been observed among the Iban of Sarawak, the Semai of the Malay peninsula, the Balinese, Malay immigrants, and most prominently among people of Malay-Javanese culture proper. It has not been noted among the aristocracy, however, nor among Chinese residents unless they have been fully acculturated. Thus, *latah* occurs solely within a single interrelated cultural milieu, and, as such, exemplifies a culture-bound syndrome. This is not to imply total cultural or social homogeneity in Malaya and Indonesia (Kenny, 1978:212).

Orang gila. *Orang gila* is a reactive syndrome characteristic of the inhabitants of many societies of New Guinea. The term itself means "madperson" or "madman" and is used only in certain areas of Indonesian New Guinea (Irian Jaya) where Malay-Indonesian trade words have penetrated. As manifested among the Asmat, it is considered an "acute illness," with identifiable periods of onset, climax, and disappearance. Usually, the period of hyperactivity lasts no more than 2 to 4 hours, and all manifestations of an episode disappear within 2 to 3 days.

Orang gila activities, as seen among the Asmat of New Guinea, typically have a relatively sudden onset. Informants state that this is caused by "sudden spirit possession," often thought to take place while one is working in a sago grove, where malevolent spirits are thought to lurk. Actual *orang gila* behavior is not manifested in the grove, but in the presence of onlookers back in the village.

Typically, the victim grabs a spear, or bow and arrows, and begins dashing madly through the center of the village, seemingly bent on homicide. (The term "amok" has been applied to this type of hyperactive phase as observed in other societies [Clarke, 1973; Carr, 1978]). Injury or death is threatened to those who get in the way. Frequently a spear is thrown, but it invariably misses the intended "victim" by a wide margin. The *orang gila* yells and screams at many of those he encounters, including his wife and children. These mad dashes can continue for 2 or more hours, until exhaustion sets in. During the period of hyperactivity, at least one male onlooker follows the *orang gila* closely and is prepared to restrain the individual, should bodily harm become imminent. Other onlookers exhibit reactions of mild amusement or of genuine fear if they have been threatened.

A 27-year old man underwent this transformation one afternoon. Symbolically, the marginal nature of his social position was evidenced by his mimicry of Indonesian soldiers; their recent presence had caused tensions in the Asmat region. For nearly 3 hours, he shouted curt militarylike instructions to all he encountered as he strutted in goose-step fashion back and forth along the village's central walkway. Occasionally he would grab his spear and dash off after an unsuspecting child. That evening, after the acute phase had subsided, male "bodyguards" slept by him in the event that his possessing spirit might try to guide him into the jungle.

Langness (1965) has described this culture-bound syndrome as a manifestation of "hysterical psychosis." In this sense, in its immediacy, it can correctly be understood as a type of acute psychosomatic disease. The physical symptoms of such psychoses are similar cross-culturally: hyperactivity, glazed eyes, impaired sense of hearing, panting

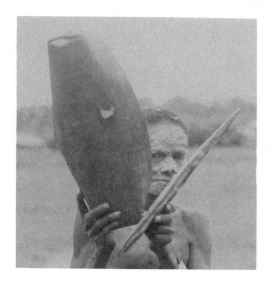

Fig. 6-5. An *orang gila* "hides" behind some of the paraphernalia used in her dashes, dances, and taunts in a coastal Asmat village. Although her behavior is considered to be deviant by fellow villagers, it is tolerated even when socially disruptive. (Photo by P. Van Arsdale.)

gasps, and skin cold to the touch. Yet the physiological manifestations can only be understood etiologically in the context of the social learning processes that take place in Asmat society.

Summary. The probable explanation for *latah* and for *orang gila* emphasizes cultural rather than psychological factors. That is, this type of patterned, reactive behavior should not be viewed as a "mental disorder." Like witchcraft, its ramifications for both actors and onlookers alike can be understood from the perspective of social learning theory. The *latah* or *orang gila* responds to cues in the sociocultural environment, and in so doing actively and symbolically expresses a situation of stress, marginality, or emotional release. The syndrome cannot be understood apart from the behavior of all relevant people in the social environment. In fact, some who observe an episode soon thereafter become *latah* or *orang gila* themselves. Clarke (1973) quite appropriately describes this type of activity as "theatre."

THE ROLES OF PRACTITIONERS AND PATIENTS

The examples presented here and in previous chapters of various forms of sickness and abnormal behavior suggest that both the patient and the curer assume a special role in relation to one another and to the given society. However, the degree to which this role and status differ from others within the society depends to a great extent on that society's system of beliefs, which govern the parameters of all social relationships. Numerous considerations must be made in analyzing illness. For example, to what degree are sick individuals given special statuses and roles? Do they wear special clothing designating their position in society? Do they have special rights and privileges, or have their ordinary rights been removed or changed? When and who decides what their role is and when it is to change? Are there special rites of passage to ease the transition from one status and role to another? In turn, what are the roles and statuses of the curers?

Although more information is available on the role of the curer than on that of the client (Landy, 1977:385), one approach to the study of role relationships and health beliefs is proposed by sociologist Talcott Parsons (1951). His model addresses the dyadic relationship between the physician and the patient. Parsons views the physician's role as being parent-like and that of the patient as weak and dependent. This model is well known and is widely applied, but it has limitations, especially when it is applied to the interactions of healers and patients cross-culturally and cross-class. In fact, Parsons' model is based on an ideal type of middle-class American society rather than on health beliefs and behaviors observed cross-cul-

turally (see Landy 1977:385-388). However, as Parsons implies (1951:428), his intent was not to develop a universal model.

A cogent critique of the Parsonian model has recently been provided by Foster and Anderson (1978:154-156). Of primary heuristic value to medical anthropologists is Parsons' delineation of a patient's rights (expectations) and duties (responsibilities). The patient has the right to be exempted from normal social responsibilities and the right to receive care until recovery (or death) is reached. Duties include the patient's acknowledgment of the sick role as undesirable, hence an obligation to recover as soon as possible, and enactment of an effort to seek competent medical assistance. These aspects of the model have wide cross-cultural applicability, especially when applied to people suffering from acute forms of illness. They have less applicability in cases of chronic disease or terminal illness, when the sick role may be severely modified or abandoned. Our brief survey of recent literature that describes a number of band, tribal, and peasant peoples and that provides enough information on the sick role to permit some general inferences demonstrates that these duties and responsibilities pertain in each instance. Specifically, the surveyed societies were the general Australian aboriginal population (Elkin, 1977); the Fore of New Guinea (Lindenbaum, 1978; 1975); the Asmat of New Guinea (see the case study, pp. 216 to 220); the Mnong Gar of Vietnam (Condominas, 1977); the "folk Buddhists" of Burma (Spiro, 1977); the adherents to traditional Chinese medicine (Kleinman, 1978c; DHEW, 1974; Davis and Yin, 1973); the adherents to the Ayurvedic medical tradition of southern Asia (Obeyesekere, 1976, 1977); the !Kung of Botswana (Lee, 1978); the Zulu of South Africa (Sibisi, 1977); the Sidamo of Ethiopia (Hamer and Hamer, 1977); the Eskimos of North Alaska (Foulks, 1972); the Navajo of the American southwest (Sandner, 1978); and the Ladinos of Guatemala (Glittenberg, 1976; Woods, 1977). Thus, although restricted in certain of its cross-cultural applications, Parsons' model provides a useful springboard for the comparative study of the role of the patient.

Landy (1977) has developed the idea of role adaptation in relation to the study of practitioner roles, in which emphasis is placed on changes in the curing role as society itself undergoes acculturative stress. "Adaptive curing roles" are those in which a traditional healer selectively adopts elements of Western medicine while continuing to emphasize key traditional practices. Recent activities in northern India are cited to support the validity of this type of role concept. "Attenuated curing roles" are seen in those instances where, in the face of powerful scientific and medical advances, the curer continues in the traditional role, even at the expense of attrition among the clientele; an example of this phenomenon can be found among the Anang of Nigeria. "Emergent curing roles" can appear in situations where no such specialized role previously existed. Landy cites the emergence of "doctor boys" among the Manus of New Guinea to support this role concept.

To illustrate the significance of curative role relationships in a belief system, we present the following three case studies. The first two are brief synopses, based on the research of one of the authors (Glittenberg, 1977). The third is intended to cover a broader range of phenomena. It is also based on the work of another of the authors (Van Arsdale, 1978).

Cakchiquel

Although expressing concern about the health of another, a person may not always realize the role that he or she plays in that process. Many of the *curanderas* of Guatemala are skilled in deciphering role relationships and relating the cause of illness to associated frictions. The anthropologist's assessment of roles must take into account the abilities that traditional curers themselves have in the area of role assessment.

Jorge was a bright, 27-year-old Cakchiquel Indian in the small village of Xajaxac in highland Guatemala. Although he was illiterate, he was eager to gain a new economic foothold in the cash market by selling personal items such as combs, shoestrings, and the like at the weekend market in the larger neighboring town of Solola. His wife, Margarita, objected to these efforts because they put her husband in contact with an outside world of which she was not a part. She wanted him to continue cultivating their small plot of native corn and beans. Selling foreign items such as combs and brushes was not the custom in their village. After continuing a strained relationship for approximately 6 months, the couple discovered that one of their five children (aged 3 months) began exhibiting symptoms of *mal ojo* (the evil eye). The only known source of cure was a *curandera*. Jorge, a devoted father, accompanied his wife and child to consult her. After completing a session of ritualized inquiry, the *curandera* indeed confirmed that the child was suffering from *mal ojo*, but she could not immediately identify who had cast the evil eye. After several additional sessions, Jorge himself was identified. The market articles, belonging to foreigners, had been a bad influence on him. The only "treatment" was for Jorge to stop his marketing practices immediately (although his continued sale of traditional products was still condoned). This Jorge did, the strained relationship was eased, and the infant recovered.

Mexican-American

Traditional healers and their practices are of interest as they emerge within the modern medical system. For example, *curanderos* or *curanderas* are recognized as traditional healers in the Mexican-American culture (see Chapter 2). In Denver, Colorado, a locally respected *curandera* is employed as a cultural specialist in a state-supported mental health clinic. In her role as a psychotherapist, she primarily serves the city's Hispanic population. Often her functions and treatments blend her skills as a modern therapist with her traditional skills as a *curandera*. To illustrate this point, she described the course of illness and treatment of one of her clients.

Lillie, a 24-year-old woman, migrated 3 years ago from a southwestern town in the United States to Denver. She came alone and without resources but very soon found a low-paying job as a carhop in a quick-service drive-in restaurant. Attractive and ambitious, Lillie wanted to attend college with the hope of some day becoming a lawyer. Finding little hope of ever achieving this goal on her limited salary, she began to supplement her income by working as a prostitute. Some of her clients were neighbors living near her in a lower-income area of the city.

After continuing her life-style for several years, Lillie fell in love with a young orthodontist, and they planned to be married. For unexplained reasons, she became increasingly depressed as the wedding date approached. She believed people were accusing her of lying and cheating. Gradually Lillie became more depressed and soon attempted suicide. It was the attempted suicide that precipitated Lillie's seeking help at a mental health center. Because of her Hispanic background, she was referred to the cultural specialist, the *curandera*.

Following several therapy sessions, the *curandera* came to believe that the source, or predisposing factor, to Lillie's depressions was the guilt she felt concerning her life as a prostitute. Strained role relationships can bring about illness, and Lillie's strained relationships with her neighbors were important factors in her depression. The *curandera* recognized the need to act as an intermediary in reestablishing some social equilibrium with the group; thus she asked Lillie to go to each house in the neighborhood in which she was known and to give each family two newspapers. Lillie also was to ask the family to come to the home of the *curandera* on a certain evening. Lillie went willingly; that evening she and the neighbor-

hood group assembled in the living room of the *curandera*. The *curandera* instructed each neighbor to crumble the newspapers into small balls. Next Lillie was instructed to get down on her knees in the middle of the room. With Lillie in that position, the *curandera* commanded, "Now each of you throw the balls of newspaper at Lillie and say 'Liar, cheat!'" A chorus of shouts was accompanied by a shower of flying newspaper balls. Following the pelting, the *curandera* instructed, "Now each of you say, 'I forgive you Lillie.'" Another chorus was heard. Slowly Lillie got up; she was crying. Spontaneously, the neighbors began to reach out, to touch, and then to hug the depressed client. Thus the first steps toward relieving the guilt of a client as well as reestablishing equilibrium in the social group had been initiated by blending the technique of psychodrama with the traditional skills of the *curandera*. Lillie had begun to reestablish herself as a member of the group, and the guilt that had precipitated the depression was lessened.

In summary, this case study illustrates the complexity of illness causation and its subsequent treatment. Broken relationships cause a multitude of physical and psychological symptoms, such as depression. Healers with the knowledge and skill needed to treat illnesses within the cultural context are critical to the healing process.

Asmat

Among the Asmat of Indonesian New Guinea, beliefs regarding health and illness can generally be described as personalistic. Human misfortunes are viewed as being manifested in illness, disrupted social relationships, the malevolent acts of spirits of the dead, or such socioeconomic difficulties as lack of a sufficient amount of fish. Illness as we have defined the term can be applied to virtually all of the prominent health maladies—psychosocial, psychosomatic, and physiological. Disease as a term may also be applied, but only to certain "superficial" ailments, such as boils and open sores. The

Asmat themselves do not have terms precisely translatable into such a dichotomy. Their terminology focuses on external causes of illness within an overarching cosmological framework. As Van Amelsvoort (1964) discovered, in addition to strong emphases on supernatural, spirit-oriented equilibrium factors, there is recognition of the need to restore bodily balance. A type of hot-cold conceptualization pertains to this. The application of heat via a smoldering wooden rod can at one and the same time "drive out the cause" of pneumonia and rectify bodily imbalance. As with the !Kung of the Kalahari Desert, fire is seen as the source of the heat necessary to activate medicine (Lee, 1978: 198).

The possession and "hysterical psychosis" of the *orang gila* of the Asmat, discussed earlier in this chapter, is conceptualized by villagers as a form of "illness," but unlike some other maladies, it is one from which total recovery is expected. This is considered probable whether or not a *namer-o* (traditional curer) or nontraditional curer intervenes. One of the authors (Van Arsdale, 1978:455) established a small clinic in the village of Owus, and for this reason was viewed as something of a nontraditional curer (albeit inexperienced). It was in Owus that the primary observations of *orang gila* reported here were made. Thus it was that Ambesu, one of the village Big Men, came seeking a pill to assist in the cure of his wife's state of possession. On one level of analysis, his behavior was a reflection of a belief in her illness; on another level, it reflected his concern that social relationships, with the author as well as other villagers, needed to be rectified. During her possession she had acted in a way deemed to be socially unacceptable having demanded tobacco from every male she encountered.

This case serves not only to exemplify one form of illness, but to illustrate certain roles and statuses of people involved in both receipt and ministration of curative services. The sick person, in any society, takes on a role and its associated status, which respectively serve as a partial guide to social interactions during the period of illness and to delineate the sick individual from others. In some instances, as Foster and Anderson note (1978:148-153), acceptance of this role can have far-reaching consequences. For example, an illness such as that associated with *orang gila* can be used to gain attention. That the author was perceived in the role of nontraditional curer and was consulted as such can best be appreciated when it is recalled that possession of this sort is thought to be followed by total recovery regardless of efforts at curative intervention. The author was not viewed as having a curative role of importance; in all but one other instance he was asked to help only in cases he categorized as representing disease rather than illness. The important factor was that the woman, in her new role as *orang gila*, had disrupted key relationships.

The curer. The role of *namer-o* in Asmat society can be assessed from two perspectives: how it is acquired and how it is enacted. The role of curer confers a great deal of status, particularly to a male. His ability to bring about a variety of cures (magical and otherwise), as well as influence those about him through charismatic persuasion, is highly respected and praised. In many ways the curer is more important than the cure. He must be able to maintain favorable communication with spirits of *safan* ("the other side"). Among the diverse spirits thought to inhabit the cosmos, some derived from nonhuman entities and others from the deceased (both friend and foe), the spirit that is responsible for visiting a potential curer to invest him or her with a "calling" is perhaps the most complex. This spirit—also known as *namer-o*—is thought to be of such magnitude that it is associated with an entire village. It is somewhat less humanlike than many other spirits and is thought to reside in the mud directly below the settlement. On occasion the spirit *namer-o* visits an individual during a dream. The Asmat believe that such a visitation is unexpected but also suggest that certain men or women may be predisposed to receive a "calling," which is never rejected. Observations indicate that those who are called usually have shown some prior interest in curing, perhaps having even informally assisted an established *namer-o* in curing sessions. Society does not consider them aberrant.

The number of people actively serving as *namer-o* in a village at any one time can vary widely. Early in 1974 in the village of Syuru (population 942) the number doubled within a few months, reaching fifteen. This was attributed in large part to a rumor that had spread concerning the deaths of several children; these were believed to have been caused by clinic immunizations in the neighboring town of Agats. As Syuru's clinic attendance for all forms of treatment ground to a virtual halt there was a resurgence in actively practicing *namer-o* (Van Arsdale, 1978: 446).

The primary enactment of the role of *namer-o* involves rectification of disrupted social relationships. In the village of Yepem, for example, a man was observed whose illness might best be described as malaise. As other villagers engaged in a session of recreational drumming and chanting near his house one evening, he and his wife could be heard wailing. Those drumming initially paid little attention. However, upon the urgings of a *namer-o*, the entire group suspended their activities and entered his house. There, under extremely crowded but socially amenable conditions, a cure was enacted. It involved no herbal remedies. It focused entirely on chanting and massage as adminis-

tered by the *namer-o* and his apprentice. A reconstruction of events surrounding the acquisition of the illness indicated that the man in question had become alienated from a portion of the village. He had sought to reestablish his bonds of friendship, only to be thwarted. The curing ceremony at last succeeded where other types of activity had failed; the *namer-o* had wisely guided a large group of villagers into his house at a time when all had initially assembled for a different purpose. Many of those present had been among the alienated individuals.

The enactment of the role of *namer-o* as curer is also exemplified in the following case of exorcism. A boy 16 years of age became very ill one morning after having dreamed that his dead brother had returned to visit him during the night. To him the dream was an extension of reality. The brother had been accompanied by a powerful spirit, and both of them had entered the boy's body in order to implant two snakes in his abdomen. Soon after relating his dream to his family, the boy began complaining of cramps and quickly passed into a dazed, comatose state. Of Syuru's fifteen male and female curers one of the most important was summoned, a man about 50 years old. He instructed the family to hold the boy in place, gently but firmly, on a mat in the center of their large hut. As numerous other people gathered around in a subdued yet casual mood, the *namer-o* began his curing ritual.

With the help of an apprentice, the *namer-o* passed a small shell over the boy's abdomen. By sleight of hand, he made the shell appear to emerge from the patient's navel. Next, the assistant was instructed to bring out his two special wooden rods, each about a foot long, which were wrapped and stored in a piece of colorful old cloth. The tip of one rod was heated with a burning ember and carefully was placed on certain vital points of the body—first on the ankles, then

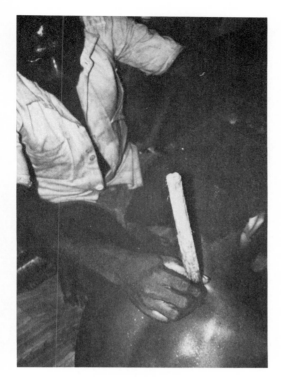

Fig. 6-6. The apprentice to an important Asmat curer, this young man applies heat to selected spots on the body by means of a special wooden rod. Heat is thought to restore internal equilibrium, and thus one's health. (Photo by P. Van Arsdale.)

on the backs of the knees, then on the lower back, the neck, and the temples (Fig. 6-6)—the curer in this case making certain never to cause a burn.

In Asmat the use of a shell and the application of heat are the first phases of exorcism. The purpose is to induce or force evil spirits, in this case two snakes, to leave the body, whereupon the patient is completely cured. Among people who believe in its efficacy, exorcism is one of the most powerful curative practices in existence. Consequently, the exorcist is viewed as an extremely influential person, someone whose personality traits are to be emulated (see Spiro, 1977).

Some 20 minutes after the curing ritual

had begun, the boy regained consciousness. However, the snakes had not yet left his body. The *namer-o* and his assistant tugged at the boy's head, arms, and legs in order to ease any cramps. Using a strong, circular motion, the curer then began to massage the entire abdomen as he initiated the third and final phase of the cure. It quickly became apparent that through a deft manipulation of the skin, he was making it appear as though one of the snakes was being drawn to the surface. Suddenly he cupped his hands together and ran out of the house. He had been able to "grab" the snake as it "emerged" magically through the skin and had run out in order to throw it into the swamp. After a few moments he returned. The same technique of massage was used to exorcise the second snake, and it also was thrown into the swamp. After a brief chat with his patient, the *namer-o* assured all concerned that the boy was completely recovered—and he was. The entire ritual had lasted about 30 minutes.

As in other societies (such as the Zulu), the curer also may serve as a sorcerer. Malevolent acts are performed in the hopes of altering the behavior of the enemy or occasionally the behavior of another person in the same village (usually a member of a different men's house group). For example, invisible arrows are sometimes shot in the direction of the victim to effect the desired change.

On assumption of the new (and, in virtually all cases, part-time) role, the individual can be expected to become an apprentice to an established curer. He or she is responsible for handling certain of the ritual paraphernalia and readying it for the *namer-o's* use. Soothsaying activities may also be performed by the apprentice. Learning thus takes place in three ways:

1. Some knowledge of herbal lore and ritual has usually been acquired prior to the calling

2. Instruction is provided through the apprenticeship

3. Additional dreams and visions involving the spirit *namer-o* can be expected

While the Asmat patient may, depending on the illness, ingest a medicinal substance prepared by the curer, it is important to note that the *namer-o* uses no hallucinogenic substances, nor are alcoholic beverages employed. In contrast to most other societies, only one prominent drug is found in Asmat—tobacco. It is smoked liberally by adults and older children alike and is occasionally smoked by the *namer-o* in preparation for a curing ritual. Tobacco is also used as a medicinal application. Festering, painful flesh wounds are treated with a liberal application of wet tobacco, which is left in place and bound with fiber and leaves. The pain of the wound seems to be deadened dramatically.

A headache is treated by tying a palm fiber firmly around the forehead. The efficacy of this practice is unclear. Similarly, a muscular ache in the lower leg is treated by tying such a fiber around the calf. The therapy for a severe fever, such as that caused by malaria, usually involves smearing the patient with clay. Physiologically this may act to gradually dissipate body heat. An alternate treatment (often followed by pneumonia) involves prolonged dousing with cold water or placement in a draft.

The patient. The role of the patient, or client, can be understood from a sociological perspective, as the above examples imply. A person's illness may or may not involve clearly delimited physiological symptoms, but it always involves impact on or disruption of the social-kinship network. Disruptions can often be rectified quickly; illness is not always "traumatic and dramatic." At times disruption of curer-client interaction patterns occurs as well; stress occasionally develops in the course of therapy or because a desired cure is not achieved. Yet among the Asmat, even in those instances where success is

attained, a curer-client dependency relationship, such as that outlined by Parsons (1951), is not present.

Especially in cases of severe illness or imminent death, close relatives stay with the sick person around the clock. Although occasional crying is not discouraged, if it becomes persistent, relatives try to persuade the patient to be quiet. Spirits thought to be involved are admonished to "go away and leave the living alone." Upon the patient's death, free emotional expression is encouraged among relatives and nonrelatives alike, although little formal attention is given the death of an infant, for it is not considered to have reached complete personhood. The most intense mourning surrounds the death of a Big Man, who in same cases may be a *namer-o*. His thatch house is permanently abandoned for fear of potentially malevolent supernatural acts; his as yet unsettled spirit may cause havoc in that vicinity. Other Big Men wail extensively, while at the same time casting themselves in the mud of the riverbank. Big Men also roll in the mud on the death of an adult of lesser status, but in that case this gesture of social support may last less than a minute. Close relatives express their grief in the same way, rolling in the mud until they are exhausted. Not only does the mud serve as a welcome way to release emotion, but it also is thought to enable relatives to mask their own body scent and so keep the spirit of the deceased at bay (see Fig. 5-12). Prior to the suppression of cannibalism in most of the Asmat region in the late 1950s, the skull of one's mother or father was worn on a string around the neck as another means to fend off the unpredictable spirit.

THE EFFICACY OF NON-WESTERN CURES

For some it would be easy to dismiss many of the non-Western cures and practices discussed in this and previous chapters too lightly as unscientific and ineffective. On the other hand, an adamant position of cultural relativity could be adopted. Radical adherents to this view would claim that traditional curers are remarkably successful, and that in fact, modern Western physicians should abandon certain of their biomedical techniques in favor of those practiced by shamans. While this text makes it clear that various types of Western and non-Western systems have much to offer, we have not yet directly addressed the crucial issue of the comparative efficacy of cures. Do traditional cures work? Is there a universal comparative criterion that can be employed?

These questions lead to what should become the next major thrust of medical anthropology inquiry in the decades ahead. Some have successfully addressed the smaller subset of questions dealing with the efficacy of herbal cures (for example, Ortiz de Montellano, 1975), but few have tackled the larger issue, which might encompass all forms of diagnostic and therapeutic activity within a society. One anthropologist who has confronted this problem is Young (1976). He stresses that curative activities can be considered successful—which is not to say that they work in all cases—if they meet the expectations of the patient and those close to the patient. Expectations imply predictability, and predictability implies the ability of a curer to effectively utilize acquired medical knowledge. If viewed from this perspective, traditional cures are frequently successful. Other research (like that on Taiwanese shamans and their clients [Kleinman and Sung, 1979]) supports this view.

Obviously one difficulty is that disease and illness take many forms. Acute self-limiting ailments usually run brief courses that result either in total recovery or death. Since, for most people, there is likely to have been some sort of medical intervention during the course of the ailment, it is difficult to determine its actual efficacy (Young, 1976:8). A principle of behavioral modification theory

would seem to be applicable for helping understand a non-Western society's evaluation of its own curing effectiveness: an activity reinforced intermittently is more powerful than one reinforced continuously (Burgess and Bushell, 1969:31-32). Success does not have to be absolute. Much additional, specific corroborative data is still needed in this area, however.

Waxler proceeds along these lines in her assessment of the efficacy of traditional cures of mental illness. Using a variant of social labeling theory, she suggests that "each society, through the responses of its members to the mentally ill person, succeeds in molding the patient to meet its own expectations about what a mentally ill person should be" (1977:233). The curative success rate is high in those instances where the act of treatment itself serves to create or strengthen ties of obligation. It is high where therapy includes socially reintegrative activities.

In cases of, for example, severe infectious diseases, such as smallpox or measles, Western biomedical techniques have enabled medical personnel to reduce mortality dramatically. The efficacy of such treatments in terms of survival is very high, especially when compared with treatments offered by traditional curers whose efforts focus on illness and social relationships rather than on disease. Efficacy therefore also must be assessed in terms of the biological survival of the population, which in turn relates to long-term adaptation.

In conclusion, possible universal comparative criteria should continue to be explored and tested along two non–mutually exclusive dimensions. As of now these are incompletely understood and integrated. The first is the sociopsychological, by which shamans and other non-Western curers have utilized techniques that demonstrate substantial efficacy. The second is the biomedical dimension, in which Western medicine has made unparalleled advances. Together, developments integrated along these dimensions will contribute to a fuller biocultural understanding of health. The new "theory of disease" suggested by Fabrega (1975) incorporates these dimensions, and if implemented would help provide medical practitioners cross-culturally with guidelines to more effective practice of preventive and curative biocultural medicine.

ALTERNATIVE CURES AND CHANGING BELIEF SYSTEMS

It is possible that exploration of universal criteria for the effectiveness of curing systems would have a long-term effect on the current foundations and organizations of Western medicine. This expectation, of course, is based on the assumption that belief systems can change. If this is true, the next important question is, what stimulates the change and in what areas are changes made? There has been a strong tradition in American anthropology to support the premise that changes in the technological sphere of a society precede changes in the ideological sphere (see, for example, White, 1959), but there also is a contrary view that changes in the ideological sphere are fundamental to changes of other sorts. Belief systems, thus, would have to change before technological

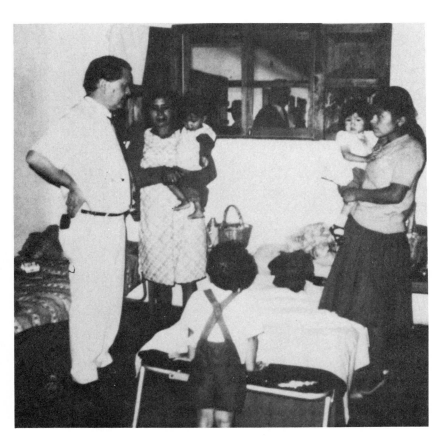

Fig. 6-7. Dr. Behrhorst and families in a typical hospital room. (Photo by J. E. Glittenberg.)

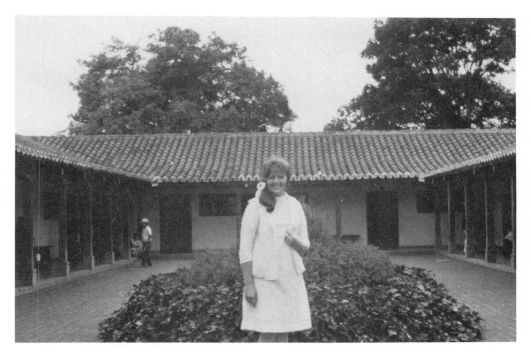

Fig. 6-8. Nurse Glittenberg in courtyard of Behrhorst Cakchiquel Hospital. (Photo by J. E. Glittenberg.)

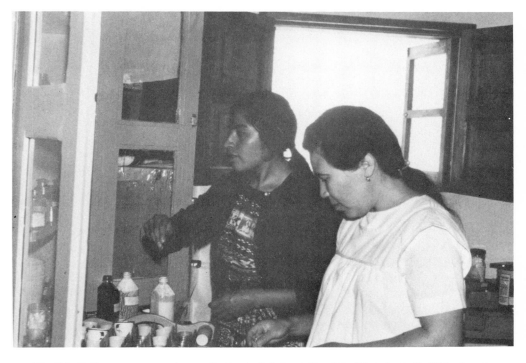

Fig. 6-9. Native nurses preparing medication in Behrhorst Hospital. (Photo by J. E. Glittenberg.)

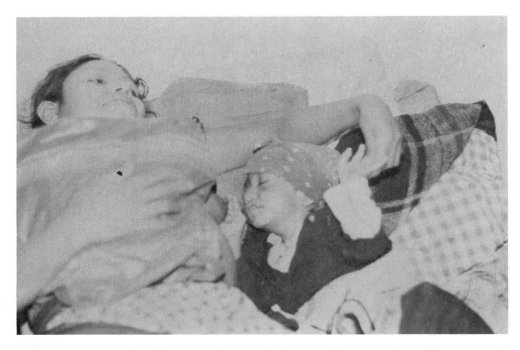

Fig. 6-10. Four-year-old child breast-feeding from his hospitalized mother in the Behrhorst Hospital. (Photo by J. E. Glittenberg.)

alterations are incorporated. We favor the first position.

Moore (1963:75), however, believes that changes can take place within certain elements of a culture quite independently of other changes within that culture. His theory is supported through a study done by Clyde Woods (1975) in highland Guatemala. Woods found that Mayan Indians showed relatively little "resistance" to the use of modern medicine while resisting other forms of modernization. In fact, he found modern medical treatments were accepted in spite of the fact that concepts of disease causation were based on other, quite different, beliefs. The primary stimulator of change, according to Woods, was the opportunity that individuals actually had to observe certain of the advantages of modern medicine. Acculturation does influence health beliefs and practices, and exposure to new ideas indeed brings

changes in perception by practice (Fig. 6-7 to 6-10).

A study by Vivian Garrison (1977) helps illustrate what may happen to an individual caught between two systems of treatment. It also illustrates the conceptual underpinnings of the respective treatments. Garrison bases her study on the premise that folk and modern medical systems are antithetical, although not mutually exclusive. When the patient is caught at the interface of the two systems, she concludes, the result is antitherapeutic. To reach this conclusion, a detailed case study of the treatment of a Puerto Rican woman in New York who had an *ataque de nervios* (nervous attack) was conducted. It was interpreted by the *espiritualista*, from whom she sought treatment, as "obsession" (possession) by three misguided spirits sent against her via the medium of witchcraft. The woman was also diagnosed by

Assumptions of the allopathic model	Assumptions of the holistic model
Treatment of symptoms.	Search for patterns, causes.
Specialized.	Integrated, concerned with the whole patient.
Emphasis on efficiency.	Emphasis on human values.
Professional should be emotionally neutral.	Professional's caring is a component of healing.
Pain and disease are wholly negative.	Pain and disease may be valuable signals of internal conflicts.
Primary intervention with drugs, surgery.	Minimal intervention with Appropriate Technology, complemented with full armamentarium of noninvasive techniques (psychotechnologies, diet, exercise).
Body seen as machine in good or bad repair.	Body seen as dynamic system, a complex energy field within fields (family, workplace, environment, culture, life history).
Disease or disability seen as entity.	Disease or disability seen as process.
Emphasis on eliminating symptoms, disease.	Emphasis on achieving maximum bodymind health.
Patient is dependent.	Patient is (or should be) autonomous.
Professional is authority.	Professional is therapeutic partner.
Body and mind are separate; psychosomatic illnesses seen as mental; may refer to psychiatrist.	Bodymind perspective; psychosomatic illness is the province of all health-care professionals.
Mind is secondary factor in organic illness.	Mind is primary or co-equal factor in all illness.
Placebo effect is evidence of power of suggestion.	Placebo effect is evidence of mind's role in disease and healing.
Primary reliance on quantitative information (charts, tests, dates).	Primary reliance on qualitative information, including patient reports and professional's intuition; quantitative data an adjunct.
"Prevention" seen as largely environmental: vitamins, rest, exercise, immunization, not smoking.	"Prevention" synonymous with wholeness: in work, relationships, goals, body-mind-spirit.

From Ferguson, M. *The Aquarian Conspiracy: Personal and Social Transformation in the 1980's,* Los Angeles: J. P. Tarcher, Inc., 1979.)

a psychiatric staff at a modern hospital as being a paranoid schizophrenic.

In comparing the two systems of belief and practices of curing, Garrison analyzes the two modes of treatment in depth. One treatment is reflected in hospitalization, the other in contacts with the *espiritualista.* There are similarities and differences between the two. In the belief system of the psychotherapist, which uses a psychodynamic theory of causation, the "self" is divided into three components: the "id," "ego," and "superego." Each of these components is "located" inside the individual. The *espiritualista* system also divides the ele-

ments influencing the "self" into three categories: "ignorant/molesting spirits," "wise and/or punishing spirits," and "one's own spirit." However, in the *espiritualista* world view, the causal elements are thought to be located outside the individual. The locus of causation is different. It is in the attempt to cope with two distinct belief systems that the patient encounters difficulties.

. . . the two types of healers (folk and professional) interpret the same feelings and behavior in similar ways . . . [they have] similar treatment techniques; but they talk about what they see and do within very different systems of conceptualizations of the self and the world (Garrison, 1977:423).

Thus Garrison systematically identifies the conceptual bases for the treatment regimens of two belief systems (see boxed material, p. 225).

This example serves to remind us again that Western medicine, although it is certainly the dominant curing system in the United States, is by no means the only system. Since there is great diversity among subcultures in this country, there is also great diversity among the types of healers on whom people depend for health care. Any attempt to modify the Western system in such a way that it can adopt the holistic approach to curing that prevails in many traditional systems must begin with an understanding of the evolution of Western medical thought.

WESTERN WAYS OF CURING: AN HISTORICAL SURVEY
The Classical and Hellenistic era

Western curing does not have its roots in a single narrow tradition, but rather in an intricate complex of trends, beliefs, and practices that date back over thousands of years. If a single broad, underlying, and unifying thread can be singled out, it might best be traced from Classical and Hellenistic Greece. What we now know as Western beliefs began in the Mediterranean countries and arrived in the United States nearly 2500 years later with the early European explorers, conquerors, and colonists. Along the way these beliefs became intermingled with information and beliefs from Egypt, the Middle East, Persia, Byzantium, and of course Europe. Western scientific medicine became a curious synthesis of knowledge from varied sources—from Pliny's *Historia Naturalis* of the first century A.D. to the Arabic writings of Abucalsis during the height of the Moorish empire. As it developed, Western medicine incorporated information on traditional "folk remedies" and herbal medicines as well as analytical information in other key subdis-

ciplines, such as anatomy, chemistry, and physiology (Fig. 6-11). In recent decades these subdisciplines have been complemented by such emergent fields as molecular biology, biostatistics, and medical economics. In all, the Western medical complex has proved itself one of the most influential macroinstitutions the world has yet witnessed.

If Western medicine's roots can be traced from the Classical and Hellenistic eras, then it must be kept clearly in mind that even this is a somewhat arbitrary choice of starting points. Folk medical practitioners and herbalists had undoubtedly developed their conceptions of health and disease fairly extensively in the Mediterranean area before this time; the classical Greeks by no means "started from scratch." In addition, trade routes had already been established among the Greeks and other societies of the Mediterranean basin from Egypt to Scythia, and along these routes traveled information as well as trade items. During the Classical and Hellenistic eras, the Greek population was expanding. Accompanying this demographic shift was colonialist expansionism, which not only brought additional territory and resources under Greek jurisdiction but also provided further channels for the dissemination and receipt of information, much of which was medically related.

Ecological concerns, basic to this text's orientation, have a Greek origin. Hughes (1975) notes that during the Hellenistic period humanpower and resources were mobilized to drain swamps and lakes for conversion into farm land. Mediterranean forests were once extensive and relatively diverse, including evergreen oaks and certain drought-resistant pines, as well as cypress, cedar, and other species (1975:15). Yet even then deforestation was a severe problem, to the point that certain groves were set aside as sacred preserves. Theophrastus, a student of Aristotle, used what would now be termed an ecological approach in that he gathered information on local temperature changes caused by the draining of marshes, alteration of river courses, and deforestation (1975: 66).

Before Aristotle's time, one innovative individual stands out—Hippocrates. Presumably some of the medical insights attributed to him were the work of others, and presumably activities and travels he is said to have engaged in are more myth than reality. Nevertheless, Hippocrates studied and worked in a society that was medically and to some extent ecologically attuned, and one

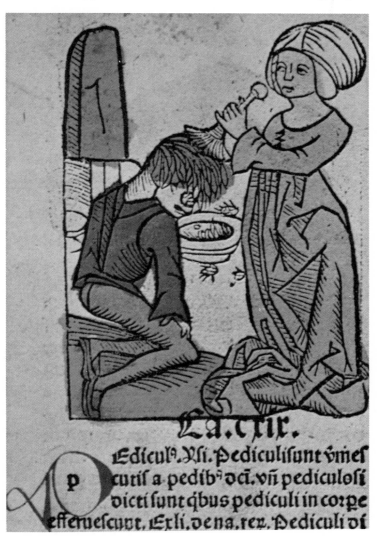

Fig. 6-11. Certain practices can contribute to health whether or not scientific principles are understood. This woodcut, from the 1491 edition of von Caub's *Hortis Sanitatis*, illustrates delousing practices of the Middle Ages. (From *Hortis Sanitatis*. Used by permission of the Trustees of the British Museum of Natural History).

that was clearly involved in significant alteration of resources and environment. Ancient biographies state that Hippocrates was born on the Island of Cos in 460 B.C.; he studied under Herodicus, Gorgias, Democritus, and others, and served (according to Plato) as "a professional trainer of medical students" (Clendening, 1942:13; Kelly, 1964). Hippocrates, the "father of medicine," contributed greatly to the sociocultural evolution of Western medicine and to the understanding of the ecological ramifications of disease.

The works of Hippocrates—or, more probably, the works of the school to which he belonged—are varied. Books in the corpus include "The Sacred Disease," a refutation of the idea that disease was sent by God; "On Airs, Waters and Places"; "Epidemics"; "Aphorisms"; and others. In "Aphorisms" can be seen a highly developed concern for the interplay of philosophical, sociocultural, ecological, and disease-related factors.

Life is short, and the Art long; the occasion fleeting; experience fallacious, and judgement difficult. The physician must not only be prepared to do what is right himself, but also to make the patient, the attendants, and externals co-operate. The exacerbations and remissions will be indicated by the diseases, the seasons of the year, the reciprocation of the periods, whether they occur every day, every alternate day, or after a longer period, and by the supervening symptoms. . . . The summer quartans [intermittent fevers] are, for the most part, of short duration; but the autumnal are protracted, especially those occurring near the approach of winter (quoted in Clendening, 1942:15-16).

Other of the aphorisms indicate concern for the interplay of diet and disease, for physiological cause-effect relationships, and for differential disease susceptibility among different age cohorts. The Hippocratic scholars attempted to minimize beliefs in magical disease causation and to discover more rational causes. For the Greeks, nature was ordered, not from without, but rationally from within. Nature was seen to have unity and harmony in all its parts, a belief common to many cultures throughout the world. Aristotle's brief comment makes this rational ordering clear: "Nature does nothing in vain" (quoted in Hughes, 1975:59). Not all Greek scholars were in agreement; some, such as Democritus, saw the world purely as a physical entity without purpose or design. However, Hippocrates believed in environmental determinism; that is, that the natural environment molds the people who live within it. While narrow in explanatory scope, this deterministic perspective has served as a basis for certain ecological perspectives of the nineteenth and twentieth centuries.

Hippocrates' ideas about determinants of health seem contemporary. He viewed climate and physical environment as important determinants; for example, an eastward-facing city generally was best for the health of its inhabitants, he thought, as were homes whose rooms opened onto an inner court (Hughes, 1975:82). Hippocrates went on to point out the importance of environment in enabling the physician to better assess the cause, diagnosis, and treatment of illness. In the treatise "On Airs, Waters and Places," Hippocrates shows Greek concern for water supply and quality:

. . . for as [waters] differ from one another in taste and weight, so also do they differ much in their qualities . . . whether they be marshy and soft, or hard, and running from elevated and rocky situations, and then if saltish and unfit for cooking . . .

In another example, he notes that, in cities exposed to cold winds during summer nights, water tends to be "hard and cold"; consequently, pleurisy and acute diseases are prevalent. Such environmental analyses tie in with the broader concern Greek physicians had for detailed diagnosis and prognosis.

To Hippocrates and his associates, medicine was an art, at which some were adept and others were not. This art arose through necessity in attempts to alleviate suffering from disease, pain, and improper diet. Yet this art could also involve persuasion and deception. An example of deception appeared at Asklepieion (a healing site at Pergamon, Turkey) where patients ran through a human-made tunnel of stone, as voices echoed in the tunnel and assured them of a cure. These voices were in fact those of Greek physicians; it was a clever deception (Fig. 6-12).

Greeks of the Classical and Hellenistic periods believed that medicine was a set of phenomena to be discovered by physicians of that period. These discoveries were intended to enable human beings to live in harmony with nature. Physicians were to record these discoveries as their role in contributing to the natural order of things. These writings were kept in the museum library at Alexandria, and proved to be rich resources.

One topic frequently pondered by the Greeks is known as the humoural doctrine. Clendening (1942:39-40) believed the Sicilian philosopher Empedocles may have been the first to suggest that four humours exist and that shortly thereafter Hippocrates applied the idea to medicine. As seen in the Hippocratic essay "On the Constitution of Man," the four elementary qualities—cold, dry, moist, hot—correspond to the four universal elements—earth, air, water, and fire. A balance of humours—blood, phlegm, yellow bile (or choler), black bile—results in good health. Imbalance results when one

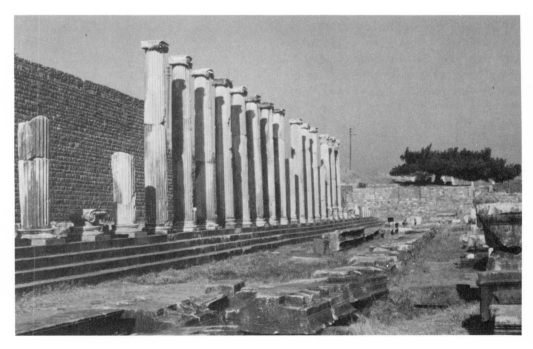

Fig. 6-12. Pergamum, the nominal homeland of Galen, was the center of the cult of Aesculapius, god of medicine. The Asklepieion, part of which is pictured here, was built in his honor. (Photo by L. G. Moore.)

humour has become predominant (see Chapter 5). Balance is restored by applying its opposite, although the doctrine holds that each individual tends to show a propensity toward one humour, resulting in a constitution that is either sanguine, phlegmatic, choleric, or melancholy. The belief system is crucial in understanding some aspects of Western curing. The doctrine maintains that the imbalance in nature is reflected in the imbalance within the system of the human body. For example, blood was considered as hot and moist, phlegm was cold and moist, yellow bile as hot and dry, and black bile as cold and dry. Treatments were aimed at reestablishing a balance.

Early centuries of the Christian era

The museum library at Alexandria assumed leadership in promoting scholarship from the third century B.C. through the early centuries of the Christian era. Galen studied there, and other scholars continued to produce manuscripts. In a tradition that was to continue through the Middle Ages and to some extent into the Renaissance and Enlightment periods, much emphasis was placed on the systematic refinement, recording, and translation of earlier knowledge, especially that of the Greeks. For example, Dioscorides, a Greek who served in the Roman armies as a surgeon during the first century A.D., wrote a detailed work on herbal medicine. In the *Herbal*, or *Materia Medica*, not only did Dioscorides systematically record information compiled by others, but he also collected plant specimens as he traveled with the armies, described them in detail, and listed all the diseases that each would cure.

The tradition of scholarly manuscript translation that emerged served Dioscorides' *Herbal* well. A Byzantine version added illustrations of plants in 512 A.D., and later, in 1655 A.D., an English version was published (see Gunther, 1934). Although the *Herbal* does not contain the ecological insights of the Hippocratic school, it does demonstrate a thorough understanding of the medicinal properties of hundreds of plant species and of their effects on people; for example (from the 1655 version of John Goodyer):

Sesamum [sesame] is hurtful for the stomach, and causes a stinking breath of ye mouth, if after it be eaten it abide between the teeth. Being applyed it doth discusse the thicknesses in the nerues; and the fractures, and inflammations in the eares, and Ambusta, and the griefs of ye Colon and ye biting of the Cerastes, it doth heale (see Gunther, 1934:132).

Roman contributions. Roman contributions, which emerged from a continuum of thought traceable to the Greeks and to Alexandria, were made in a sociopolitical context by which Rome was considered the center of the world, and Romans themselves believed they were superior (Hughes, 1975: 96). Pliny the Elder, writing in the first century A.D., was an astute naturalist who also attempted certain ecological assessments. Of particular importance to the development of Western medicine is his *Historia Naturalis*. Much like the *Herbal* of Dioscorides, this work focuses in detail on the medicinal-pharmaceutical properties of plants. Mint, for example, is claimed to aid in the cure of thirty ailments. Again through the tedious process of recording and translation, much of the *Historia Naturalis* was preserved, and it appeared in the West in the eleventh century, known as *Macer Floridus de Viribus Herbarum*. It contains a list of nearly 100 plants and herbs along with their medicinal properties (Flood, 1977).

One of the most prolific medical researchers and writers in the history of Western curing was Galen. In combining much of the medical knowledge of his predecessors with his own findings, Galen wrote an encyclopedic work equivalent to nearly 10,000 pages of Greek text (Siegel, 1968:1). Galen lived during the second century A.D. Most of his books were written from his base in Rome. There, he attempted to analyze the functions of the human body, developing definitions, some of which are still with us today in modified form. Physiology he defined as the study of "the predominant and regulating forces of the organism." Anatomy was a part of his definition of physiology, so his anatomical treatises include observations on organ functioning. His own extensive dissections and physiological experiments were conducted on numerous animals, such as monkeys, goats, sheep, and even an elephant. Galen defined pathology as the "general and individual affections and diseases, causes, symptoms and all their variations . . . and the study of the affected parts of the body" (Siegel, 1968:2). He was concerned with psychology, psychiatry, neurology, and hygiene as we know them today (Green, 1951).

Above all, Galen was a disciple of the Hippocratic school. He has been described as a humoural pathologist, but one who did not hesitate to apply alternate treatments if they would benefit his patients (Sigerist, 1951: viii). As a researcher, Galen's observations were thorough and for the most part accurate if judged by today's Western standards. His work on circulation was very detailed, serving as an impetus for William Harvey's crucial research in the seventeenth century. Some of Galen's interpretations concerning blood flow have been shown to be incorrect, but even these have proved to be of heuristic significance (Siegel, 1968:78-83).

Judeo-Christian influences. Contemporaneous with Galenic medical philosophy and likewise contributing to the ultimate development of certain aspects of modern Western

curing was early Christian ideology. This tradition is traced from classical Jewish sources, such as the Bible and the Talmud. Rosner (1977) stresses that a wealth of historical data as well as knowledge of religious mystical health beliefs and socio physiological viewpoints are to be found in these writings. For example, the book of Genesis states that Sarah, the wife of Abraham, at the age of 90 gave birth to Isaac. Many issues are raised of how birth procedures were conducted in early Hebraic societies, what taboos surrounded them, and how a 90 year old woman could bear a child. Physiologically, the latter issue is resolved if it is accepted that this is a legend, without basis in fact. Culturally, passages of this sort yield a great deal of information, shedding light on a belief that early human beings were superhuman in certain of their physical abilities. Apart from healings listed as "miracles," one of the most extraordinary of all such events would have to be the life of Methuselah, a man who was said to have lived 969 years.

Judeo-Christian ideology emerged with strong ethical and moral implications. The Hebrew term *rofe* can best be translated "healer," not physician (Rosner, 1977:151), and can best be placed in a religious rather than scientific context. Sickness increasingly came to be seen in this "moral milieu." As Christian influence strengthened during the first centuries A.D., so did the philosophy of purification. Those who were sick could be purified and made whole. Out of sickness also could come an eternal benefit, with the purification of the soul and the promise of eternal life (Wain, 1970:39). Thus the role of the sick took on an expanded status that not only affected individuals but also the social network of which they were a part. Those healers who ministered to the sick during their illnesses also benefitted, for they were viewed as substitutes for, or representatives of Christ, the "great physician." As the Christian medical-religious system assumed more clear-cut form and expanded in power, the healers assumed roles of "little gods" (substituting for the great physician), while the nurses became known as "angels of mercy." The intrusion of Galenic philosophy also crystalized. Health and disease came to be seen as analogous to lightness and darkness, with aging representing an intermediate phase—a flickering of life's flame. The loss of moisture, analogous to humoural wetness, was believed to lead to death (see Chapter 5).

Certain of the Jewish and Christian healers did have a fairly simplistic understanding of internal functions of some of the organs, such as the gallbladder; this knowledge is traceable to classical Jewish sources. Such classical works related organ functioning to human emotions—the gallbladder was associated with jealousy, for example. In the case of an animal, the Talmud states that diseased or injured internal organs can render it unfit for human consumption (Rosner, 1977:93). Dietary restrictions related to the eating of animal flesh are further refined in the Jewish Code, written during the Middle Ages by Moses Maimonides.

Some of the scholars who attempted to study mechanisms of the body and disease processes in more detail were persecuted in various ways. During the time of Galen, 200 Christian students were excommunicated because of their research into "pagan medicine." Church leaders of that time believed that any medical intrusion into the body was based on a pagan belief, because Christ had healed without medicine or surgery. (Even today vestiges of this viewpoint are perpetuated in such groups as the Christian Science Church). However, through time, leaders of the Christian church gradually modified their views, coming to believe that scholars should attempt to learn as much as they could about pagan medicine in order to rid it of any of the devil's influence.

Byzantines, Arabs, and Europeans through the Middle Ages

Constantinople, the center of Byzantium, had served as an outpost in the eastern Roman Empire. With the fall of Rome in 476 A.D., it assumed an even more important role. For the next 1000 years, the outgrowths of Greek and Roman scholarship were focused here. Some of the works of Jewish and Christian scholars also were given serious consideration. However, through the Middle Ages Galenic medical practice and philosophy predominated (Rosner, 1977:20). Certain Jewish scholars even contributed to this emphasis with their textual translations. And, historians translated Hellenic works into Syriac, the predominant language of Christian Byzantines. In Constantinople the doctrine of *humanitas* was kept alive. Byzantine medicine was based on compilation rather than investigation, thus preserving the lore of the ancient Greeks. Christian influence was seen in the socioreligious role a sick person was thought to occupy (Marti-Ibañez, 1967:11-12). The sick were regarded as potential saints. Prayer was adopted as the best "medicine." The Church was regarded as the best "hospital." Christianity's more ardent believers were everyday laborers and peasants; many of the well-to-do were engaged in other belief systems and cult activities.

Syntheses of medical knowledge and philosophy form an integral part of the history of Western curing. Europeans did not contribute substantially to the expansion of knowledge during the Dark Ages, but others, such as the Arabs, did. The conquest of the Iberian peninsula by Moors in 711 A.D. initiated an intense blending of Arabic and European beliefs, not the least of which was in the area of medicine. The surgical treatise of the Spanish-Moorish physician Abucalsis, for example, became a leading text in European medicine during the late Middle Ages. By way of contrast, in 948 A.D. a Byzantine emperor sent a set of an illustrated *Materia Medica* of Dioscorides (in the original Greek) to the caliph of Cordoba. The caliph's Moslem physicians and herbalists, in concert with a Jewish court physician and others, proceeded to translate all the plant and drug names into Arabic (Anonymous, 1969:139). Galen's writings also were translated and utilized by Arabic scholars.

The ecological impetus of Hippocrates, Theophrastus, and other early scholars went through a dormant state in Europe during the Dark Ages. (By the twelfth century, however, a germ theory of disease was being recognized.) European monks did see to the task of manuscript preservation, recording, and translation; for example, St. Benedict made manuscript copying a mandatory assignment for the Benedictine order he founded in the sixth century. A certain ecological emphasis, again with the thrust of environmental determinism, is seen in the writings of medieval Arabic scholars. Ibn Khaldun presented a theory of the origin, nature, and diversity of human civilization that is couched in some environmental statements. His work is of interest to students of the history of anthropology in general because it indicates recognition of the importance of studying different ways of life and different patterns of behavior.

Toward a Renaissance

A glimmer of the Renaissance, still then several centuries in the future, is seen retrospectively in a key development of the ninth century. At Salerno, Italy, the first secular medical center in Christian Europe was established. The students' first texts focused on Greek and Latin sources. Over the course of the following centuries Salerno attracted some of the Western world's most famous medical teachers; for example, Benvenuto Grafeo, an oculist, and Rolando Capelluti, a surgeon. Eventually the school moved beyond mere devotion to past medical works into new areas of physiological research. However, one of its most well-known products remains a relatively simplistic Latin poem, "Regimen Sanitatis Salernitanum," wherein rules for hygiene and medical treatment are set forth (Clendening, 1942:76-79). In 1607, well over a century after it was first printed, it was translated into popular English prose by Sir John Harington. The new title became "The Englishmans Doctor, or Physicall Observations for the Perfect Preserving of the Body of Man in Continuall Health" (see Anonymous, 1969:142).

The period between 1100 and 1600 A.D., much like the preceding eras, had exhibited a complex relationship among science, philosophy, and theology, making any attempt at analytical separation nearly impossible even by twentieth-century standards (Wallace, 1978:85). But by the 1600s the foundations of modern Western medicine had solidified. William Harvey's analysis of circulation and heart function, published during the seventeenth century, helped usher in the new era of physiology and medicine. In the rigid hierarchy of the seventeenth century, surgeons and apothecaries were still considered somewhat inferior to physicians because they used their hands, as did those engaged in manual occupations. Surgery was considered an "art," while medicine per se was deemed a "science" and, therefore, superior (Brockliss, 1978:224). Nor is this the only area where boundaries were unclear; for example, faith healing was popular in France as well as in England. King Charles II supposedly touched and cured 22,982 people in the 4 years after his restoration in 1660 (Laver, 1978:35). The emergence of science was not accompanied directly by a decline in the importance of witchcraft and demonology. Although during the early part of the Middle Ages church records indicate a general denial of witchcraft, it had a renewed sociocultural impact again in the sixteenth and seventeenth centuries (Kirsch, 1978).

COMPETING AND COMPLEMENTING TREATMENTS IN WESTERN CURING

From the diverse historical roots of the Classical and Hellenistic eras through the time of the Byzantine Empire, Western curing became an eclectic science. Balance in bodily functions, such as the humours (blood, phlegm, yellow bile, and black bile), and balance in nature were characterized by harmony; and rational order was the basis for empirical observation and thinking, cornerstones of scientific inquiry. The Judeo-Christian ideology also merged or, at times, conflicted with the pursuit of medical knowledge. Illness had come to be viewed not in an empirical context but rather in a moral light. Mind (or soul) and body became dichotomous units, the soul being purifiable and eternal while the body was temporal. Thus, opposing views were a chief characteristic in the development of the science of medicine. These basic assumptions are still the foundation for different schools of thought in contemporary curing.

Two major assumptions of modern scientific medicine

Modern scientific medicine has been accused of being monopolistic. This monopoly is not new; as far back as 1224 A.D. it was decreed that no one should practice medicine without having passed an examination before the masters of the medical school at Salerno (Osborne, 1977:2). Such trends of exclusivity have continued to the present. Yet this same monopolistic medicine, supposedly characterized in part by an inability

to tolerate alternative health care systems, is in fact an outgrowth of the contributions of multiple (and at times disparate) belief systems and medical studies over the centuries, as we have just described.

The first major assumption of modern scientific medicine is the germ theory of disease. Today it is most clearly represented by the modern medical belief in the process of infection. Current conceptual understanding can be traced to the bacteriological studies of Louis Pasteur, who in the mid to late nineteenth century demonstrated (to cite his own words) "the presence and multiplication of organic beings," that is, bacteria (Clendening, 1942:388). He attributed the process of fermentation to bacterial activity, thus helping to dispel long held notions of spontaneous generation. Pasteur's research also helped dispel the idea that reproduction in organisms had to be solely sexual. However, it would not have been possible for Pasteur to register the success he did without an earlier recognition of the general concept of contagion, which can be traced to authorities such as Galen. Galen had recognized the problem of contagion with tuberculosis, yet apparently not with "plagues and pestilences" (Wain, 1970:20). As mentioned earlier, the germ theory gained some ascendance in Western medicine by the twelfth century. The French surgeon Guy de Chauliac wrote of the contagious aspects of the plague as it scourged France in 1348 A.D. Yet, like those before him and for some centuries after him, he did not understand the mechanisms involved. In the writings of both de Chauliac and Fracastorius (b. 1478, d. 1553) can be seen a belief that the mere sight of an infected person could cause the disease to spread instantaneously to the onlooker (Wain, 1970:59; Clendening, 1942:107ff). Had subsequent Western curing been exclusive, the general social notion of contagion might have been dismissed too lightly. The contagion concept, despite underlying flaws, proved to be of great heuristic importance.

The second major assumption of scientific medicine is that of preventive medicine, which has ancient roots and did not emerge as a true Western scientific assumption until after Pasteur's discoveries. Early concern with hygiene and public sanitation was found in Rome during the time of Christ. Drains and sewers were continually being extended under the city. Sewage was thus diverted into the River Tiber (Wain, 1970:23). Quarantines have also served for centuries as preventive health measures, although mechanisms of infectious disease transmission were not entirely understood. The plague that invaded fourteenth-century Europe was countered, albeit to little avail, through the use of quarantine (Wain, 1970:61-62). Again, the point is that modern Western curing owes much to certain of the innovations that accompanied the advent of preventive medicine.

Diversity among treatment systems

It is of little wonder that in contemporary Western treatment systems, diversity exists. The three major systems of treatment—allopathy, homeopathy and naturopathy—have in common the belief that a disease may be caused by germs but that illnesses also can be prevented. Each of these major systems has other specific basic assumptions. The other systems ("minor" as defined by the number of known clients as well as the incorporation of their beliefs into the dominant medical social institution) have a basic assumption that a life force or energy within the human body needs release, redirection, or balance. The minor systems include osteopathy, chiropractic, acupuncture, and autosuggestion (such as hypnosis and biofeedback).

Allopathic medicine. The most prominent treatment modality within the Western medical complex is allopathy, which grew out of the doctrine of contraries that began to flourish in Asia Minor in the first century B.C. The principle on which it is founded is simple: when a substance deviates from the normal, a counteracting procedure should be applied. Utilizing an outgrowth of this principle in the case of illness, healers have sought to rid the body of its poisonous or disturbing substances by various methods, such as bleedings, cuppings, and enemas. Purgings of this sort can in turn be traced to outgrowths of humoural doctrines, specifically in the attempt to reestablish balance among bodily humours through evacuation of corrupt substances (see, for example, Clendening, 1942: 285-287).

The principle seemingly had little underlying validity at first because disease causality in this belief system fell into the general category of witchcraft, cosmic forces, and miasmas (vapors arising from decaying substances). However, with the discoveries of Pasteur, allopathy found a scientific explanation for the doctrine of contraries. With the discovery of "germs" and their relationship to disease carried by outside agents, drugs could be found to counteract the germs and thus eliminate the disease as well. Since that time, Western medicine has largely been identified with allopathic medicine, so much so that analysis of its other multiple roots has been somewhat neglected.

Along with recognition of the germ theory of disease causality came a new revolution in chemistry. New pharmacological discoveries based on hitherto unknown chemical compounds resulted in the eventual proliferation of life-saving drugs, such as the sulphur drugs and antibiotics. However, as useful as these allopathic drugs have been against infectious diseases, they are virtually ineffective in treating degenerative diseases. Extensive reliance on drug therapies has also spawned a new problem, that of drug resistance. At first it was not known why certain strains of microorganisms became resistant to previously successful regimens of treatment. However, it was discovered that bacteria, like other living organisms, are also governed by principles of evolution and adaptation; mutations present new advantages within an ecological niche. The mutational strains may be drug-resistant and more powerful than their parent generations.

Other problems have resulted from the use of certain drugs in treatment. Unexpected drug reactions, sometimes representing highly individual allergic responses, have left the use of some "wonder drugs" quite questionable. One such example is that of cortisone, a hormone that can be used for the treatment of various types of arthritis. This hormone therapy encourages the proliferation of microorganisms such as streptococci and staphylococci in the body. Other side effects that have been observed are obesity, "moon face," facial hair in women and children, and a dangerous softening of the bones. Clearly, the cure at times is a greater risk than the disease.

In spite of drug-related problems, the association between allopathy and modern drug therapies is a powerful relationship. A long list of diseases with specific allopathic treatments constitute the major healing approach to illnesses in modern Western societies. The economic interdependency between the pharmaceutical companies and the medical society in the United States is a recognized phenomenon.

Homeopathy. Homeopathy is a system of contemporary medicine that relies on philosophical premises similar to those of allopathy. Homeopathy has several roots, two of which are found in early Arab records and Hippocratic writings. Hippocrates wrote, "Illness arises by similar things, and by similar things can the sick be made well." It basically refers to a belief that "likes cure likes."

The term "homeopathy" derives from the Greek words *homeos* ("similar") and *pathos* ("suffering"). For example, if a sick person had a fever, the cure as generally applied would involve a treatment that would likewise invoke a fever. In certain instances, the belief also included use of a medicine that resembled in form the locus of illness (for example, if one had an earache, the medicine produced from a flower shaped like an ear would be the treatment of choice).

A more systematic approach was promoted by Samuel Hahnemann, an orthodox German physician of the early nineteenth century. Hahnemann sought treatments that would enhance the body's natural healing activity. Rather than giving massive doses of drugs, Hahnemann proposed giving small dosages to stimulate biochemical and biological activity within the body and to let the "life force" within the patient do the rest. The homeopathic physician sees signs and symptoms of disease as reactions of the body in its attempts to restore homeostasis. Such signs are viewed as products of a disturbance in function. Thus, the homeopath conceptualizes his practice as involving the treatment of sick individuals rather than the treatment of disease. In this respect it affirms the underlying concept of holistic health (discussed previously). Illness is seen as a deviation from "normal functions"; thus, the body must be stimulated so that it can play the major role in its own cure.

Hahnemann's research was significant from another perspective as well (Menolascino, 1978). Much like some of his forebears in medicine, he prepared a type of *materia medica*, containing the results of extensive series of tests and trials. His administration of small doses of plant, mineral, and animal substances was accompanied by precise self-report records of physical and psychological changes in a large number of human subjects. Hahnemann's systematic observations led him to the conclusion that a diluted curative substance was more effective than a nondiluted one, because of the smaller dose's ability to stimulate (but not overwhelm) the body's own curative forces. He also concluded that only one drug should be used at a time, thus avoiding "interference" (Coulter, 1973:14).

Contemporary homeopaths rely on many *materia medica* and prescription manuals. For instance, William Boericke (a translator of some of Hahnemann's works) wrote the popular *Pocket Manual of Homeopathic Materia Medica* in the early twentieth century, and it is still in use today. Using this text in conjunction with a manual such as Clarke's *The Prescriber* (1972), homeopaths believed that effective cures can be enacted. The symptoms that a patient exhibits are keys and through use of a manual can be related to symptoms produced in the patient by the drug of choice. Following Hahnemann, these are categorized according to region of the body. Clarke (1972:18) refers to homeopathic categories as more than mere clinical repertories—they are repertories of localities. Furthermore, the nature of pain and the manner in which it is aggravated (its "condition") must be carefully assessed. To state that a patient is suffering from a particular disease (and thus to categorize and treat simply by disease name, such as "arthritis") is insufficient for the homeopath. The total person and activity patterns must be assessed.

The challenge such practitioners present today can be summarized by the remarks of Dana Ullman, a Berkeley homeopathic teacher: "Homeopathy is about to explode into the public awareness" (quoted in Fager, 1977). The interest in homeopathy today must be viewed as a U.S. resurgence. In the nineteenth century, homeopathic medicine flourished in this country as well as through much of Europe. It formed one

basis for Mary Baker Eddy's work, which led to the development of the Christian Science Church. Don Gerrard, a medical historian, claims that prior to 1910 as many as one out of five American physicians was a homeopathic practitioner (quoted in Fager, 1977). The Flexnor Report of 1910,* which attempted to identify medical schools that graduated poorly trained, often incompetent practitioners, was aimed at the suppression of quackery, which included homeopathy in the minds of many (Kaufman, 1971). Hahnemann's practice of administering very small dosages was said to offer nothing more than a placebo effect.

Researchers such as C. E. Wheeler and Rudolph Arndt, biologists, have provided an explanation of the workings of homeopathy. The human body's cells react differently to given thermal, chemical, or electrical stimuli and also react according to dosage. These authors point out that small doses impede and very large doses destroy cellular activity. Variations of this explanatory theory are interwoven throughout the modern Western medical system, as exemplified by the formulation of the theory of the immunological response of the cells. The practice of immunizing human beings against a variety of infectious diseases using small doses of either live, attenuated, or dead bacteria, or the antigens from such, is basic to building up the human body to resist such illness on a temporary or long-term basis.

Naturopathy and herbalism. There is a growing notion in the United States—known as naturopathy—that the body is nourished only by the natural ingredients it needs and that if these substances are used routinely, disease can be avoided; if disease should occur, the body is capable of throwing off its

---

*Flexner, A. *Medical Education in the United States and Canada.* New York: Carnegie Foundation for Advancement of Teaching, 1910.

effects without the use of drugs or operations. To naturopaths, hospitals ("places of the sick") should be replaced by a type of clinic that exposes people to regimens of unadulterated foods. For the most part, these foods are to be eaten raw or in unrefined states. Health regimes that include exercise, "natural life," fresh air, and meditation to free oneself from worry are all part of this holistic regimen.

Roots of this growing movement may be traced historically in the United States to a social distrust and dissatisfaction with orthodox medicine, especially with such treatments as bloodletting and certain drugs made popular by Benjamin Rush. A New Hampshire farmer named Samuel Thomson (b.1769, d.1843) became interested in medicinal plants and applied his knowledge to the treatment of his family. His son, John, said:

Shall we give medicine that will assist nature in throwing off the disease? Or shall we administer such medicine as she must be compelled to throw off with the disease, and that with a double exertion if she should prove strong enough? The metals and minerals are in the earth and being extracted from the depths of the earth have a tendency to carry all down into the earth . . . the grave. The tendency of all vegetables is to spring up . . . to invigorate . . . uphold mankind from the grave (Coulter, 1973:92.)

The Thomsonians eventually founded a medical society but later became part of a larger anti–orthodox medicine movement, the Eclectic Medical Institute. What united the 133 graduates in 1852 and about 10,000 practitioners in 1880 was an admiration for vegetable remedies and a hatred of orthodox medicine (Coulter, 1973:93). The beliefs of the Thomson followers and the Eclectics and of today's popular health-food movement is striking. The eventual demise of the Eclectics as a recognized group can be traced to the activities of a private body, the American Medical Association (Coulter, 1973:218).

However, the naturopathic movement and its beliefs still exist in the United States in various forms; for example, in the United States, many communes practice naturopathy. Some well-known, expensive health spas also espouse the philosophy. The natural-food movement is a form of this belief system and supports the popular notion of eating grains, legumes (such as bean and alfalfa sprouts), and natural sweeteners (such as honey). Interestingly, this impetus began in the cereal industry with such famous names as Kellogg and Post early in the twentieth century. Both these companies were founded in Battlecreek, Michigan by advertisers and promoters who motivated the population to relate how they felt to what they ate (Deutsch, 1971). Recently people in the United States also have been influenced by the investigative reports of such people as Choate who in 1970 exposed the nonnutritive value of most American breakfast cereals. Choate coined the phrase "empty calories" in describing the highly processed foods that cost more and more and provide less and less nutritional value in the American diet. Others reinforced the belief that natural foods were more beneficial, as exposure to adulterated foods became something of a national scandal with such writings as Rachel Carson's *Silent Spring*.

The simple network of associating diet with health is not universal, although some forms are found in other parts of the world. However, the health-food movement in the United States has taken on the semblance of a cult in which an increasingly complex network of patrons, practitioners, publications, and political lobbyists operate in conflict with the medical system. Within the movement, a continuum exists, from those who adhere to good nutrition to those who espouse a total life-style of health foods, supplements, and meditation. Not only are local health products sold in specialty stores, but a whole industry geared to the production of nationally marketed natural vitamins, natural cosmetics, and natural foods has sprung up. In addition, companies such as Water-Pik were quick to capitalize on the health-promotion fad by marketing, for example, a nicotine-filtering device that is intended to wean people off cigarettes. The health food stores were the first to introduce such specialized equipment as food grinders and sprout growers.

The health food stores found in metropolitan areas in many ways resemble naturopathic health centers. Here one may find libraries of literature with descriptions of a variety of health concerns that can be resolved through naturopathic practices. Some of the literature found in one suburban health store included titles in the following areas: proper eating, health products, and the management of problems (the latter category including hemorrhoids, kidney stones, menopause, high blood pressure, anxiety, insomnia, low blood sugar, impotency, arthritis, anemia, diabetes, colitis, and cancer). Most of the products recommended in the literature can be bought in the store, but others must be obtained from an informal supply network (Glittenberg, 1977). Thus the health-food movement is expressed in our society as a category of health-seeking behavior that is aimed at promoting holistic health as well as solving health problems.

The movement has been advanced through the publication of a popular book, *Folk Medicine*, by D. C. Jarvis (1958). The book, written by a distinguished Vermont physician, has sold more than 3 million copies. It was found on the best-seller, non-fiction "top ten list" for over a year. Its popularity bespoke the felt need of many Americans to "get back to nature." Jarvis describes the "natural secrets" of honey, apple cider vinegar, and other health foods. He believes that American pioneers, partially relying on their observations of animal behavior, evolved a system of folk healing. Animals,

for example, first seek absolute relaxation; and by close observation one can then learn how they obtain natural herbs to correct the deficiency present. Jarvis states, "Folk medicine reaches very far back in time . . . Primitive man and the animals depended on preventive use of [nature's] stock of plants and herbs to avoid disease and to maintain health and vigor" (1958:9). Jarvis believes ". . . the doctor of the future will be a teacher as well as a physician. His real job will be to teach people how to be healthy. Doctors will be even busier than they are now because it is a lot harder to keep people well than it is just to get them over a sickness" (Jarvis, 1958:ii). Among other Western publications that have served to advance this viewpoint are those of Edward Bach (as in *The Twelve Healers and Other Remedies* [1933]). By using appropriate wild flowers and herbs, Bach laid out "a simple and natural method of healing through the personality."

Herbalism can be viewed as a specialty in the belief system of naturopathy, but it also includes some features of allopathy. Many of its aspects are Eastern in origin; herbal treatment appeared in China as a system of healing around 3000 B.C. Papyrus writings dating from 1550 B.C. list some 700 different herbs that were used throughout Egypt. When Pliny wrote his natural history, he believed that herbalism was so standardized that there was to be found an herb remedy specific for every disorder (Inglis, 1964:67).

During the Middle Ages herbalism lost some of its acceptance as a gradual transition toward what eventually emerged as allopathy and internal medicine began to take place. When, in the middle seventeenth century, a book on healing herbs made their trade secrets public, practitioners of herbalism lost still more of their power and status.

In order to regain their status, certain physicians began to suggest their herbs had special magical powers because of their secret acquisition of them or because of potency invoked through an astrological event. Thus the actual potency of the herb was lessened unless the magical powers were also present; to maintain the knowledge of the biological-magical efficacy of these herbs, the "secret magical powers" were only held in the hands of the physicians or healers (Inglis, 1964:67). Only in recent decades in the United States has the general interest in herbal cures again been aroused along with the movement toward self-care and natural foods. Herbal teas have been adopted by the general public. The new herbalists are less narrow in approach and have adopted eclectic methods from the naturopaths, potencies from the homeopaths, manipulations from the osteopaths and chiropractors (see next section on other Western curing systems), and the use of radiesthesia for diagnosis.

Cosmopolitan medicine. Although the definition and explanations of these three systems of curing—allopathy, homeopathy, and naturopathy—appear to be mutually exclusive, they are frequently interwoven in a single practitioner's curing practices. The name that appears most appropriate for this union is "cosmopolitan medicine" (Leslie, 1976). This term, coined by Fred Dunn (1976), incorporates the major characteristics of professionalization, scientific objectivity, and advanced technology. Cosmopolitan medicine is a recently evolved system, although, through its various elements, it has roots in the Renaissance and Reformation. All too frequently, the term "allopathic medicine" has been used synonymously with this system (Montgomery, 1976) when in fact cosmopolitan medicine combines the basic assumptions of these three major approaches to healing.

For example, a physician in the United States who practices within a cosmopolitan system might prescribe an antibiotic (allopathy), a polio vaccination (homeopathy), and a natural food diet (naturopathy). The physician may further include in the treatment plan primary care for a sickness as well as a preventive plan to ward off future disease. Each concept would be a part of cosmopolitan medicine.

Other features of cosmopolitan medicine may include professionalization and preeminence. Professionalization includes certification and legalization through accredited college courses, a supervised apprenticeship, rigid examinations, and clinical practice. The major professional groups in cosmopolitan medicine are those of physicians and nurses, although large numbers of allied health professionals also are included, among them midwives, pharmacists, physical and occupational therapists, social workers, and psychologists. New statuses and roles continue to emerge among these groups in the dynamic process of adapting the system to meet society's health needs.

Parallel to the formal or cosmopolitan system of medicine is the informal system. A variety of roles and statuses also exist within this system, such as family members who are skilled in caring and curing. For example, "grandma's remedies" are found cross-culturally and throughout time, such as "grandma's remedy" for the common cold, which includes such traditions as hot teas, broths and chicken soup, chest rubs, steamers, soaking the sufferer's feet in hot water, and hot water bottles. This informal system of healing is an important parallel and complement to the formal cosmopolitan system and is certainly complemented by the natural-food and health-food movement of past decade.

Other Western curing systems

A number of other Western curing systems share a basic assumption: that health and healing depend on activating or releasing a life force or energy from within the individual. This assumption is part of the healing treatments of osteopathy, chiropractic, acupuncture, biofeedback, and hypnotherapy.

Osteopathy. The development of osteopathy is credited to two men. One was an Englishman, Herbert Barker, famous for his bone-setting techniques. He believed that when the body is out of alignment, either from chronic misuse or injury, bones need to be realigned to work at their fullest capacity. Andrew Taylor Steel, an American, developed the theory that a structurally sound body is a healthy body. If the body is out of balance, it cannot function properly. Consequently disorders were traced to structural disturbances, such as malpositions of bones and strains and slips in the skeletal form. Once the body was realigned, Steel believed, its own internal life force could be released and would do the healing. With such an all-encompassing holistic theory, a wide variety of symptoms were thought to be treatable, including tuberculosis, epilepsy, and gallstones. Spinal adjustments were made in these cases for the purpose of reestablishing a normal blood supply to the ailing organs.

Chiropractic. Another group of practitioners who base their treatments on releasing a life force is chiropractors. Long resisted by the orthodox Western medical system, chiropractors, under the initial leadership of Daniel David Palmer, have come to focus on the belief that minor spinal displacements cause nerve irritation and subsequent illness. Thus, the process of life is interfered with, and illness occurs because of this interference. By 1960, 35 million Americans were seeking chiropractic treatment, and in most states workmen's compensation laws recognized chiropractors. In many instances, chiropractors have been allowed to sign death certificates (Inglis, 1964:122).

Acupuncture. Acupuncture and manipulative surgery share similar underlying beliefs. Although a standard form of treatment

in China and other Eastern countries for more than 5000 years, in the 1950s acupuncture still was unknown in the United States except to a very few readers, physicians, and world travelers. Early in the 1960s, articles began to appear and an interest arose; by the 1970s, interest had climbed, and acupuncture continues to attract response from both medical authorities and the general public. (Despite the longevity of the general practice of acupuncture in China, it is instructive to note that it was not used to produce analgesia for surgical operations until 1958.)

Acupuncture is based on a belief that the body contains channels through which energy *(chi)* flows and that if these channels are interrupted the life force is impaired. In order to establish equilibrium among *yin* and *yang* forces and restore normal functioning, a fine needle is stuck into the flesh at very specific, relevant meridian points (Fig. 6-13). These needles are believed to act as "spurs on a horse's flank" and electrically stimulate the autonomic nervous system. The impulse travels to the lower centers of the brain, thus stimulating the diseased organ to restore equilibrium. Empirical evidence supports the belief that human beings have been thus relieved if not healed of physical ailments (see Davis and Yin, 1973). The science of locating the exact meridian points into which needles can be inserted was given fresh impetus with the discovery that an electrical machine similar to the chiropractor's neurokilometer is capable of measuring the variation in electrical resistance on the skin around the insertion points. This reaffirmed the accuracy of ancient Chinese charts illustrating meridian points (Inglis, 1964:125).

Several theories have been espoused as to how acupuncture works. One is the "spinal-gate" theory of Melzack and Wall. In 1965 they suggested that the key lies in the analysis of pain and its arousal, suppression, and transmission in the human body.

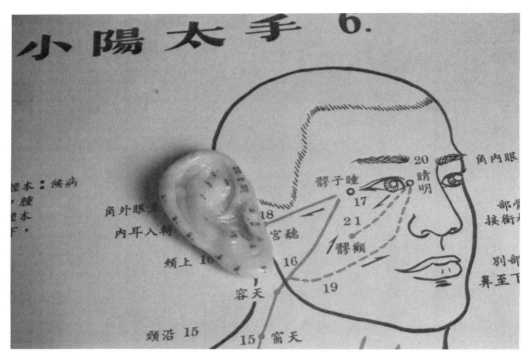

Fig. 6-13. Acupuncture focuses on energy paths that are thought by Chinese practitioners to interconnect parts of the body. The ear is thought to be a focal point wherein proper needle placement can affect any of dozens of other body locations. (Photo courtesy Food and Drug Administration, Department of Health, Education and Welfare.)

They believe that stimulation of certain large "A-delta" fibers in the sensory nerves closes a hypothetical "gate" in the spinal cord, which in turn blocks pain impulses traveling along a different set of smaller nerve fibers from reaching the brain (Davis and Yin, 1973:18). But as Man and Chen pointed out in a separate investigation, this "below the neck" theory does not account for the observation that acupuncture needles struck in the face reduce surgical pain in the abdomen. Man and Chen suggest that a second "gate" exists as well. Professor Chang Hsiang-tung of Shanghai's Academy of Sciences has gone still further, theorizing on the existence of "gates" at four levels: in the spinal cord, the brainstem, the thalamus, and the cerebral cortex (Davis and Yin, 1973:

18-19). The discovery of beta-endorphins, opiatelike substances that are produced by the body, has also been linked to acupuncture. Believed to be stimulated by acupuncture, beta-endorphins are more potent painkillers than morphine and may, thus, be responsible for producing the analgesic effects attributed to acupuncture.

Biofeedback. Studies done on biofeedback also reveal the close interrelationship between electrical resistance on the skin and human brain-wave response. While there is agreement that further extensive research is needed to clarify the physiological mechanisms involved, it must be recognized that the possibility of psychological processes as intervening variables in acupuncture and other treatments is likely: there is little support for the lingering notion among some in the West of the existence of a "mind-body dichotomy."

Hypnotherapy. Hypnotherapy has been long associated with curing, having been used by Egyptians and Greeks as well as in the New World by the Incas. In the West it was Charcot in the 1880s who began to use hypnotism in treating patients with hysteria. He is given credit for having made hypnotism a respectable part of medicine, although he did not use it as the sole means of treatment (Inglis, 1964). In 1880 Coué suggested that hypnotism was a liberation of the subject's own potential rather than the power of the hypnotist. This led to recognition of the concept of autosuggestion.

The belief that through either self-hypnosis or autosuggestion the power of healing residing within the subject can be released, is a forceful one. Recognition of the active potential of the individual vis-à-vis his or her own health, before a concept such as that of autosuggestion had been scientifically delineated, was attained early by Christian Scientists. One foundation of this religion came to be that of health-mindedness, tied to the potential of the individual to effect its activation. Historically this can be traced to the middle of the nineteenth century when Quimby, having been attracted to the mesmeric idea of animal magnetism, began putting his hands on the heads of sick patients (much like King Charles II and others before him). He claimed to be able to draw the illnesses out of his patients with a magnetic force that he believed came from God's spiritual power. Autosuggestion was also advocated. He had the patients think positively because he believed negative, festering thoughts could contribute to conditions of illness.

It was Mary Baker Glover, later Mary Baker Eddy, (originally one of Quimby's patients) who became the leader of the Christian Science movement. Following mesmeric philosophy, Quimby's inspiration, and Christian doctrine, she came to advocate the interactive powers of the individual and God. Converts entrust themselves not merely to their own suggestive powers but also to the divine will. Thus what came to be called autosuggestion is mediated and made easier by the belief that an outside being is responsible; the mind acts as a transformer of divine energy into physical energy (Inglis, 1964: 205).

Noted throughout history and in contemporary accounts as well are healings that have been described as miracles. Western scientists have suggested that such healings can be traced to the interplay of psychosomatic illnesses and autosuggestion. Studies such as that done by Nolen (1974) support the claim that in some spiritual or psychic healings, fraud does exist; in others autosuggestion seems to be evidenced. It is only within the past few years that a more "scientific" physiological explanation is beginning to take form, although much more empirical research is needed.

The holistic health movement. The holistic health movement grew out of the humanism of the late 1960s, and today is widely recognized as a vital change in the basic concept of human beings as whole, biocultural creatures. The major assumption is that health can be promoted actively not only within the individual but rather within and outside of the individual. The biomedical model defines sickness and health at the microbiological level; in contrast the holistic health movement acknowledges the social restructuring that is necessary to effectively achieve and maintain an acceptable level of health. In contrast to biomedical models of health care, where the individual is treated separately, in the holistic movement efforts are directed at promoting and maintaining the health of the individual as well as of so-

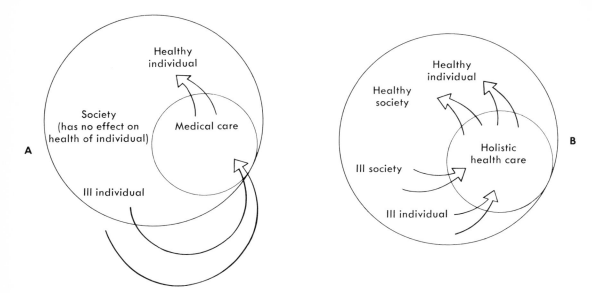

Fig. 6-14. A, Medical model. Look for illness and health at microbiological level. Heal individual to return to normal functions in society. **B,** Holistic health model. Look for illness and health at the societal level. Question of society is structured to provide a healthful living environment. An ill society produces ill members. (From Hayes-Bautista and Harveston, 1977:9.)

ciety. Hayes-Bautista and Harveston have compared the medical model and the holistic health model diagrammatically as viewed in Fig. 6-14.

As we described in Chapter 1, medicine is in a state of crisis. Engel (1977:133) claims a new medical model is needed. His use of a general systems approach for looking at the important variables beyond the somatic experience of the patient has yielded a biopsychosocial model. Our test is an endeavor to develop an analogous model, viewing health as bioculturally based. Our definition of a healthy human being, regardless of age, is one whose mind and body are in a state of dynamic equilibrium. We agree with Jerome D. Frank that "Healing, then, is the process by which a health equilibrium is restored; it may occur spontaneously or with the aid of a medical or nonmedical healer" (Frank, 1978:42).

The causes and treatment for disequilib-

rium are many. Richard Miles has developed a useful health modality matrix from which we have adapted some elements. He cautions that, as treatment modalities have proliferated, so has the need for consumers to become aware of the quality of each (see Table 9).

In sum the holistic health movement encompasses numerous treatment modalities, each with diverse means of diagnosis and techniques for achieving dynamic equilibrium. Their goals are similar in that they help the individual to achieve a higher level of functioning. The movement is significant, and it is growing. It has deep historical roots, with similar health modalities being found cross-culturally. However, within the biomedical model of health care in the United States, major changes will have to occur before the holistic movement can become a formal part of the medical-social institution.

Table 9. Health modality matrix

Modality	Diagnosis	Technique for achieving equilibrium	Goals
Spiritual	Recognize mind/body pat-	Focus, posture	Integrate life energy
Yoga	terns		
Psychological			
Behavior modifica-	Behavior analysis		New behavior
tion			
Psychoanalysis	Identification of patterns		New behavior
Physical disciplines			
Chiropractic	Spinal alignment	Alignment	Improved neural functioning
Osteopathy	Structural alignment	Adjust structure	Improve function
Biofeedback	Awareness of action patterns	Relaxation techniques	New patterns
Emotional/physical			
Gestalt	Identify parts and wholes	Resolution of conflict	Experience here/now
Rolfing	Structural alignment	Adjust structure	Released tension
Bio-chemical			
Homeopathy	Case analysis	Remedy matching symptoms	Facilitate self-teaching
Allopathy	Case analysis	Remedy opposing symptoms	Eliminate disease symptoms
Etheric (body energy)			
Acupuncture	Pulse diagnosis	Rebalance energy	Homeostasis of energy
Psychic	Aura/energy visualization	Rebalance energy	Homeostasis of energy

Adapted from Miles, R. B., 1978.

Summary

Thus an understanding of the development of Western beliefs and curing clarifies the existence of competing and complementary treatments in the Western curing system. The present system has been developing for nearly 2500 years, and diversity has sprung from such widespread influences as Middle Eastern (the Arabic world) as well as Western cultures (Greek and Roman).

Presently, diverse treatment modalities in the United States are based on various basic assumptions about illness and disease causation. No longer faced with the epidemic spread of germ-caused disease, new models of treatment have arisen to deal with stress-related sicknesses. Health may be restored by a variety of new healers, and much of the treatment seems to be shifting into the hands of the people themselves. Certainly throughout human history, individuals have been responsible in various ways for their own care, but today we are experiencing a trend toward institutionalization of this form of health care. Each of us has a stake in this cultural change, and these issues are addressed further in the next chapter.

REFERENCES

Aamodt, A. M. The care component in a health and healing system. In Bauwens, E. E. (ed.). *The Anthropology of Health*. St. Louis: The C. V. Mosby Co., 1978.

Ackerknecht, E. H. Paleopathology. In Landy, D. (ed.). *Culture, Disease, and Healing: Studies in Medical Anthropology*. New York: The Macmillan Co., 1977.

Alland, A., Jr. *Adaptation in Cultural Evolution: An Approach to Medical Anthropology*. New York: Columbia University Press, 1970.

Anonymous. Translations and science. *MD: Medical Newsmagazine*, 1969, *13*(10), 136-148.

Bach, E. *The Twelve Healers and Other Remedies*. London: The C. W. Daniel Co. Ltd., 1933.

Barnouw, V. *Culture and Personality*, revised ed. Homewood, Ill.: Dorsey Press, 1973.

Benedict, R. *Patterns of Culture.* New York: Houghton Mifflin Co., 1934.

Boericke, W. *Pocket Manual of Homeopathic Materia Medica.* Philadelphia: Boericke & Runyon, 1927.

Boyer, P., and Nissenbaum, S. *Salem Possessed: The Social Origins of Witchcraft.* Cambridge, Mass.: Harvard University Press, 1974.

Brockliss, L. W. B. Medical teaching at the University of Paris, 1600-1720. *Annals of Science,* 1978, *35*(3), 221-251.

Bromberg, W. *From Shaman to Psychotherapist.* Chicago: Henry Regnery Co., 1975.

Bronowski, J. *Magic, Science, and Civilization.* New York: Columbia University Press, 1978.

Burgess, R. L., and Bushell, D., Jr. *Behavioral Sociology: The Experimental Analysis of Social Processes.* New York: Columbia University Press, 1969.

Butzer, K. W. *Early Hydraulic Civilization in Egypt: A Study in Cultural Ecology.* Chicago: University of Chicago Press, 1976.

Byrne, P. F. *Witchcraft in Ireland.* Cork, Ireland: The Mercier Press Ltd., 1967.

Caporael, L. R. Ergotism: the Satan loosed in Salem? *Science,* 1976, *192,* 21-26.

Carr, J. E. Ethno-behaviorism and the culture-bound syndromes: the case of *amok. Culture, Medicine and Psychiatry,* 1978, *2*(3), 269-293.

Carson, R. L. *Silent Spring.* Boston: Houghton Mifflin Co., 1962.

Clarke, J. H. *The Prescriber: A Dictionary of the New Therapeutics.* Devon, England: Health Science Press, 1972.

Clarke, W. C. Temporary madness as theatre: wildman behavior in New Guinea. *Oceania,* 1973, *43*(3), 198-214.

Clements, F. E. Primitive concepts of disease. *University of California Publications in American Archaeology and Ethnology,* 1932, *32,* 185-252.

Clendening, L. *Source Book of Medical History.* New York: Dover Publications, Inc., 1942.

Condominas, G. *We Have Eaten the Forest: The Story of a Montagnard Village in the Central Highlands of Vietnam.* New York: Hill & Wang, 1977.

Coulter, H. *Divided Legacy: A History of the Schism in Medical Thought,* vol. 3. Washington, D.C.: Wehawken Book Co., 1973.

Currier, R. L. The hot-cold syndrome and symbolic balance in Mexican and Spanish American folk medicine. *Ethnology,* 1966, *5,* 251-263.

Davis, J. B., and Yin, L. Acupuncture: past and present. *FDA Consumer,* U.S. Department of Health, Education and Welfare, Publication no. (FDA) 74-4001, Washington, D.C., May 1973, pp. 17-23.

Deutsch, R. M. *Nuts Among the Berries.* New York: Random House, 1971.

DHEW. *A Barefoot Doctor's Manual.* (Translation of a Chinese Instruction to Certain Chinese Health Personnel). U.S. Department of Health, Education and Welfare, no. (NIH) 75-695, Washington, D.C., 1974.

Dunn, F. L. Traditional Asian medicine and cosmopolitan medicine as adaptive systems. In Leslie, C. (ed.). *Asian Medical Systems: A Comparative Study,* Berkeley: University of California Press, 1976.

Elkin, A. P. *Aboriginal Men of High Degree,* ed. 2. New York: St. Martin's Press, Inc., 1977.

Engel, G. L. The need for a new medical model: a challenge for biomedicine. *Science,* 1977, *196,* 129-136.

Epstein, S. A sociological analysis of witch beliefs in a Mysore village. In Middleton, J. (ed.). *Magic, Witchcraft and Curing.* Austin, Tex.: University of Texas Press, 1967.

Fabrega, H., Jr. *Disease and Social Behavior: An Interdisciplinary Perspective.* Cambridge, Mass.: The M.I.T. Press, 1974.

Fabrega, H., Jr. The need for an ethnomedical science. *Science,* 1975, *189,* 969-975.

Fabrega, H., Jr. The scope of ethnomedical science. *Culture, Medicine and Psychiatry,* 1977, *1*(2), 201-228.

Fager, C. A new age for homeopathy? *San Francisco Bay Guardian,* 1977, *11*(26).

Flood, B. P., Jr. Pliny and the medieval "Macer" medical text. *Journal of the History of Medicine and Allied Sciences,* 1977, *32*(4), 395-402.

Fortune, R. F. Sorcery and sickness in Dobu. In Landy, D. (ed.). *Culture, Disease, and Healing: Studies in Medical Anthropology.* New York: The Macmillan Co., 1977. (First printed, 1932.)

Foster, G. M. *Applied Anthropology.* Boston: Little, Brown and Co., 1969.

Foster, G. M. Disease etiologies in non-Western medical systems. *American Anthropologist,* 1976, *78*(4), 773-782.

Foster, G. M. Peasant society and the image of limited good. In Potter, J. M., and others (eds.). *Peasant Society: A Reader.* Boston: Little, Brown and Co., 1967.

Foster, G. M., and Anderson, B. G. *Medical Anthropology.* New York: John Wiley & Sons, Inc., 1978.

Foulks, E. F. *The Arctic Hysterias of the North Alaskan Eskimo.* Anthropological Studies no. 10, Washington, D.C.: American Anthropological Association, 1972.

Frank, J. D., The medical power of faith. *Human Nature,* 1978, *1*(8), 40-45.

Frazer, J. G. *The New Golden Bough.* (New abridgement by Theodor H. Gaster). New York: New American Library, 1959. (First printed, 1890.)

Gajdusek, D. C. Unconventional viruses and the origin and disappearance of kuru. *Science,* 1977, *197,* 943-960.

Garrett, C. Women and witches: patterns of analysis. *Signs: Journal of Women in Culture and Society*, 1977, 3(2), 461-470.

Garrison, V. The "Puerto Rican syndrome" in psychiatry and *espiritismo*. In Crapanzano, V., and Garrison, V. (eds.). *Case Studies in Spirit Possession*. New York: John Wiley & Sons, Inc., 1977.

Gilbert, W. H. Religions of the world. In Hunter, D. E., and Whitten, P. (eds.). *Encyclopedia of Anthropology*. New York: Harper & Row, Publishers, 1976.

Glittenberg, J. E. *A Comparative Study of Fertility in Highland Guatemala: A Ladino and an Indian Town*. Unpublished doctoral dissertation, University of Colorado, Boulder, Colo. 1976.

Glittenberg, J. E. *Shamans, Exorcists, and Psychotherapists: Common Healers?* Unpublished paper, University of Colorado School of Nursing, Denver, Colo., 1977.

Glock, C. Y., and Bellah, R. N. (eds.). *The New Religious Consciousness*. Berkeley, Calif.: University of California Press, 1976.

Green, R. M. *A Translation of Galen's Hygiene (De Sanitate Tuenda)*. Springfield, Ill.: Charles C Thomas, Publisher, 1951.

Gunther, R. T. *The Greek Herbal of Dioscorides*. New York: Hafner Publishing Co., Inc., 1934.

Hackenberg, R. A., Gerber, L., and Hackenberg, B. H. Cardiovascular disease mortality among Filipinos in Hawaii: rates, trends, and associated factors. *R & S Report*, no. 24, Research and Statistics Office, Hawaii State Department of Health, 1978.

Hamer, J., and Hamer, I. Spirit possession and its sociopsychological implications among the Sidamo of southwest Ethiopia. In Landy, D. (ed.). *Culture, Disease, and Healing: Studies in Medical Anthropology*. New York: The Macmillan Co., 1977.

Harner, M. J. The sound of rushing water. In Logan, M. H., and Hunt, E. E., Jr. (eds.). *Health and the Human Condition: Perspectives on Medical Anthropology*. North Scituate, Mass.: Duxbury Press, 1978.

Harris, M. *Cows, Pigs, Wars, and Witches: The Riddles of Culture*. New York: Vintage Books, 1974.

Harwood, A. The hot-cold theory of disease. Implications for treatment of Puerto Rican patients. *Journal of the American Medical Association*, 1971, 216, 1153-1158.

Hays-Bautista, D., and Harveston, D. S., Holistic health care. *Social Policy*, 1977, 7(6).

Hippocrates. *The Theory and Practice of Medicine*. (With an introduction by Emerson Crosby Kelly.) New York: Philosophical Library, Inc., 1964.

Hughes, J. D. *Ecology in Ancient Civilizations*. Albuquerque, N.M.: University of New Mexico Press, 1975.

Hunt, E. E., Jr. Ecological frameworks and hypothesis testing in medical anthropology. In Logan, M. H., and Hunt, E. E., Jr. (eds.). *Health and the Human Condition: Perspectives on Medical Anthropology*. North Scituate, Mass.: Duxbury Press, Inc., 1978.

Illich, I. *Medical Nemesis: The Expropriation of Health*. New York: Pantheon Books, Inc., 1976.

Inglis, B. *Fringe Medicine*. London: Faber & Faber Ltd., 1964.

Jarvis, D. C. *Folk Medicine: A Vermont Doctor's Guide to Good Health*. New York: Henry Holt, 1958.

Karlsen, C. Book review of *Salem Possessed* by Paul Boyer and Stephen Nissenbaum. *Signs: Journal of Women in Culture and Society*, 1978, 3(3), 703-704.

Kaufman, M. *Homeopathy in America: The Rise and Fall of a Medical Heresy*. Baltimore: The Johns Hopkins University Press, 1971.

Kay, M. A. Health and illness in a Mexican American barrio. In Spicer, E. H. (ed.). *Ethnic Medicine in the Southwest*. Tucson: University of Arizona Press, 1977.

Kelly, E. C. Introduction. In Hippocrates. *The Theory and Practice of Medicine*. New York: Philosophical Library, Inc., 1964.

Kenny, M. G. *Latah:* the symbolism of a putative mental disorder. *Culture, Medicine and Psychiatry*, 1978, 2(3), 209-231.

Kenny, M. G. Religion. In Hunter, D. E., and Whitten, P. (eds.). *Encyclopedia of Anthropology*. New York: Harper & Row, Publishers, 1976.

Kirsch, I. Demonology and the rise of science: an example of the misconception of historical data. *Journal of the History of the Behavioral Sciences*, 1978, 14(2), 149-157.

Kleinman, A. M. Concepts and a model for the comparison of medical systems as cultural systems. *Social Science & Medicine*, 1978a, 12(2B), 85-93.

Kleinman, A. M. Editorial: three faces of culture-bound syndromes: their implications for cross-cultural research. *Culture, Medicine and Psychiatry*, 1978b, 2(3), 207-208.

Kleinman, A. M. The failure of Western medicine. *Human Nature*, 1978c, 1(11), 63-68.

Kleinman, A. M., and Sung, L. H. Why do indigenous practitioners successfully heal? *Social Science & Medicine*, 1979, 1(13B), 7-26.

Landy, D. Role adaptation: traditional curers under the impact of Western medicine. In Landy, D. (ed.). *Culture, Disease, and Healing: Studies in Medical Anthropology*. New York: The Macmillan Co., 1977.

Langness, L. L. Hysterical psychosis in the New Guinea highlands: a Bena Bena example. *Psychiatry*, 1965, 28, 258-277.

Laughlin, W. S. Acquisition of anatomical knowledge by ancient man. In Landy, D. (ed.). *Culture, Disease, and Healing: Studies in Medical Anthropology.* New York: The Macmillan Co., 1977.

Laver, A. B. Miracles no wonder! The mesmeric phenomena and organic cures of Valentine Greatrakes. *Journal of the History of Medicine and Allied Sciences,* 1978, *33*(1), 35-46.

Lee, R. B. Trance cure of the !Kung bushmen. In Logan, M. H., and Hunt, E. E., Jr. (eds.). *Health and the Human Condition: Perspectives on Medical Anthropology.* North Scituate, Mass.: Duxbury Press, Inc., 1978.

Leininger, M. *Transcultural Nursing: Concepts, Theories, and Practices.* New York: John Wiley & Sons, Inc., 1978.

Leininger, M. Witchcraft practices and psychocultural therapy with urban United States families. *Human Organization,* 1973, *32*(1), 73-83.

Leslie, C. Introduction. *Asian Medical Systems: A Comparative Study,* Berkeley: University of California Press, 1976.

Lindenbaum, S. *Kuru Sorcery: Disease and Danger in the New Guinea Highlands.* Palo Alto, Calif.: Mayfield, 1978.

Lindenbaum, S. Sorcery and danger. *Oceania,* 1975, *46*(1), 68-75.

Logan, M. H. Anthropological research on the hot-cold theory of disease: some methodological suggestions. *Medical Anthropology,* 1977, *1*(4), 87-112.

Logan, M. H. Humoral medicine in Guatemala and peasant acceptance of modern medicine. In Logan, M. H., and Hunt, E. E., Jr. (eds.). *Health and the Human Condition: Perspectives on Medical Anthropology.* North Scituate, Mass.: Duxbury Press, Inc., 1978.

Logan, M. H., and Hunt, E. E., Jr. (eds.). *Health and the Human Condition: Perspectives on Medical Anthropology.* North Scituate, Mass.: Duxbury Press, Inc., 1978.

Malinowski, B. *Magic, Science and Religion.* New York: The Free Press, 1948.

Marti-Ibañez, F. Magic and drama of Byzantium. *MD: Medical Newsmagazine,* 1967, *11*(2), 9-12.

Mattson, P. H. Holistic health: an overview. *Phoenix: New Directions in the Study of Man,* 1977, *1*(2), 36-43.

McQueen, D. V. The history of science and medicine as theoretical sources for the comparative study of contemporary medical systems. *Social Science & Medicine,* 1978, *12*(2B), 69-74.

Medawar, P. B. Book review of *Magic, Science, and Civilization* by Jacob Bronowski. *Nature,* 1978, *276*, 124-125.

Menolascino, S. *Homeopathy.* Unpublished paper, University of Denver Department of Anthropology, Denver, Colo., 1978.

Miles, R. B. *Health Modality Maitrix.* Paper for Commonweal OTA Conference on New Technologies and Health, Bolinas, Calif., Nov. 19-20, 1978.

Montgomery, E. Systems and the medical practitioners of a Tomil town. In Leslie, C. (ed.). *Asian Medical Systems: A Comparative Study.* Berkeley: University of California Press, 1976.

Moore, W. E. *Social Change.* Englewood Cliffs, N.J.: Prentice Hall, Inc., 1963.

Neuenswander, H. L., and Souder, S. D. The hot-cold wet-dry syndrome among the Quiche of Joyabaj: two alternative cognitive models. In Neuenswander, H. L., and Arnold, D. E. (eds.). *Cognitive Studies of Southern Mesoamerica.* Dallas: SIL Museum of Anthropology, 1977.

Nolen, W. A. *Healing: A Doctor in Search of a Miracle.* New York: Random House, 1974.

Obeyesekere, G. The impact of Ayurvedic ideas on the culture and the individual in Sri Lanka. In Leslie, C. (ed.). *Asian Medical Systems: A Comparative Study.* Berkeley: University of California Press, 1976.

Obeyesekere, G. The theory and practice of psychological medicine in the Ayurvedic tradition. *Culture, Medicine and Psychiatry,* 1977, *1*(2), 155-181.

Olien, M. D. *The Human Myth: An Introduction to Anthropology.* New York: Harper & Row, Publishers, 1978.

Ortiz de Montellano, B. Empirical Aztec medicine. *Science,* 1975, *188*, 215-220.

Osborne, O. H. *Merging Traditional and Scientific Health Care Systems: Conceptual and Pragmatic Issues.* Paper presented at the Annual Meeting of the Society for Applied Anthropology,, San Diego, 1977.

Parsons, T. *The Social System.* New York: The Free Press, 1951.

Paul, B. D. (ed.). *Health, Culture and Community: Case Studies of Public Reactions to Health Programs.* New York: Russell Sage Foundation, 1955.

Polgar, S. Evolution and the ills of mankind. In Tax, S. (ed.). *Horizons of Anthropology.* Chicago: Aldine-Atherton, Inc., 1964.

Polgar, S. Population history and population policies from an anthropological perspective. *Current Anthropology,* 1972, *13*(2), 203-211.

Rapoport, A. Foreword. In Buckley, W. (ed.). *Modern Systems Research for the Behavioral Scientist.* Chicago: Aldine-Atherton, Inc., 1968.

Rappaport, R. A. *Pigs for the Ancestors: Ritual in the Ecology of a New Guinea People.* New Haven, Conn.: Yale University Press, 1968.

Rivers, W. H. R. *Medicine, Magic, and Religion.* London: Kogan Paul Ltd. 1924.

Rogers, S. L. *The Shaman's Healing Way.* Ramona, Calif.: Acoma Books, 1976.

Rosen, G. *From Medical Police to Social Medicine: Essays on the History of Health Care.* New York: Science History Publications, 1974.

Rosner, F. *Medicine in the Bible and the Talmud: Selections from Classical Jewish Sources.* New York: Ktav Publishing House, Inc., 1977.

Sandner, D. F. Navaho medicine. *Human Nature,* 1978, *1*(7), 54-62.

Scheper-Hughes, N. Saints, scholars and schizophrenics—madness and badness in western Ireland. *Medical Anthropology,* 1978, *2*(3), 59-93.

Sibisi, H. How African women cope with migrant labor in South Africa. *Signs: Journal of Women in Culture and Society,* 1977, 3(1), 167-177.

Siegel, R. E. *Galen's System of Physiology and Medicine: An Analysis of His Doctrines and Observations on Bloodflow, Respiration, Humors and Internal Diseases.* Basel: S. Karger AG, 1968.

Sigerist, H. E. Introduction. In Green, R. M. *A Translation of Galen's Hygiene (De Sanitate Tuenda).* Springfield, Ill.: Charles C Thomas, Publisher, 1951.

Sorenson, E. R., and Gajdusek, D. C. *A Catalogue of Research Films in Ethnopediatrics.* Bethesda, Md.: National Institutes of Health.

Spanos, N. P. Witchcraft in histories of psychiatry: a critical analysis and an alternative conceptualization. *Psychological Bulletin,* 1978, 85(2), 417-439.

Spanos, N. P., and Gottlieb, J. Ergotism and the Salem Village witchcraft trials. *Science,* 1976, *194,* 1360-1394.

Spiro, M. E. The exorcist in Burma. In Landy, D. (ed.). *Culture, Disease, and Healing: Studies in Medical Anthropology.* New York: The Macmillan Co., 1977.

Steward, J. C. *Theory of Culture Change.* Urbana, Ill.: University of Illinois Press, 1955.

Stone, D. The human potential movement. In Glock, C. Y., and Bellah, R. N. (eds.). *The New Religious Consciousness.* Berkeley: University of California Press, 1976.

Tobey, A. The summer solstice of the Healthy-Happy-Holy Organization. In Glock, C. Y., and Bellah, R. N. (eds.). *The New Religious Consciousness.* Berkeley: University of California Press, 1976.

Unschuld, P. U. Discussion on David McQueen's paper. *Social Science & Medicine,* 1978, *12*(2B), 75-77.

Van Amelsvoort, V. F. P. M. *Early Introduction of Integrated Rural Health into a Primitive Society.* Assen: Van Gorcum, 1964.

Van Arsdale, P. W. Population dynamics among Asmat hunter-gatherers of New Guinea: data, methods, comparisons. *Human Ecology,* 1978, *6*(4), 435-467.

Vayda, A. P. Ecology: cultural and non-cultural. In Clifton, J. A. (ed.). *Introduction to Cultural Anthropology: Essays in the Scope and Methods of the Science of Man.* New York: Houghton Mifflin Co., 1968.

Wain, H. *A History of Preventive Medicine.* Springfield, Ill.: Charles C Thomas, Publisher, 1970.

Wallace, W. A. Book review of *The Cultural Context of Medieval Learning,* edited by J. E. Murdoch and E. D. Sylla. *Annals of Science,* 1978, 35(1), 84-86.

Ward, R. *Magic, Myth, Medicine: Theories of Disease Causation in Aboriginal Cultures.* Unpublished paper, University of Colorado School of Nursing, Denver, Colo., 1977.

Waxler, N. E. Is mental illness cured in traditional societies? A theoretical analysis. *Culture, Medicine and Psychiatry,* 1977, *1*(3), 233-253.

Wellin, E. Theoretical orientations in medical anthropology: continuity and change over the past half century. In Landy, D. (ed.). *Culture, Disease, and Healing: Studies in Medical Anthropology.* New York: The Macmillan Co., 1977.

White, L. *The Evolution of Culture: The Development of Civilization to the Fall of Rome.* New York: McGraw-Hill Book Co., 1959.

White, R. W. *The Abnormal Personality,* ed. 3. New York: The Ronald Press Co., 1964.

Whiting, B. B. *Paiute-Sorcery.* Viking Fund Publications in Anthropology no. 15. New York: Wenner-Gren Foundation, 1950.

Wilk, S. Magic and science. In Hunter, D. E., and Whitten, P. (eds.). *Encyclopedia of Anthropology.* New York: Harper & Row, Publishers, 1976.

Woods, C. M. Alternative curing strategies in a changing medical situation. *Medical Anthropology,* 1977, *1*(3), 25-54.

Woods, C. M. *Culture Change.* Dubuque, Iowa: William C. Brown, 1975.

Yap, P. M. The culture-bound reactive syndromes. In Landy, D. (ed.). *Culture, Disease, and Healing: Studies in Medical Anthropology.* New York: The Macmillan Co., 1977.

Young, A. Some implications of medical beliefs and practices for social anthropology. *American Anthropologist,* 1976, 78(1), 5-24.

CHAPTER 7

The future of health: an interpretation

Throughout the preceding chapters, three major themes are inseparably entwined and continually influence each other. One is the process of human adaptation—a set of strategies inherited or transmitted from the past but continually being modified in response to ongoing challenges of the present. Another is the theme of the human life cycle—the setting in which the interplay between biological and cultural adaptive strategies translates into states of health or sickness for the individual. The third theme stresses the importance of the cultural belief system for the basis of practices used to effect curing. These themes are built on the past as well as the present. In this concluding chapter, we ask where these factors that influence health are likely to lead us in the future and attempt to forecast the principles and policies that promise to foster health and wellbeing. We are witnessing today transitions of whole societies in many parts of the world. These changes are rapid in some, creating enormous stresses for values held for centuries that, within only decades, have been supplanted by different ways of thinking. Jonas Salk clearly describes the kinds of value shifts that may be induced in an industrialized culture as it moves from the contemporary era he calls epoch A into the future, epoch B (Salk, 1973). He uses the classical sigmoid-shaped curve to suggest how past and present trends may be projected into the future (Fig. 7-1). Epoch A encompasses the lower section of the curve in which stability translates into rapid, exponential growth and expansion. Epoch B is said to begin after the inflection point in the curve where growth tapers to reach a new period of comparative stability. The future of health too can be viewed this way. In fact, in some segments of the American population, new approaches are already becoming visible when one compares the past 3 decades (epoch A) with the late 1970s.

We seem to be moving from an era of "medicine" to one of "health" in the United States. In the opening chapter of this book, we considered the crisis in health care in this country, concluding that Americans are paying more money than ever before for health care but are not getting healthier as a result. Increasing the expenditures for episodic acute care benefits the health care industry but has not improved significantly the overall health of the American population. As stated by the late John Knowles, President of the Rockefeller Foundation, "The next major advances in the health of the American people will result from the assumption of individual responsibility for one's own health and a necessary change in life style for the majority of Americans" (Knowles, 1977). Changing the emphasis from medicine to health carries with it the requirement to understand the basis of health and disease and the treatment of illness. Thus, Chapters 2 through 6 developed such a basis. Through the presentation of a model of the human ecosystem and application of it to the hu-

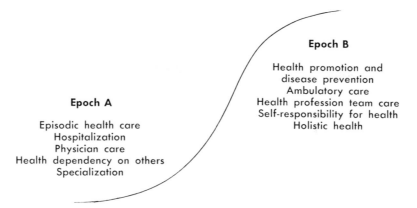

Epoch B

Health promotion and
disease prevention
Ambulatory care
Health profession team care
Self-responsibility for health
Holistic health

Epoch A

Episodic health care
Hospitalization
Physician care
Health dependency on others
Specialization

Fig. 7-1. The sigmoid-shaped curve as applied to changes affecting health. Epoch A refers to a time just ending in which features pertaining to health care differ from those of the coming Epoch B.

man evolutionary and historical record, a perspective has been developed in which health is seen to result from adaptation and sickness from the failure of adaptation to occur. Both biological and cultural factors are integral to this evolutionary process and to the attainment of states of health or sickness. The determinants of health and sickness throughout the human life cycle point, on the one hand, to the distinctiveness of each stage of the life cycle for the particular biological developments and for the cultural context in which the developments occur. On the other hand, the behaviors and developments of one age influence health and sickness at subsequent ages. The cultural belief system also exerts considerable influence on the means and efficacy of the curative strategies available.

Challenges for the future of health derive from continuing developments of the present as well as from new features. Problems that stem from a loss of human scale in the technological advances—employed for adaptive ends but that generate unforeseen, maladaptive consequences—threaten health. The example of the near meltdown at the Three Mile Island, Pennsylvania, nuclear power plant illustrates the fragile relationship be-

tween technological advancement and unforeseen maladaptive consequences for health. Health-related exports of Western culture, such as industrialization and urbanization, have the potential for generating sickness through the effects of noise, crowding, traffic, and pollution of air, food, and water. Modification and adaptation of such features by local cultures may or may not occur, as demonstrated by the examples of retention of cultural customs affecting older-aged people in Japan and the adoption of Spanish-style houses in Guatemala respectively. Health care systems also may be expected to change, for they too are part of a dynamic adaptive process. Demands for new forms of health care personnel, such as the nurse-practitioner, the "generalist specialty" in family medicine, and paramedical personnel reflect the dynamic nature of the health care system. The impact of alternative curing systems, such as biofeedback, folk healers, and holistic health and the growing participation of health care clients in the decision-making process through citizen advisory boards and regulatory groups may reinforce tendencies toward a health care system that exhibits greater cultural diversity than does the present arrangement. Changes in the economic and political spheres affecting inflation, the existence of national health insurance, and environmental threats also can exert important influences on the future of health.

To develop further our view of the future challenges affecting health on both a worldwide and national scale, the remaining pages focus on international health, particularly in developing countries, and finally examine patterns of health in the United States.

THE INTERNATIONAL PREDICAMENT

The international predicament concerning health is based on two factors: first, the unequal distribution and consumption of resources necessary for health, and second, the identification and implementation of culturally appropriate health care systems.

In earlier chapters, reference was made to world population dynamics and the accumulating evidence that the rate of population growth has begun to decline. Nevertheless, world population continues to race ahead, placing great demands on the limited world resources that are required for health in the future. Several industrialized nations have reduced their birth rates to the point that they have fallen to replacement levels or even below. Developing countries in many instances are showing sharp decreases in their birth rates, but this is not at all uniform. There has been little decline on the continent of Africa and in parts of southeast Asia.

While population growth has slowed in

Table 10. Major military spenders and their rank in economic-social indicators, 1975*

	Military expenditures		Rank among 140 nations			
			Economic-social standing (avg. rank)	GNP (per capita)	Education	
	Million US $	Rank among 140 nations			Public expend. per capita	School-age population per teacher
USSR	94,000	1	17	27	25	23
United States	90,948	2	6	6	7	12
China	18,000	3	79	103	97	55
West Germany	15,299	4	9	9	15	30
France	13,093	5	4	11	15	12
United Kingdom	11,477	6	16	23	18	8
Iran	7,742	7	65	44	46	71
Egypt	5,368	8	88	100	82	90
Italy	4,656	9	24	28	29	23
Japan	4,640	10	24	21	21	44
Saudi Arabia	4,260	11	63	20	3	79
Israel	3,517	12	22	25	24	2
Canada	3,074	13	4	10	4	8
India	3,008	14	111	125	121	90
Netherlands	2,869	15	15	15	5	39
East Germany	2,644	16	13	24	26	17
Poland	2,384	17	28	31	35	41
Sweden	2,344	18	1	4	2	1
Spain	2,200	19	31	30	48	39
Turkey	1,971	20	70	59	72	83

*From Sivard, 1978.

developed countries, consumption on a per capita basis continues to rise in the developed compared to the developing countries. For example, the Western countries plus the Soviet Union and Japan contain one-fourth of the world's population but consume 80% to 90% of the world's resources (Miller, 1975: 13). Thus, demands from industrialized countries that developing nations slow their population growth can be countered by demands for decreased consumption and increased resource sharing in the developed world.

Within developed countries, such as the United States, resources are not evenly distributed across all segments of the population or of the economy. One set of comparisons concerns military versus social-eco-

nomic expenditures. Table 10 summarizes the world's major military spenders and their ranks according to social-economic indicators. Clearly, the strongest military powers make a relatively poor showing in social-economic terms, yet there is considerable resistance to decreased military spending. As stated by John Kenneth Galbraith,

There can be few more seemingly unequal political contests in the world than those over military spending and its claims against social needs. On the one side, powerful military bureaucracies, influential and richly financed weapons industries, their lobbies, their captive legislators, those for whom paranoia or past wars are a way of life. On the other side, only reason, the will to survive, the inarticulate poor. (Quoted in Sivard, 1978.)

Rank among 140 nations							
Education			Health				
School-age population in school	Women in total university enrollment	Lit-eracy rate	Public expend. per capita	Popula-tion per physician	Popula-tion per hosp. bed	Infant mortality rate	Life expec-tancy
46	7	1	27	1	6	34	29
4	22	1	13	18	33	13	7
43	7	26	97	93	117	51	56
28	45	1	3	9	4	21	18
23	15	1	6	23	17	8	10
5	61	16	15	26	20	13	10
92	78	85	46	69	105	106	77
96	70	80	76	52	78	71	84
41	37	30	18	11	14	26	10
20	92	1	16	33	16	2	3
117	112	114	31	72	102	113	104
41	22	37	24	2	40	25	10
3	27	26	4	19	21	13	7
100	78	86	118	83	132	95	88
43	74	16	7	22	4	2	1
32	17	1	23	13	11	13	15
66	12	16	26	17	29	29	29
10	37	1	1	20	1	1	1
32	53	32	25	25	44	10	10
85	94	72	79	59	79	83	70

Clearly, the competition for resources within the United States is intense and the prospect of decreasing overall consumption so as to increase the availability of resources for developing nations is not encouraging. A strategy that the developing countries have used and will likely continue to use is to withhold or reduce the supply of the raw materials that are exported to the developed world.

Adapting or readapting to a human scale entails use of a less energy-intensive technology for ends judged to be in the best interests of the population as a whole, not just for certain individuals. As applied to health, examination of other cultures demonstrates the strength of indigenous traditions and beliefs regarding health care. The continuation of what we have termed alternative health care systems is one means of addressing health care needs within a culturally diverse population, such as that of the United States. Increasing diversity within the established health care system by stressing admission standards and programs in medical and nursing school education that accommodate a range of backgrounds and goals is another means of making health care resources accessible and appropriate to the settings where they are needed. Flexibility in the orientation of health care systems in other countries is also desirable. For example, small-scale, perhaps mobile, clinic systems may be better suited to serve populations where transportation and communication are difficult than are facilities located in urban centers. In cultures where family attendance to the sick is important, hospitals could be built in ways that permitted family members to stay with the patient.

A more general issue is of an ethical nature. Matters affecting health on an international scale are part of a broader set of issues that are intricately linked with trade and development. For example, the United Nations Conference on Science and Technol-

ogy convened in Vienna in August 1979, addressed topics such as "technology transfer" from the industrialized to the less-developed countries in order to improve access to scientific information and technological capacity. A major point of disagreement concerned the assertion of some less-developed countries that technology was a common heritage and, therefore, should be freely shared; in contrast, Western business corporations claimed that technology, while it can be shared, is the intellectual property of the originator (Walsh, 1979). Ethical concern for the survival and wellbeing of the world population must accompany and modify what would otherwise result in advancing the goals of only one group. We are both the research director and the guinea pig on planet Earth; if we are to survive as a species, we must be wise enough to address health as an international human issue of common concern.

Health in developing countries

The discussion in the preceding chapters of the factors that influence health and health care in developing countries pointed to their several advantages as well as disadvantages regarding health. In traditional settings, cultural homogeneity acts to increase familiarity with and acceptance of the healing practices in use, even though the healer occupies an elevated, somewhat removed status. In the absence of any major influences of advanced technology, such as are felt in Western nations, many features of life in these countries remain within the boundaries of a more human scale. In some areas, however, human scale is growing rapidly in response to the forces of urbanization and industrialization.

Individual health benefits from cultural traditions such as the couvade, rites of passage, and kinship networks. For example, mechanisms that ensure support for families are of assistance during times of sickness. The elderly benefit where they are accorded honor and respect from society.

Health problems in the developing world center on the diseases and conditions that cause infant and child mortality. The facts of high infant mortality, a large number of children in the population (as much as 40% of the total), and causes that stem primarily from the related disorders of infectious disease and nutritional deficiency distinguish mortality patterns in developing countries from those of developed regions. Deaths before the age of 5 years range from 25 per 1000 live births in the industrialized world to 170 in Africa, 107 in Asia, and 70 in Latin America. One-half million childhood deaths occur per year in the developed countries compared to 15 million in the developing world. Because of these high rates, life expectancy is shortened to an estimated 45 years in Africa, 56 years in Asia, and 62 years in Latin America, figures that do not compare well with the industrialized world's 72 years (Fig. 4-7).

Obstacles to the improvement of infant and child health do not include a lack of means for curing the responsible disorders. It has been estimated that 90% of all child deaths could be avoided by safe water and adequate sanitation (Fig. 4-7). Rather, obstacles lie in the scarcity of available resources and their distribution and in the orientation of health care workers. An average of one dollar is available per person for health care in the developing countries compared to 100 dollars per person in developed countries. In some countries such as Bangladesh, amounts available averaged fifteen cents per person (Morley, 1973). Future trends are not likely to augment resources substantially because of slow rates of economic growth and high rates of population growth. The distribution and deployment of scarce resources creates additional obstacles.

Three-fourths of the population resides in rural areas, but three-fourths of the health care services are urban in location. Three-fourths of childhood deaths could be prevented at low cost, but three-fourths of the medical budget is spent on curative services at high cost (Morley, 1973). Health care workers tend to be recruited from urban areas where higher education is available. Training cast in the model of Western medicine emphasizes centralized, teaching hospital–based health care systems in urban centers. Education tends to be strictly medical, to the exclusion of familiarization with the characteristics of the local culture, including health belief systems, organization of communities, and operation of economic constraints. One frequent result is the "medical brain drain" by which personnel leave for industrialized countries, higher salaries, and more modern facilities. Another result is perpetration of the colonial system in which the elite have access to specialized, Western-style health care services, but the remainder of the population goes largely unserved (Morley, 1973).

To improve health in developing countries, policies must be adapted to respond to the existing circumstances that affect health care and not to the directives of a system based on a foreign culture, which itself is undergoing revision (Fig. 7-2). An understanding of the culture is critical. The educated, urban physician or nurse may regard the beliefs and practices of their compatriots as "backward" and, therefore, may not realize the significance of these beliefs to their patients. Traditional healers can be a source of valuable information if their assistance is sought and efforts are made toward cooperation (Fig. 7-3). Existing social networks in the community must be recognized, for they can be critical for ensuring distribution of health care resources and the winning of people's cooperation. Health care workers in concert

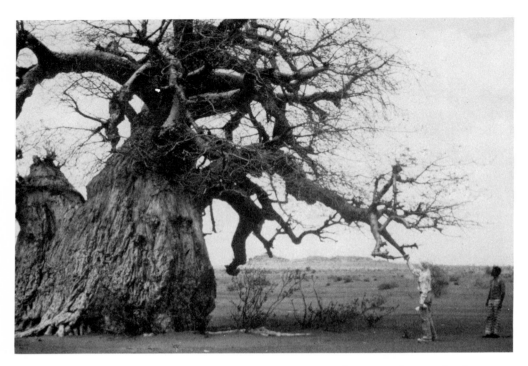

Fig. 7-2. Scientists inspect drought-resistant vegetation in western Sudan as part of a water development project funded by the World Bank. During the dry season villagers in this area of Acacia savannah have to travel as far as 20 km to obtain well water. Surface water is frequently stagnant and contaminated with animal excrement. If used for drinking, such surface supplies can transmit typhoid, cholera, and dysentery. Bathing can result in the transmission of "washable" (through-the-skin) diseases such as trachoma. (Photo by P. Van Arsdale.)

with people in the community can serve as health educators to train villagers, in the manner of the "barefoot doctors" in China and the village medical helpers in Tanzania. Industrialized nations should reassess their aid to developing countries, perhaps reducing military materials and increasing food supplies as well as technical assistance for maintaining sanitation and clean water. When one views the future worldwide, it is evident that the developed and developing nations cannot continue to exist peacefully with two-thirds of the world hungry and one-third affluent.

The preceding discussion has emphasized factors that affect infant and child health. Its ramifications extend beyond childhood, how-ever, since the health of the adolescent, adult, and older person is partly determined by their preexisting condition. The infant and child are more susceptible to sickness stemming from infectious diseases and nutritional deficiencies, but the adolescent, adult, or older person is not immune to their effects. Food deficiencies also are particularly stressful for pregnant or lactating women and for the elderly. Undernourished adults cannot perform work and other tasks as effectively as they could if adequately fed; this contributes to the continuing cycle of impoverishment, hunger, and poor health. An additional relationship concerns the possible link between infant and child survival and the birth rate. Currently, in India, for exam-

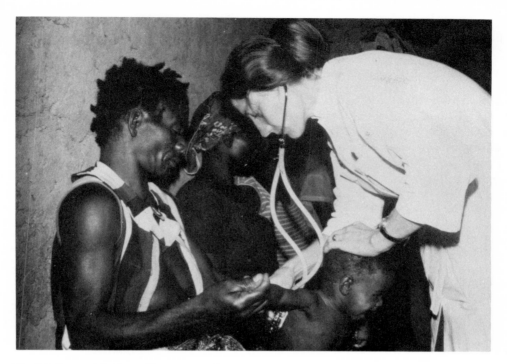

Fig. 7-3. In parts of Africa, Western-trained personnel have made efforts to preserve traditional curing practices alongside more modern techniques. (Photo by Kooperation Evangelischer Kirchen and Missionen.)

ple, a family must have six or seven children to be certain of having a surviving son (Fig. 4-7). If infant and child mortality were reduced, families might voluntarily limit the number of future births; thus, available resources would not be distributed among as large an infant or child population.

Health in the United States

In the United States, health problems increasingly reflect a different set of causes than was true in the past. Infant mortality continues to decline, but the present rate remains higher than in other developed countries. The reasons appear to reside in factors that affect the availability of health care rather than on such intrinsic factors as more intractable disease problems. While many childhood diseases have succumbed to impressive advances in medical science, new causes of childhood deaths, such as automobile accidents, have arisen. Mortality from these causes, while lower than in developing countries, is on the increase. Accidents now constitute the leading cause of death among children as well as among adolescents. The growing proportion of deaths from chronic disease, chiefly cardiovascular diseases and cancers, is perhaps the most remarkable twentieth-century health-related change in the United States. Such diseases existed in the past (see Chapter 3), but their increasing prevalence, in part resulting from the culturally mediated increase in the proportion of the elderly in the population and from the role of environmental factors and life-style in the etiology of chronic disease, suggests that modern culture has played an important role in their rise.

Concern has grown in recent years about

the ineffectiveness and rising cost of our health care system, a concern that many view as a health care crisis (see Chapter 1). A leader in health economics has stated, "Changes in health are much more dependent on non-medical factors than on the quantity of medical care" (Fuchs, 1978:2), and that "Personal behavior and genetic endowment are far more important to health than is medical care." Clearly, a new strategy is needed for the control of modern-day epidemics, one that educates about the nature of self-imposed risks and adds to our understanding of factors that enhance health and prevent illness. The influences on health of the social and physical environment are major nonmedical factors.

These views are being expressed by political leaders and, thus, clearly reflect the public demand for more than disease control. Given the importance of the biological and cultural basis for health, the remedy for existing problems and the challenge for future health care in the United States lies in modifying the practices used to restore health in accordance with knowledge about the range of biological and cultural factors involved. In other words, future health care policies must take into account influences on health that stem from all levels of environmental influences as well as from the individual's adaptive capacity and means for coping and repair (see Chapter 2). To meet the goals of health promotion and disease prevention, the lessons of this book translate into recommendations that individuals be informed about health determinants throughout the life cycle and that cultural variation be accepted in the health care system.

PROMOTING LIFETIME HEALTH

Health promotion as a goal that should accompany sickness control entails its prevention by facilitating both biological and cultural adaptive processes. Such a goal

is operative throughout the world, although attention is directed here toward the United States. Health promotion is also a concern that extends from the time of conception until the moment of death and even involves those processes that determine conception and the influences that stem from death.

The health and sickness determinants traced throughout the human life cycle (see Chapters 4 and 5) point to a number of particular issues that were highlighted by the contrasts between middle-class American culture and non-Western cultures. For example, the concern voiced over birthing and the call for "natural" childbirth in a setting that facilitates parent-infant bonding are supported by the recognition that, throughout most of human history, mothers were not anesthetized and were likely to have immediate contact with their infants. Cultural practices, such as the couvade described for the Wai Wai of Venezuela, appeared to ensure that opportunity for bonding was available. In a similar vein, the American experiences of adolescence contrast with those in other cultures, where rites of passage eliminate social and psychological ambiguity that is an important contributor to health problems in the American adolescent. Networks that link families with relatives and other groups in society are also a cultural mechanism for ensuring support that could be instrumental for coping with acute as well as chronic illness in a family member.

Health promotion thus entails addressing the biological and cultural factors that contribute to sickness. For example, prevention of death or injury from accidents, the leading cause of mortality in children in the United States, involves the use of emergency facilities once injury has occurred; but prevention requires precautions on the part of the child, parents, and other caretakers. Observations on the distribution of traffic fatalities among children in Denver point to the importance of social, economic, and environmental forces. Fatalities clustered in five areas, each of which contained a public housing complex located on busy streets that permitted curbside parking. Children's play areas in some instances were across the street from the housing complex (Nicholson and Huska, 1976).

Concern over factors that determine health and disease continues during the adult years and, as was mentioned in Chapter 5, extends into areas of work or career, body, and family. The costs of poor health—whether measured in economic, personal, or social terms—are considerable, as was demonstrated by the National Longitudinal Survey. Middle-aged men (45 to 52 years old) were followed over a 5-year period (1966 to 1971) in order to describe the consequences of health limitations for them. Men whose health affected their work were more likely to die during the next 1 to 5 years than men whose work was unaffected by their health; but, interestingly, the type of health limitation was generally not the cause of death. The greatest effects of health limitations were to reduce annual earnings and/or to encourage early retirement. Health limitations were not distributed evenly across the survey sample. Mortality among middle-aged black men was twice as high as for their white counterparts during the 5-year period. Among occupational groups, non–farm laborers and service workers had higher-than-average mortality; mortality was lower than average among white-collar workers, and craftsmen. White, white-collar, semiskilled and skilled workers and professionals missed fewer days from work because of health limitations than did blacks, blue-collar, unskilled and semiskilled workers, and laborers. While a great many factors affect absences from work, the parallels between these findings and the mortality differentials suggest that morbidity as well as mortality is lower among skilled, semi-skilled, and white-collar workers (Andrisaani and Parnes, 1978).

Health promotion through education

Are there ways of bridging the gap in understanding the biocultural basis of health throughout the life cycle and in meeting people's health care needs? One way is through increased knowledge. It is hoped that having read this book, the readers have a better understanding of the biocultural basis of health and the ways in which biocultural factors bear on their own health.

Current health education programs in primary and secondary schools vary widely. Some are oriented toward personal hygiene. Sex education is sometimes taught under the rubric of health education but often concerns only selected aspects of health-determining factors. In general, comparatively little attention is devoted to the bases of health and disease at the primary- and secondary-school levels.

The bases of health are compartmentalized at the prebaccalaureate and baccalaureate levels among a number of fields of study. For example, in the usual liberal arts and sciences college curriculum information about health is distributed in departments of biology, chemistry, anthropology, psychology, and sociology. Economics, English, history, physics, and other departments may have curricula of interest, such as health economics, history of medicine, and biophysics.

The diversity in departments dealing with health reflects its multicausal nature (see Chapter 2). Yet, traditionally, only the premedical or prenursing student has had access to and the opportunity to integrate the full range of health-related curricula. Health has not been considered a part of the general education that a college student is expected to acquire. Realizing the interest of the individual in his or her own health, as well as the individual's influence on other people's health, points to the need for the general liberal arts and sciences student as well as for the pre–health professional student to acquire an integrated health education.

Anthropology, in particular medical anthropology, offers one way of providing access to health education. Other departments with multidisciplinary orientations in the behavioral and natural sciences and the humanities could also offer the liberal arts and sciences student an integrated health education. Anthropology is suited to the study of health for reasons that should be apparent from the preceding chapters of this book. Anthropology offers a holistic approach to studying human beings. As its subdisciplines reflect, anthropology is concerned with the cultural and the biological and with the present and past dimensions of human experience. Even more importantly, anthropology's goal is to put human beings, or rather the information about human beings, back together again. The multidisciplinary and integrating aspects of anthropology make it unique among liberal arts and sciences disciplines and, hence, in our view, make anthropology eminently well suited to integrating information for general liberal arts and sciences students seeking health education.

Graduate training in medical anthropology has begun at both the master's and doctoral levels at a number of institutions across the country.* A listing of course outlines and reference materials for teaching medical anthropology has also been published (Todd and Ruffini, 1979). Graduate programs in medical anthropology have become increasingly attractive to students preparing for careers and to those with established careers in the medical and nursing sciences

---

*The Medical Anthropology Newsletter, published by the American Anthropological Association, 1703 New Hampshire Avenue, N.W., Washington, D.C. 20009, contains listings and periodic updates about such programs.

as well as in related health fields. Students pursuing careers in community development, business administration, planning, and architecture also may benefit from training in medical anthropology, since decisions made in these fields have health consequences and health policy implications.

Health promotion through disease prevention

In addition to education, what other means are available for promoting health throughout the life cycle? For many years, the periodic health examination has been a standard procedure, although not one that a majority or even large sectors of the population utilize regularly. It is intended to establish a medical base and a continuing relationship between patient and physician that will make it possible to identify sickness earlier and more easily. These periodic encounters usually include the performance of laboratory procedures, a physical examination, and an interview dealing with how the patient feels about his or her health (Dales, Friedman, and Collen, 1974). This time-honored approach is in demand by professional groups, and there is evidence of growing interest by other groups in the labor community (Delbanco, 1975).

Questions about the efficacy of such programs and their cost effectiveness have been raised repeatedly, thus provoking an increasing number of studies that point toward using more discriminating procedures that improve both the effectiveness and the economic efficiency of these examinations. One such effort involved a study of 20,648 men, almost all white and in upper socioeconomic circumstances, and suggested but did not conclusively prove that periodic, employer-sponsored health examinations favorably influenced survival (Roberts, 1969).

The periodic health examination should include assessment of personal and cultural circumstances. "We should give more attention to the old English definition of the word 'health' which connoted 'safety and soundness' of an individual in his or her life situation, and we should spend less time and money searching for what is all too often a non-disease" (Bates, Parker, and Riefler, 1971:930). Preexisting psychological experiences and individual characteristics were shown to differ significantly in a prospective study made of medical students' health that extended over 30 years. Those dying of hypertension, coronary occlusion, malignant tumor, mental illness, and suicide differed in youthful habits and family attitudes from their healthy classmates; personal attributes also differed among those dying from each category of disease (Thomas, 1976).

A system based on use of knowledge about life experience, clinical evaluation, and laboratory analysis has been proposed by Lester Breslow and Ann Somers. They have outlined, stage by stage, a lifetime health-monitoring program by identifying ten age groups and then attaching to each some specific health goals and the desirable professional services for each age group (Breslow and Somers, 1977). In the interest of giving the practical and useful substance of their work, the plan they recommend is given in the Appendix. One effort to estimate the costs of the Breslow-Somers program was made by the Department of Health, Education and Welfare for Congress. This figure came to $15 per capita per year on the assumption that there would be 100% participation. This is a great deal lower than the average per capita health care expenditures of $547 in the United States in fiscal year 1975. Cultural diversity among the U.S. population is not addressed by this plan; however, it would be constructive to make suitable modifications that would adapt lifetime monitoring to different cultures without losing the valuable

concepts that Breslow and Somers have proposed.

HUMANISTIC HEALTH CARE

Discussion thus far of recommendations for health in the United States has centered on steps to be taken by individuals, in some instances in conjunction with members of the health care community. Our concern with humanistic health care is directed primarily toward health care sytems and the means by which they might maximize opportunities for achieving health. An important element in the humanistic approach is that alluded to previously in this chapter, namely incorporation of a concern for cultural tradition and practice and their effect on health.

By "humanistic health care," we further refer to the need for a system that asserts the dignity and worth of the individual. Health care is given and received on a personal basis. A scalpel in the hands of a skilled surgeon touches one human being at a time, not a population pyramid or a subculture. Bureaucracy, with its proliferation of fixed rules and red tape, often leads the individual who seeks treatment into an incomprehensible maze. The restoration of humanistic health care harks back in some respects to the by-gone days of the "country doctor." However, it is not realistic nor particularly useful to propose turning back the clock. Rather, we suggest that the incorporation of diverse cultural concepts and community factors is a means of achieving such care.

Current populist movements in the health care field suggest the widespread nature of forces for change. These alternative healing systems were discussed in Chapter 6. Some of the fuel for these movements is based on the inadequacies, such as ineffective treatment and inequitable services, and on the bureaucratic insensitivity of the present system (Knowles, 1977). In response to these gaps, holistic health care centers are springing up throughout the states. One such center in Arizona, for example, offers diagnosis and treatment by a "new" health team that includes a physician, nurse, psychologist, herbalist, naturopath, and astrologer. At the same time, there is a move toward acceptance of responsibility for one's own health and a desire for greater control over factors that affect personal health. Not all current movements in health care are necessarily equally effective; nevertheless, the very fact that they have come into being and have generated interest is perhaps the main point.

Concurrent with a rise in consumer concern in the health field has been a trend toward examining one's cultural roots. The Civil Rights Movement of the 1960s as well as the great social unrest that followed the assassinations of the two Kennedys and Martin Luther King, Jr., and the war in Viet Nam left us a nation looking to our heritage. At the same time, we began questioning the nature of that heritage. One direction this self-examination took was to focus on the inequality of minority groups' access to important resources, such as jobs, education, and health care. Affirmative action programs thus began to influence the health care field. Programs in schools of nursing and medicine dealt with the rights and needs of minority students. Many schools altered enrollment policies and provided needed tutoring for students whose previous education was of poor quality in order to equalize access to professional status. Means for providing quality health care for ethnic minority groups also became an issue. For example, it was recognized that standard procedures, such as checking for dark blue coloration of the skin as a sign of cyanosis (brought about by a shortage of oxygen) required modification for black or other dark-skinned patients.

Understanding and applying diverse cultural concepts to the health field, however, demands a deeper appreciation of the im-

portance of culture in the life of an individual than that gained by the recognition of variation in features such as skin color. The cultural dimensions of an individual patient are as important to assess as are the physiological and psychological states. The melting pot myth obscures the diverse nature of the United States population. In each large urban center is clustered a myriad of ethnic groups with distinct ancestry, habits, and traditions. Different areas of the United States also have their own character, which reflects the particular geography, history, and cultures of that region.

The existence of cultural diversity combined with the importance of cultural factors for the basis of health and the belief systems that affect health care must be taken into account in the delivery of health care services. Some practitioners succeed in this task. How can more be encouraged to do so and how can the health care system as a whole become more responsive to cultural factors? The strategy we recommend entails the incorporation of community factors in the delivery and design of health care and reorientation in the education of health practitioners toward a consideration of the whole person.

Involvement of the community entails a broader distribution of power in which all members of the health care team, patients, and their families share in the decision-making process regarding the diagnosis and treatment of sickness. "Culture brokers" are important where differences arise between patient and practitioner regarding the basis and treatment of disease. The scientific explanation is foreign and incomprehensible to many people, although it is usually the only form of explanation given by the practitioner. The inclusion of community members on advisory boards for hospitals, clinics, and special treatment programs (such as hospice organizations providing residential or home care for terminally ill patients) are other means of ensuring community participation.

There are several reasons for community involvement in health care. The conditions that produce health and disease are, in part, localized in the community. Unsafe intersections and thoroughfares, contamination of food or water, air pollution, and radiation hazards exemplify sickness- or injury-promoting conditions within communities. Conversely, health and wellbeing are also linked to community features. Because of limited resources, community leaders may be forced to decide which of several deserving projects should be funded. Health considerations must then be considered alongside others in deciding on matters such as the construction of roads, housing projects, sewage lines, and mass transportation systems. Community support is essential for the operation of educational and other health-related institutions. Plans currently underway for national health insurance programs involve a kind of community participation that might translate into an even more direct link between communities and health care. Local boards are being considered that would establish fees in consultation with health care practitioners in advance of administering the health care services. Such strategies are being pursued as means of controlling the soaring health care costs of the present system and ensuring more equitable access to health care.

The education of health care practitioners has traditionally emphasized the acquisition of technical skills, grounded in the basic sciences (such as anatomy, biochemistry, pathology, physiology), and a repertoire of the clinical signs and symptoms for numerous diseases. While most concede this to be a useful education, it is one that tends to fragment the individual. The practitioner may lose sight of the whole person, which may in turn lead to problems in diagnosis or treatment. For example, a person from a culture

in which there are prohibitions against drawing blood, such as among some Chinese, cannot be administered "standard" treatment for hyperthyroidism or other conditions that rely on blood tests. Alternatively, the causes of iron deficiency anemia might be misdiagnosed among black women, typically from rural areas in the South, whose craving for eating clay leads to the anemia. A more common example pertains to the difficulty that people have in understanding the scientific terminology used to describe the causes of and treatments for disease and, hence, the reasons for following recommended treatment programs.

Innovative approaches—designed to acquaint students with the importance of considering the whole person—are being introduced in nursing and medical curricula. At the University of Colorado Health Sciences Center, all incoming nursing and medical students take a course entitled "Introduction to Clinical Medicine." Students are assigned to families whose homes they visit. Processes that influence health and sickness are observed firsthand rather than only viewing individuals with diseases. Courses combining nursing and medical students prior to the acquisition of professional status fosters communication otherwise inhibited by the professional hierarchy. Such courses are not equally effective for all students, for some remain tied to preconceived ideas about the utility of behavioral science as opposed to the basic sciences for addressing health problems and about the nature of the "other" (medical or nursing) profession. Another problem has been the unwillingness of faculty members to change the nature of the education that they experienced.

CONCLUSIONS

In closing this last chapter, we hope that the reader has come to appreciate the role of both biological and cultural factors in the determination of health and sickness. The importance of adaptation, continuity with the past, and distinctiveness of the present are broad features that we have stressed with reference to the United States and to other cultures of the world. Common features of today's developed and developing countries emerge that indicate the directions to be pursued in the future. The need for a more equitable distribution of resources within countries—for reaching the underserved, often in rural areas—and for sharing the world's resources among countries are common issues. Also, the recognition that health care systems need to be built from the "bottom up," beginning rather than ending with considerations of the culture and community, applies to both the developed and developing world. The need to control costs of health care also is and will increasingly become a shared problem. Financial resources available for health care on a per person basis are far more limited in the developing regions, but expansion of funds presents problems in both settings. Differences arise between the developing and developed world with respect to the kinds of diseases that exact the greatest mortality and the kinds of traditional beliefs that guide health care. Hopefully, the future will bring a partnership that will foster health in the human species as a whole. The developed world can offer assistance for preventing much of the infant and child mortality presently experienced in the developing countries. The developing regions can help to reacquaint the developed countries with the importance of cultural factors and the significance of human scale in the determination of health.

REFERENCES

Andrisaani, P. J., and Parnes, H. S. Five years in the work lives of middle aged men: findings from the National Longitudinal Surveys. In Waring, J. (ed.). *The Middle Years*. New York: Academy for Educational Development, 1978.

Bates, B., Parker, C. R., Jr., and Reifler, C. B. Clinical evaluation and multiphasic screening. *Annals of Internal Medicine*, 1971, 75, 929-931.

Breslow, L., and Somers, A. R. The lifetime health-monitoring program: a practical approach to preventive medicine. *New England Journal of Medicine*, 1977, 296(11), 601-608.

Dales, L. G., Friedman, G. D., and Collen, M. F. Evaluation of a periodic multiphasic health checkup. *Methods of Information Medicine*, 1974, 13, 140-146.

Delbanco, T. L. The periodic health examination revisited. *Annals of Internal Medicine*, 1975, 83(2), 271-272.

Fuchs, V. *Economics, Health, and Post Industrial Society*. Vancouver: University of British Columbia, 1978.

Knowles, J. H. Introduction: Doing better and feeling worse: health in the United States. *Daedalus*, 1977, 106, 1-7.

Miller, G. T. *Living in the Environment*, Belmont, Calif.: Wadsworth Publishing Co. Inc., 1975.

Morley, D. *Pediatric Priorities in The Developing World*. Kent: Butterworth & Co. (Publishers) Ltd. 1973.

Nicholson, J., and Huska, P. *Distribution of Traffic Fatalities in Denver*. Unpublished manuscript, 1976.

Roberts, N. J., Ipsen, J., Elsom, K. O., and others. Mortality among males in periodic health examination programs. *The New England Journal of Medicine*, 1969, 281(1), 20-24.

Salk, J. E. *The Survival of the Wisest*. New York: Harper and Row, Publishers, 1973.

Sivard, R. L. *World Military and Social Expenditures—1978*. Leesburg, Va.: W.M.S.E. Publications, 1978.

Thomas, C. B. Precursors of premature disease and death. The predictive potential of habits and family attitudes. *Annals of Internal Medicine*, 1976, 85, 653-658.

Todd, H., and Ruffini, J. (eds.). *Teaching Medical Anthropology*, Washington, D.C.: Society for Medical Anthropology Special Publication, 1979.

Walsh, J. UN meeting in Vienna unlikely to be a waltz. *Science*, 1979, 204, 926-927.

Appendix

Lester Breslow and Anne Somers have presented a lifetime health-monitoring program by specifying the health goals and professional services appropriate for each of ten ages. The following survey of the lifetime program and specific procedures outlined for two age groups appeared in the article, "The Lifetime Health-Monitoring Program: A Practical Approach to Preventive Medicine.*

GESTATION (CONCEPTION TO BIRTH)
Health goals

1. To provide the mother a healthy, full-term pregnancy and rapid recovery after a normal delivery.
2. To facilitate the live birth of a normal baby, free of congenital or developmental damage.
3. To help both mother and father achieve the knowledge and capacity to provide for the physical, emotional and social needs of the baby.

Professional services

1. Prior education and appropriate counseling for parents expecting their first baby in physical, emotional and social aspects of childbearing and infant care, including family planning.
2. Antenatal and postnatal care for mother and baby, education/counseling for both parents, and risk assessment throughout the perinatal period, as needed.
3. Delivery services, including specialized perinatal care, as needed.

INFANCY (FIRST YEAR)
Health goals

1. To establish immunity against specified infectious diseases.
2. To detect and prevent certain other diseases and problems before irreparable damage occurs.
3. To facilitate growth and development to the infant's optimal potential.
4. To provide a basis for lifetime emotional stability, especially through a loving relation with mother, father and other family members.

Professional services

1. Before discharge from the hospital: tests for inherited metabolic and certain other congenital disorders; parent counseling.
2. Four post-discharge professional visits with the healthy infant during the year for observation, specified immunizations and parent counseling.

PRESCHOOL CHILD (ONE TO FIVE YEARS)
Health goals

1. To facilitate the child's optimal physical, emotional and social growth and development.

*Reprinted by permission from the New England Journal of Medicine 296(11):601-608, 1977.

2. To begin the process of socialization through happy and effective family relations and gradual introduction to school and other facets of the outside world.

Professional services

1. Two professional visits with the healthy child and mother (ideally, the father also) at two to three years and at school entry for compliance with immunization schedule, and for observation and counseling about nutrition, activity, vision, hearing, speech, dental health, accident prevention and general physical, emotional and social development.
2. For special high-risk groups, blood tests for anemia, lead poisoning and tuberculosis.

SCHOOL CHILD (SIX TO 11 YEARS)
Health goals

1. To facilitate the child's optimal physical/mental/emotional/social growth and development, including a positive self-image.
2. To establish healthy behavioral patterns for nutrition, exercise, study, recreation and family life, as a foundation for a healthy lifetime life-style.

Professional services

1. Two professional visits with the healthy child (at six to seven and nine to 10 years of age), including one complete physical/mental/behavioral/social examination, with appropriate tests for, and follow-up observation of, any physical or mental impairment, including obesity, vision and hearing defects, muscular incoordination and learning disabilities, and completion of any necessary immunizations.
2. Mandatory school health education and individual counseling, as needed, for physical fitness, nutrition, exercise, study, accident prevention, sexual development and use of cigarettes, drugs and alcohol.
3. Annual dental examination and prophylaxis.

ADOLESCENCE (12 TO 17 YEARS)
Health goals

1. To continue optimal physical/mental/emotional/social growth and development.
2. To reinforce healthy behavior patterns and discourage negative ones, in physical fitness, nutrition, exercise, study, work, recreation, sex, individual relations, driving, smoking, alcohol and drugs, as foundation for healthy lifetime life style, including marriage, parenthood and career or job.

Professional services

1. Mandatory school health education and individual counseling, as needed, for the above subjects, including a course in sex, marriage and family relations as a prerequisite to graduation from high school.
2. One professional visit with the healthy adolescent (at about 13 years of age) with attention to emotional status, vision and hearing, skin, blood pressure, blood cholesterol and contraception.
3. Annual dental examination and prophylaxis.

YOUNG ADULTHOOD (18 TO 24 YEARS)
Health goals

1. To facilitate transition from dependent adolescence to mature independent adulthood with maximum physical, mental and emotional resources.
2. To achieve useful employment and maximum capacity for a healthy marriage, parenthood and social relations.

Professional services

1. One professional visit with the healthy adult, including complete physical examination, tetanus booster if not received within 10 years, texts for syphilis, gonorrhea, malnutrition, cholesterol and hypertension, and medical and behavioral history. This visit may be provided upon entrance into college, the armed forces or first full time job, but should be before marriage.
2. Health education and individual counseling, as needed, for nutrition, exercise, study, career, job, occupational hazards and problems, sex, contraception, marriage and family relations, alcohol, drugs, smoking and driving.
3. Dental examination and prophylaxis every two years.

YOUNG MIDDLE AGE (25 TO 39 YEARS)
Health goals

1. To prolong the period of maximum physical energy and to develop full mental, emotional and social potential.
2. To anticipate and guard against the onset of chronic diseases through good health habits and early detection and treatment where effective.

Professional services

1. Two professional visits with the healthy person—at about 30 and 35—including tests for hypertension, anemia, cholesterol, cervical and breast cancer, and instruction in self-examination of breasts, skin, testes, neck and mouth.
2. Professional counseling regarding nutrition, exercise, smoking, alcohol, marital, parental and other aspects of health related behavior and life style.
3. Dental examination and prophylaxis every two years.

OLDER MIDDLE AGE (40 TO 59 YEARS)
Health goals

1. To prolong the period of maximum physical energy and optimum mental and social activity, including menopausal adjustment.
2. To detect as early as possible any of the major chronic diseases, including hypertension, heart disease, diabetes and cancer, as well as vision, hearing and dental impairments.

Professional services

1. Four professional visits with the healthy person, once every five years—at about 40, 45, 50 and 55—with complete physical examination and medical history, tests for specific chronic conditions, appropriate immunizations and counseling regarding changing nutritional needs, physical activities, occupational, sex, marital and parental problems and use of cigarettes, alcohol and drugs.
2. For those over 50, annual tests for hypertension, obesity and certain cancers.
3. Annual dental prophylaxis.

THE ELDERLY (60 TO 74 YEARS)
Health goals

1. To prolong the period of optimum physical/mental/social activity.
2. To minimize handicapping and discomfort from onset of chronic conditions.
3. To prepare in advance for retirement.

Professional services

1. Professional visits with the healthy adult at 60 years of age and every two years thereafter, including the same tests for chronic conditions as in older middle age, and professional counseling regarding changing life style related to retirement, nutritional requirements, absence of chil-

dren, possible loss of spouse and probable reduction in income as well as reduced physical resources.
2. Annual immunization against influenza (unless the person is allergic to vaccine).
3. Annual dental prophylaxis.
4. Periodic podiatry treatments as needed.

OLD AGE (75 YEARS AND OVER)
Health goals

1. To prolong period of effective activity and ability to live independently, and to avoid institutionalization so far as possible.
2. To minimize inactivity and discomfort from chronic conditions.
3. When illness is terminal, to assure as little physical and mental distress as possible and to provide emotional support to patient and family.

Professional services

1. Professional visit at least once a year, including complete physical examination, medical and behavioral history, and professional counseling regarding changing nutritional requirements, limitations on activity and mobility and living arrangements.
2. Annual immunization against influenza (unless the person is allergic to vaccine).
3. Periodic dental and podiatry treatments as needed.
4. For low income and other persons not sick enough to be institutionalized but not well enough to cope entirely alone, counseling regarding sheltered housing, health visitors, home helps, day care and recreational centers, meals-on-wheels and other measures designed to help them remain in their own homes and as nearly independent as possible.
5. Professional assistance with family relations and preparations for death, if needed.

• • •

In order to further illustrate this program in their article, they spell out specific procedures to be used in two age groups, infancy and older middle age.

INFANCY (FIRST YEAR)

Specific screening procedures to be carried out before discharge from the hospital or during four post-discharge visits are as follows:

Suspected or possible condition	Procedure
Metabolic disorders	Phenylketonuria screening
Gonorrheal ophthalmia	Silver nitrate prophylaxis
Diphtheria, tetanus & pertussis	
Measles, mumps, rubella	Immunization
Poliomyelitis	
Bleeding due to hypo-prothrombinemia	Prophylactic administration of Vitamin K
Anemia	Hematocrit
Growth & development disorders, including congenital dislocation of hip	Developmental assessment, including observation for congenital disorders, height & weight

OLDER MIDDLE AGE (40 TO 59 YEARS)

Suspected or possible condition	Screening procedure
INTERVALS OF 2-3 YEARS	
Malnutrition, including obesity	Weight & height measurements—history of nutrition and activity*
Hypertension & associated conditions	Blood pressure*
Cervical cancer	Papanicolaou smear
Intestinal cancer	Stool for blood*
Breast cancer	Professional breast examination, with mammography for those over 50*
Complications from smoking	Smoking history
Endometrial cancer (post-menopausal women)	History of postmenopausal bleeding*
5-YEAR INTERVALS	
Coronary-artery disease	Cholesterol, triglycerides, electrocardiography
Alcoholism	Drinking history
Anemia	Hematocrit
Diabetes	Blood sugar test (fasting & 1-hour p.c. suggested)
Vision defect	Refraction
Hearing defect	Audiogram
HIGH-RISK GROUPS	
Add to 5-year Intervals:	
Tuberculosis	PPD
Syphilis	VDRL

*Once/year over 50.

Index*

A

Aborigines Protection Society, 8
Accidents, childhood, 132
Acheulian hunters, seasonal mobility model of, *66*
Ackerknecht, Erwin, 195
Activity theory of aging, 171
Acupuncture, 241-242
Adaptation
    evolution and historical record of, 53-91
    fertility and, 55-56
    fitness and, 55-57
    to high altitude, 24-33
        process of, 25, 27-30
    mechanisms of, 54-55
    mortality and, 56
    to natural disaster, 33-38
    patterns of, in evolution, 60-68
    to urban neighborhoods, 39-42
Adolescence, 138-142
    health considerations in, 141-142
    health goals during, 266
    nutritional problems of, 142
    pregnancy during, 141-142
Adolescent growth spurt, 138
Adulthood, young, health goals during, 266-267
Age status, cultural concepts of, 137
Age-sex distribution in demographic analysis, 76-77
Aging, 168-180; *see also* Old age
    activity theory of, 171
    cultural and behavioral factors in, 171-172
    disengagement theory of, 171
    genetic role in, 169-170
    immune system in, 170
    personality and, 171-172
    role of hormones in, 170
    theories of, 168-172
Air pollution
    effect of, on health, 18
    fetal growth and, 113

---

*An italicized page number indicates illustration; the letter T following a page number indicates table.

Albinism among Hopi Indians, 11
Alcohol, maternal use of, and fetal growth, 113
Alland, Alexander, Jr., 196
Allopathic medicine, 235-236
Altitude, high
    characteristics of, 25
    effect of, on reproduction, 30-33
    and health-sickness process, 32
    human adaptation to, 24-33
Americans, Native; *see* Native Americans
Amniocentesis, prenatal diagnosis with, 105
Andaman Islanders, rites of passage of, 140-141
Andean Indians, high-altitude adaptation of, 25, 27-32
Anemia
    pernicious, climate and, 18
    physiological, of pregnancy, 114-115
Animals, domestic, health risks from, 19
Anorexia nervosa in adolescence, 142
Anthropoidea, 60
Anthropology
    biological, dimensions of, 5
    medical; *see* Medical anthropology
    themes and methods of, 5-6
Arabs, medicine of, 232-233
Arthritis, paleopathological evidence of, 71-72
Asbestosis, 159
Asmat of New Guinea, 77, 78, 79-81
    belief system of, 216-217
    role of curer among, 217-220
    role of patient among, 220
Australia antigen, hepatitis B and, 54
Australopithecus afarensis, bipedalism in, 62
Australopithecus africanus, 62
Australopithecus boisei, 62
Australopithecus robustus, 62
Aztecs, pre-Columbian, belief system of, 202

B

Bacteria, classification of, 19
Barker, Herbert, 241
Behavior(s)
    cooperative, among people of the lake, 63

270